Parasitic Diseases

Michael Katz   Dickson D. Despommier   Robert W. Gwadz

Illustrations by   *Photography by*
John W. Karapelou   Eric V. Gravé

Parasitic Diseases

Second Edition

With a Foreword by Donald Heyneman

With 350 Illustrations Including
34 Parasite Life Cycle Drawings
and 4 Color Plates

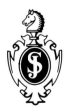

Springer-Verlag
New York Berlin Heidelberg
London Paris Tokyo

Michael Katz, M.D., Reuben S. Carpentier Professor and Chairman, Department of Pediatrics, and Professor of Public Health (Tropical Medicine), College of Physicians and Surgeons, Columbia University; Director, Pediatric Service, Babies Hospital; Parasitologist, Presbyterian Hospital; New York, New York 10032, U.S.A.

Dickson D. Despommier, PH.D., Professor of Public Health (Parasitology) and Microbiology, College of Physicians and Surgeons, Columbia University; Director, Parasitology Laboratory, Clinical Microbiological Service, Presbyterian Hospital, New York, New York 10032, U.S.A.

Robert W. Gwadz, PH.D., Senior Scientist, Laboratory of Parasitic Diseases, National Institute of Allergy and Infectious Disease, National Institutes of Health, Bethesda, Maryland 20205, U.S.A.

John W. Karapelou, Chief, Medical Illustration Department, Audio Visual Service, College of Physicians and Surgeons, Columbia University, New York, New York 10032, U.S.A.

Eric V. Gravé, F.N.Y.M.S., F.B.P.A., Medical Photographer, College of Physicians and Surgeons, Columbia University, New York, New York 10032, U.S.A.

The illustration on the front cover is a differential interference contrast photomicrograph by Eric V. Gravé of the Nurse cell–parasite complex of *Trichinella spiralis*. The original photograph was awarded First Prize in the "Small World" competition (1976), sponsored by Nikon, Inc.

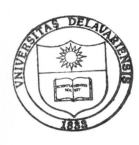

Library of Congress Cataloging-in-Publication Data
Katz, Michael, 1928–
  Parasitic diseases/Michael Katz, Dickson D. Despommier, Robert
W. Gwadz; illustrations by John W. Karapelou; photography by Eric
V. Gravé.—2nd ed.
      p.   cm.
  Includes bibliographies and index.
  ISBN 0–387–96800–8 (alk. paper)
  1. Parasitic diseases. I. Despommier, Dickson D.   II. Gwadz,
Robert W.   III. Title.
  [DNLM: 1. Parasitic Diseases.   WC 695 K19p]
QR201.P27K38   1988
616.9′6—dc19
DNLM/DLC
for Library of Congress   88-39759
                                                               CIP

Typeset by David E. Seham Associates, Inc., Metuchen, New Jersey.
Printed and bound by Arcata Graphics/Halliday, West Hanover, Massachusetts.
Printed in the United States of America.

9 8 7 6 5 4 3 2 1

ISBN 0–387–**96800**–8 Springer-Verlag New York Heidelberg Berlin
ISBN 3–540–**96800**–8 Springer-Verlag Berlin Heidelberg New York

Erratum

Parasitic Diseases, Second Edition

*Michael Katz, Dickson D. Despommier, and
Robert W. Gwadz*

P. 18: Caption for Fig. 4.2 should read: Head of adult *Ancylostoma duodenale*. Note teeth in upper region of oral cavity.

P. 78: Caption for Fig. 16.1 should read: This stage causes larval infections
in the intermediate host (pig) and in man.

P. 130: Caption for Fig. 24.2 should read: Cyst of *Giardia lamblia*. All
four nuclei are visible. × 800.

P. 153: Life cycle of Cryptosporidium: Reservoir hosts on upper right
side should show a calf, kid, and lamb.

P. 155: Fig. 28.5 should have several arrows pointing to the numerous
small round projections (trophozoites) on the surface of the
columnar epithelium.

P. 164: *Plasmodium vivax* life cycle: A single arrow leading from the
liver to the enlarged hepatocyte should replace the two arrows.
The caption should read: Exoerythrocytic phase.

P. 222: Caption for Fig. 38.11 should read: *Cordylobia anthropophaga*
abscesses in a small child.

P. 241: Reference 55 should read: Jupp PB, McElligott SE, Lecatses G: The mechanical transmission of Hepatitis B virus by the common bedbug (*Cimex lectularius* L) in South Africa. S Afr Med J 63:77–81, 1983.

P. 283: Caption for Fig. A56 should read: (Octanucleate cyst).

P. 284: Caption for Fig. A59 should read: Four nuclei are visible in this view.

PP. 283–284: Figs. A58–A60: This through-focus series of photomicrographs of an octanucleate cyst of *Entamoeba coli* is not the same as the one depicted in Figures A55–57.

The reservoir hosts in illustrations on PP. 23, 75, 97, 101, 109, 113, 117, 131, 145, 153, 183, 189, and 191 are reproduced from Despommier DD and Karapelou JW: Parasite Life Cycles. Copyright © Springer-Verlag, 1987.

This book is dedicated to the memory of

Harold W. Brown, M.D., Sc.D., Dr. P.H.
(1902–1988)
Professor of Parasitology Emeritus,
Faculty of Medicine of Columbia University

As a teacher he had few peers and his impact on generations of students
was enormous.

Foreword

One of the most compelling characteristics of parasitic infections in humans is their unbelievable number. Infection levels reach boggling proportions—one of every five humans harbors 8″-long *Ascaris* worms, nearly as many carry whipworms, especially in the tropics. Hookworms take a daily blood toll that equals the entire volume of blood in the population of a good-sized city. Blood flukes (cause of schistosomiasis) and malaria afflict a significant proportion of the population of Africa. Strange disease names soon to become familiar to the readers of this book take similar tolls: Chagas' disease, leishmaniasis, amebiasis, clonorchiasis, paragonimiasis.

These numbers tell us several things: parasites are deeply entwined in the daily lives of most people in developing and especially tropical areas. For the most part these parasites infect without causing disease—though with such huge numbers involved, even a small proportion of infected persons rendered ill can make a major impact. For example, by conservative estimate at least 200 millions harbor the agent of amebiasis, *Entamoeba histolytica*. Of these, some 15–20 millions suffer severe bouts of amebic dysentery. Malaria infects a similar number, but its 0.5–1.0% mortality levels mean 1 to 2 million infants dying each year, continuing the rule of malaria as the greatest human killer of all time. Yet, by and large, parasites are remarkably successful, parasitizing every human organ and only rarely destroying their human habitat, while infiltrating every niche and opportunity for survival in the burgeoning human population. To do so, a most remarkable set of life-cycle adaptations has evolved, each intimately keyed to specific human behavior, food habits, dwelling sites, and life style. All too often these are a product of poverty, crowding, lack of safe water or sewage disposal, or even of projects that are well-intended yet conceived in ignorance of epidemiology.

Each of these aspects of medical parasitology suggests reasons for the rising interest in the subject, e.g.:

1. Huge numbers of humans infected, especially in the developing world
2. Fascinatingly complex parasite life cycles
3. Direct relationship between the human condition and spread of infection and modification of infection patterns
4. Extended rapid travel, international interest, and involvement abroad with increased exposure to parasites heretofore rarely seen and little known to our medical practitioners.

This new edition of the book addresses these concerns through a tightly organized and well-honed presentation highlighted by a series of exceptional wash drawings of parasite life cycles. Its popularity attests to this combination, trimmed down for

medical students' impossible schedules. The book also reflects the increasing awareness of our involvement in all areas and all climes, including our own. Future physicians and other health care workers will be increasingly aware and must be re-
sponsive to this reality.

Donald Heyneman, Ph.D.
Berkeley, California

Preface

When is it time to revise a textbook? This question has been asked by most authors in the vain hope that the answer "not yet" would allow them to remain satisfied with the completion of the original task. In reality, in the case of biomedical sciences, the time to revise has grown progressively shorter. Like the massive suspension bridges whose paint jobs begin anew the moment the preceding ones are done, medical textbooks must be brought up to date as soon as they appear in print. New diagnostic techniques are developed, new drugs synthesized and—yes—new diseases identified.

In the case of parasitic infections, these new events are even more plentiful than in some other phases of medicine. This can be attributed to the application of methods of molecular biology to parasitology, which has led to a renaissance of this venerable biological discipline. In this second edition we have endeavored to bring forth those aspects of the new knowledge that relate to the main theme of our textbook, parasitic diseases.

This has resulted in an extensive re-writing of the chapters on malaria and leishmaniasis because so much new information has come to light since the publication of the first Edition. Resistance to antiparasitic drug has emerged as a major negative force and we have addressed this problem. A new chapter on Cryptosporidium was added because this parasite has emerged as an important cause of diarrhea, especially among immuno-compromised patients. A new section on diagnosis featuring specific methods and illustrated by photomicrographs of relevant stages of the organisms has been added. Other revisions reflect new information appropriate to each subject. Most important, the references have been brought up to date, retaining from the first edition only those that are still appropriate.

A new constituency of our critics has developed since the publication of the first edition. They are the students who have used the textbook and have helped us by pointing out how we could improve it. Their supportive comments have encouraged us in our work and we hope to thank them by providing to their successors a better product.

We have been helped by many colleagues whose criticism and advice have made this a better book than it otherwise would have been. They included Drs. Philip D'Alesandro, Martin Blechman, Thomas Brasitus, William Campbell, George Hillyer, Susanne Holmes-Giannini, Seymour Hutner, John Frame, Miklos Muller, Mike Schultz, William Trager, Jerry Vanderberg, and Ms. Joanne Csete. Any errors that it still contains can be attributed only to us. Dr. Benjamin Kean gave us free access to historical references. We also thank Drs. Robert Armstrong, Irene Cunningham, Gabriel Godman, Thomas Jones, Jay Lefkowitch, Donald Lindmark, David Meyers, Peter Schantz, Fred Schuster, Gerald Shad, Ralph Schlaeger, Roger Williams, Marianne Wolff, Gregory Zalar, and Mr. John Ma, who supplied us with biological materials, which we used to produce various figures.

The authors wish to acknowledge the enormous contribution of John Karapelou, whose imaginative artistic drawings of the life cycles have enriched this textbook. The help and encouragement given us by Springer-Verlag, especially the editorial and production departments, were invaluable to us.

New York, New York and   Michael Katz
Bethesda, Maryland   Dickson D. Despommier
November, 1988   Robert W. Gwadz

Contents

I
The Nematodes

Introduction

Nematodes are nonsegmented roundworms belonging to the phylum Nematoda. The members of most species of nematodes are free living and inhabit soil and fresh and salt water, as well as other, more specialized habitats. The majority of parasitic nematodes have developed a highly specific biological dependence on a particular host and are incapable of survival in any other host. A few have succeeded in adapting to a variety of hosts.

Anatomy and Physiology

The typical nematode, both larva and adult, is surrounded by a flexible, durable outer coating, the cuticle, resistant to chemicals. It is a complex structure composed of a variety of layers, each of which has many components such as structural proteins, a small number of enzymes, and lipids. The cuticle of each species has a unique structure and composition. It not only protects the worm, but can also be involved in active transport of small molecules, including water, certain electrolytes, and some organic compounds.

All nematodes move by means of a muscular system. The muscle cells form an outer ring of tissue lying just beneath the cuticle and their origins and insertions are in the cuticular processes. In addition, there is some muscle tissue surrounding the buccal cavity and esophageal and subesophageal regions of the gut tract. These muscles are particularly important elements of the feeding apparatus in a wide variety of parasitic and free-living nematodes. Each muscle cell consists of filaments, mitochondria, and cytoplasmic processes that connect it with a single nerve fiber. The nervous system consists of a dorsal nerve ring or a series of ganglia that give rise to the peripheral nerves.

The digestive system of nematodes is divided into three major regions: oral (i.e., buccal) cavity and esophagus, midgut, and hindgut and anus. The oral cavity and hindgut are usually lined by epithelial cells extending from the cuticle; the midgut consists of columnar cells, complete with microvilli. The function of the midgut is the absorption of ingested nutrients, whereas the usually muscular esophagus serves to deliver food to the midgut.

In addition, a number of specialized exocrine glands open into the lumen of the digestive tract, usually in the region of the esophagus. These glands are thought to be largely concerned with digestion, but may, indeed, be related to other functions. For example, in hookworms the cephalic glands secrete an anticoagulant. In other instances, there are rows of cells, the stichocytes, that empty their products directly into the esophagus. These cells occupy a large portion of the body mass of trichinella and trichuris. The function of these cells is unknown.

The worms excrete solid and fluid wastes. Excretion of solid wastes takes place through the digestive tract. Fluids are excreted by means of the excretory system, consisting of two or more collecting tubes connected at one end to the ventral gland (a primitive kidney-like organ) and the excretory pore at the other.

Reproductive organs, particularly in the adult female, occupy a large portion of the body cavity. In the female, one or two ovaries lead to the vagina by way of a tubular oviduct and uterus. A seminal receptacle for storage of sperm is connected to the uterus. The male has a testis connected to the vas deferens, seminal vesicle, ejaculatory duct, and the cloaca. In addition, males of many species of nematodes have specialized structures to aid in transfer of sperm to the female during mating. Identification of the species of worm is often based on the morphology of these structures. Most nematodes lay eggs, but some are viviparous.

1. *Enterobius vermicularis* (Linnaeus 1758)

Enterobius vermicularis, commonly known as pinworm, is one of the most widely prevalent parasitic nematodes of man, affecting mainly children below the age of 12 years. It has no host other than man.

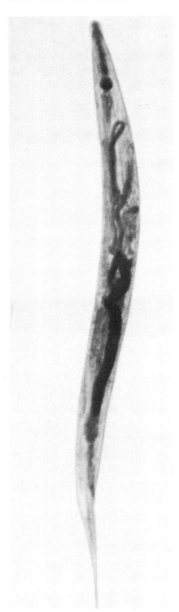

Historical Information

Early medical writings describe a worm infection that resembled in all respects infection with *E. vermicularis*, a name assigned to it by Linnaeus in 1758. Johann Bremser in 1824 distinguished this worm from the other Oxyurids and Ascarids and provided an accurate classification of it.[1]

Life Cycle

The adult pinworms live freely in the lumen of the transverse and descending colon and the rectum. The female worm (Fig. 1.1) measures 8–13 mm in length and 0.3–0.6 mm in width. The male (Fig. 1.2) is smaller, measuring 2–5 mm by 0.2 mm. The distal end of the male contains a single copulatory spicule and is quite curved, a characteristic permitting ready morphological differentiation from the female.

Although the biochemical and physiological requirements of the adult pinworms are not known, it is presumed that they use fecal matter as the source of their nutrients.

The adult worms copulate, and each female produces approximately 10,000 fertilized, no-nembryonated eggs. At night, presumably spurred by the drop in the body temperature of the host, the female migrates through the anus onto the perianal skin, where she experiences a prolapse of the uterus, expels all the eggs, and dies. This expulsion can be so intense that the eggs, which are quite light, become airborne and are distributed throughout the surrounding environment.

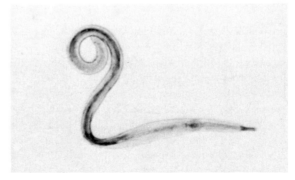

Figure 1.2. Diminutive male *Enterobius vermicularis*. ×20.

Figure 1.1. Adult female *Enterobius vermicularis*. The tail is pointed or pin-shaped, hence the common name "pinworm." ×20.

Enterobius vermicularis

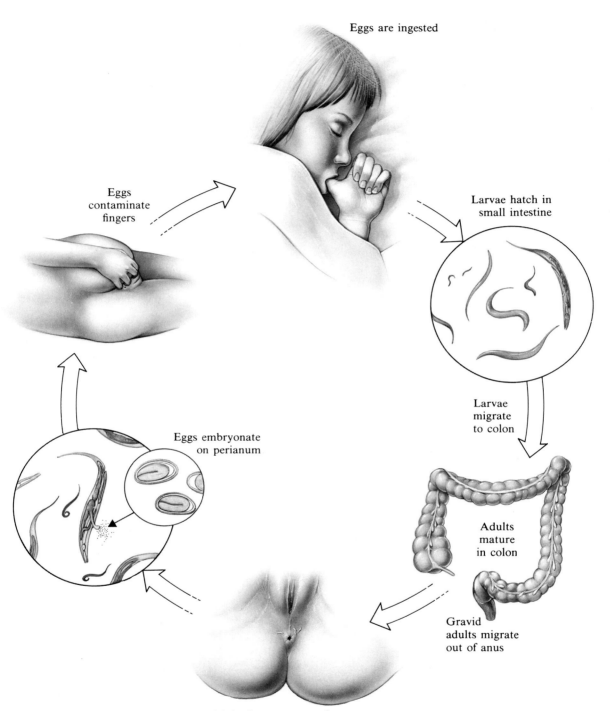

Eggs are ingested

Eggs contaminate fingers

Larvae hatch in small intestine

Larvae migrate to colon

Eggs embryonate on perianum

Adults mature in colon

Gravid adults migrate out of anus

Adults lay eggs on perianum

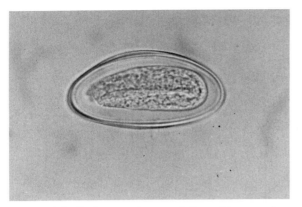

Figure 1.3. Embryonated egg of *Enterobius vermicularis* containing an infective larva. × 1000.

More often, however, they remain at the site of deposition. The eggs embryonate (Fig. 1.3) and become infective within 6 h of being laid.

The embryonated eggs are swallowed and hatch into the second-stage larvae once they reach the small intestine. Development to the third and fourth stages also occurs there. Finally, the adult worms take up residence in the large intestine. The entire cycle is completed within 4–6 weeks after the original ingestion of the egg. Alternatively, the eggs have been known to hatch on the skin at the site of the original deposition and the second-stage larvae then crawl back through the anus into the rectum and eventually the colon, where they develop into reproducing adults.

In women and girls, the larvae that hatch on the skin near the anus occasionally crawl into the vagina instead of the rectum, and there establish an aberrant infection. Even less frequently, gravid female worms make their way into the fallopian tubes. Other reported aberrant infections have included pelvic peritonitis,[2] ovarian infection,[3] and granuloma of the liver[4].

Pathogenesis

The migratory phase of the pinworm is restricted to the gastrointestinal tract and thus the host does not experience any systemic reactions. The parasite does evoke a minor inflammatory response in the intestine that may be associated with a low-grade eosinophilia, but it has not been definitively documented.

The pruritis that some patients develop results from an allergic response to the worm proteins.

Whether pinworm infection causes secondary problems, such as appendicitis or pelvic inflammatory disease, is moot. Pinworms have been found in these organs at autopsy with no evidence of an inflammatory reaction.

Although there are no comparable studies in man, there is experimental evidence that the immune status of the host does affect the infection. The mouse pinworm *Syphacia oblevata* reaches much larger numbers in nude (athymic) mice than it does in the same mice into which subcutaneous implant of thymic tissue from syngeneic donors was introduced.[5]

In man susceptibility to pinworm infection decreases with age, but the reasons for this are not clear and it remains to be determined whether this difference in susceptibility is immunologic.

Clinical Disease

The majority of infected individuals are free of symptoms. Those few who are symptomatic experience an intense itching of the perianal area; women with vaginal infection develop vaginal itching and, sometimes, serous discharge.

Although enuresis has been attributed to infection with pinworm, no causal relationship has been established.[6] Gnashing of teeth and sleep disturbances have not been definitely related to the pinworm, either, although there are myths that they are.

Diagnosis

The infection is best detected by the examination of a transparent plastic adhesive tape previously applied to the perianal region. This tape, subsequently cleared with xylol, or another suitable solvent, and attached to a glass slide, is examined microscopically at the × 100 magnification for the presence of the eggs (Fig. 1.4). The eggs can be readily detected. They are not usually found in the feces and therefore examination of a stool specimen is useless.

There are no serological tests and no known specific reactions that help to make an indirect diagnosis. Although low-grade eosinophilia has been reported in some cases, this relatively nonspecific finding is not helpful in the diagnosis.

Adult pinworms can be readily identified when they are seen on histological sections (Fig. 1.5 A and B) because of bilateral cuticular ridges

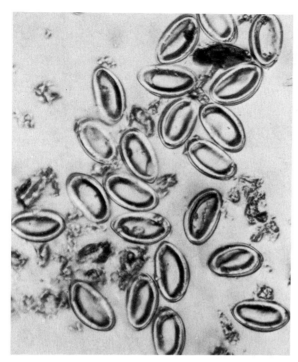

Figure 1.4. Eggs of *Enterobius vermicularis* as seen attached to a transparent plastic adhesive test tape. ×240.

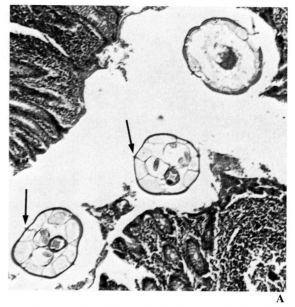

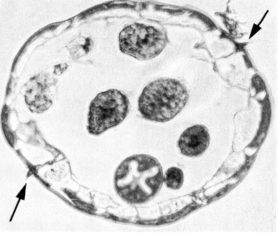

Figure 1.5. A and **B.** Cross sections of adult *Enterobius vermicularis*. Note characteristic cuticular projections, called alae (*arrows*), which help to identify this nematode in histological sections. **A,** ×90; **B,** ×270.

known as alae, which are not present in any other intestinal nematode of man.

Treatment

Of the available drugs, pyrantel pamoate,[7] in a single dose, or mebendazole,[8,9] also in a single dose is the best therapy. Neither piperazine citrate nor pyrvinium pamoate, drugs used until recently, has any place in the treatment of this parasite.

In treating the patient, one must remember that neither drug kills the eggs. Therefore, "blind" retreatment of the patient is recomended 2 or 3 weeks after the original therapy. This will destroy worms that have hatched from eggs ingested after the first treatment.

Prevention and Control

The probability of infection and reinfection is exceedingly high because of the ready transmissibility of the pinworm. Compounding the problem is the fact that the eggs can survive for several days under conditions of high humidity and intermediate to low temperatures.

The groups showing highest prevalence of infection are school children and institutionalized individuals. There are no differences in predilection on the basis of sex, race, or socioeconomic class.

No effective means for prevention are currently available. Pinworm infection should not be considered per se as evidence of poor hygiene. Any exaggerated attempts to eradicate the infection in the household should be discouraged by a rational discussion to allay anxiety.

References

1. Bremser JG: Oxyure vermiculaire. Traite zoologique et physiologique sur les vers intestinaux de l'homme. C.L.F. Panchouke, Paris, 1824, pp 149–157
2. Pearson RD, Irons Sr RP, Irons Jr RP: Chronic pelvic peritonitis due to the pinworm *Enterobius vermicularis*. JAMA 245:1340–1341, 1981
3. Beckman EN, Holland JB: Ovarian enterobiasis—a proposed pathogenesis. Am J Trop Med Hyg 30:74–76, 1981
4. Daly JJ, Baker GF: Pinworm granuloma of the liver. Am J Trop Med Hyg 33:62–64, 1984
5. Jacobson RH, Reed ND: The thymus dependency of resistance to pinworm infection in mice. J Parasitol 60:976–979, 1974
6. Weller TH, Sorenson CW: Enterobiasis: Its incidence and symptomatology in a group of 505 children. N Engl J Med 224:143–146, 1941
7. Blumenthal DS, Schultz MG: Incidence of intestinal obstruction in children infected with *Ascaris lumbricoides*. Am J Trop Med Hyg 24:801–805, 1975
8. Maqbool S, Lawrence D, Katz M: Treatment of trichuriasis with a new drug, mebendazole. J Pediatr 86:463–465, 1975
9. Aubry ML, Cowell P, Davey MJ et al.: Aspects of the pharmacology of a new anthelminthic, pyrantel. Br J Pharmacol 38:332–344, 1970

2. *Trichuris trichiura* (Linnaeus 1771)

Trichuris trichiura, popularly known as whipworm because of its characteristic shape, is distributed throughout the world in the same areas where ascaris and hookworm are found. It is estimated that there are at present some 500 million infections.

There are no reservoir hosts for *T. trichiura*, but other species of trichuris are found in a wide range of mammals (e.g., *T. vulpis* in the dog; *T. muris* in the mouse; and *T. suis* in the pig). Host specificity is the rule, but one case of *T. vulpis* in a child has been reported.

Although trichuris infections are usually not serious clinically, overwhelming infections leading to death have been reported in children.

Historical Information

Linnaeus, in 1771, classified this organism as a nematode, then called "Teretes." In 1740, Morgagni[1] described the location of *T. trichiura* in the caecum and transverse colon. This description was followed by an accurate report, in 1761, by Roederer[2] of the external morphology of *T. trichiura*. Roederer's report was accompanied by drawings that are considered accurate by current standards.

Human infection with trichuris has been identified in coprolites of prehistoric man.

Life Cycle

The adult worms (Figs. 2.1, 2.2A and B) live in the transverse and descending colon. The anterior

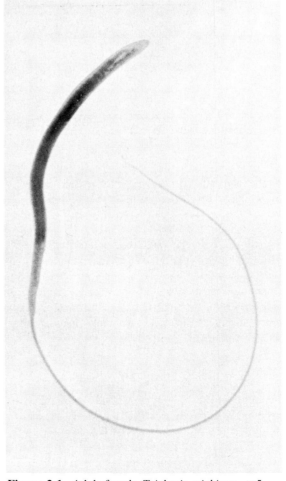

Figure 2.1. Adult female *Trichuris trichiura*. ×5.

Trichuris trichiura

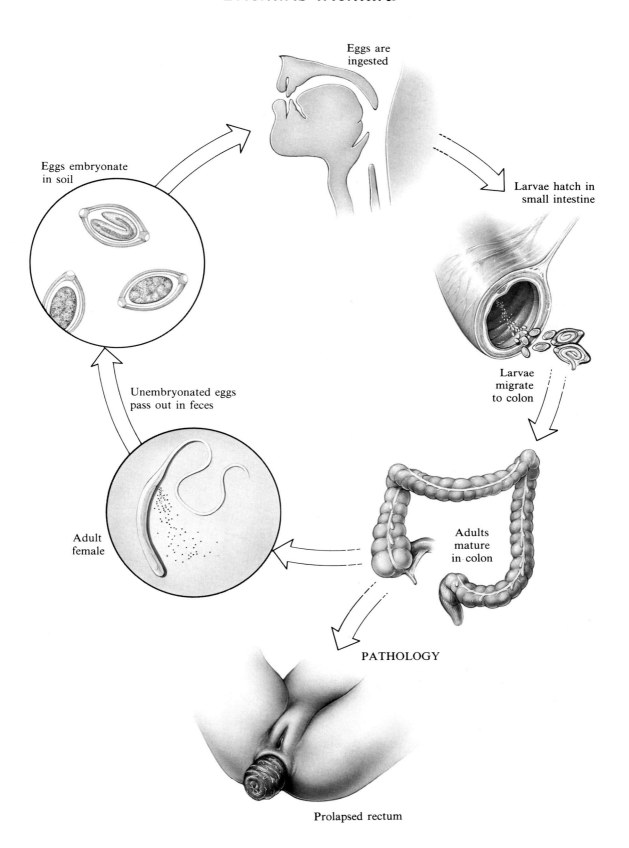

Eggs are ingested

Eggs embryonate in soil

Larvae hatch in small intestine

Larvae migrate to colon

Unembryonated eggs pass out in feces

Adult female

Adults mature in colon

PATHOLOGY

Prolapsed rectum

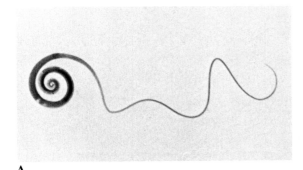

A

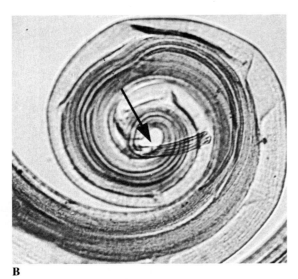

B

Figure 2.2. A. Adult male *Trichuris trichiura*. **B.** Enlarged view of male *Trichuris trichiura* showing the copulatory spicules (*arrow*). **A,** ×5; **B,** ×36.

narrow portion of their bodies is embedded within the columnar epithelium (Fig. 2.3); the posterior end protrudes into the lumen.

Nothing is known about the nutritional requirements of the adult worms, but experimental evidence on related species suggests that they do not ingest blood.[3]

The worms mature in the large intestine, mate, and lay eggs. Females produce 3000–5000 eggs per day,[4] and live 1.5–2 years.[5] Fertilized eggs (Fig. 2.4), deposited in the soil with feces, are undeveloped and must embryonate before becoming infectious. For this they require a favorable environment. Such external factors as high humidity, sandy or loamy soil, and a warm temperature (i.e., 20°–30°C) favor embryonation,

which, under optimal conditions, takes place within 18–25 days.[6]

Infection is acquired by swallowing the embryonated egg. The larva hatches in the small intestine, penetrates the columnar epithelium, and comes to lie just above the lamina propria. Four molts later, the immature adult emerges and is passively carried to the large intestine. The time required for a new infection to become patent (i.e., for mature worms to begin laying eggs passed into the feces) is about 90 days after ingestion of the egg.

Pathogenesis

The mechanism by which trichuris causes diarrhea remains unknown, although a number of theories have been suggested. These include intoxication with various products of metabolism of the worm and direct mechanical damage to the intestinal mucosa.

Clinical Disease

Only heavily infected patients develop clinical disease,[7] which presents itself as chronic diarrhea, characterized by mucous stools, and associated with tenesmus. If the diarrhea is protracted, the patient may develop rectal prolapse, more likely to occur in small children. Many individuals infected with trichuris—symptomatic, or not—tend to be malnourished and anemic. Nevertheless, no direct causal relationships have ever been established between trichuris infection and malnutrition and anemia. In view of the fact that trichuris is widely prevalent and that in the area where it is found there is a high frequency of anemia, malnutrition, and infection, the correlation may not be causal. In an experimental animal study using labeled erythrocytes, no evidence of intestinal loss of blood due to trichuris was demonstrated.[3] Severe diarrhea in association with trichuris infection is not necessarily attributable to trichuris; other causes for it must be sought (see Diagnosis).

Diagnosis

Identification of the characteristic eggs of trichuris (Fig. 2.4) in the stool establishes the diagnosis of

Figure 2.3. Scanning electron micrograph of an adult *Trichuris* in the large intestine. Note that the entire head of the worm is "woven" into the columnar epithelium, with the tail exposed to the lumen. ×100. (From Lee TDG, Wright KA: The morphology of attachment and probable feeding site of the nematode *Trichuris muris*. Can J Zool 56:1889–1905, 1978. Reproduced with permission.)

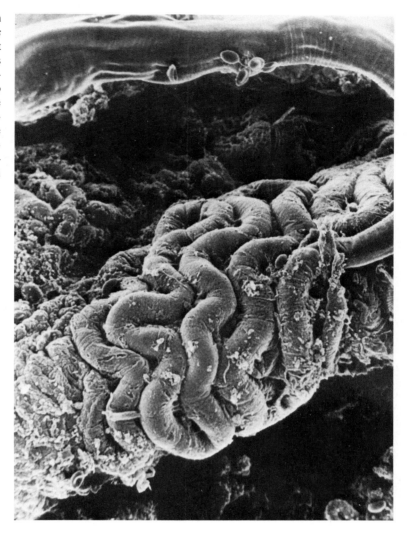

infection. Presence of Charcot-Leyden crystals (see Figs. 25.8A and B) strongly suggests that there is colitis due to trichuris and therefore implies in the particular patient a causal relationship between this organism and diarrhea. In any case, search for pathogenic protozoa such as *Entamoeba histolytica* or *Giardia lamblia* is indicated in view of the high frequency of multiple infections. It must be noted that identification of eggs of trichuris is relatively easy, whereas finding giardia or entamoeba is difficult and requires an experienced observer. When doubt exists, it would be reasonable to treat the patient for trichuris infection and request expert advice only if the patient's symptoms do not abate. Failure to control diarrhea after trichuris has been eradicated man-

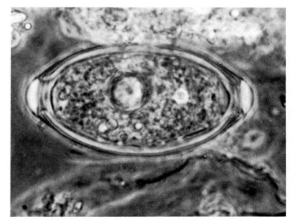

Figure 2.4. Fertilized, nonembryonated egg of *Trichuris trichiura.* ×1000.

dates a more thorough evaluation of the cause of the diarrhea. Stool cultures should be used to determine the possible presence of enteric pathogens.

In histological preparations trichuris can be readily identified by the characteristic variability of its diameter in different sections (Fig. 2.5).

Treatment

Mebendazole is effective in about 90% of cases. Retreatment is recommended if the first attempt at therapy is unsuccessful. Dose need not be adjusted to the weight of the patient because the drug is poorly absorbed.[8]

Prevention and Control

The infection is most common in tropical areas, where prevalence as high as 80% has been documented. Most infections tend to be light and therefore are asymptomatic. Warm, moist soil in tropical and subtropical regions favors the infection; direct sunlight for 12 h, or exposure to temperatures in excess of 40°C for 1 h or to temperatures below −80°C destroys the eggs. The eggs are relatively resistant to chemical disinfectants.

Proper disposal of feces is, of course, the primary means of prevention. In areas of the world where untreated human feces are used to fertilize crops, control of this infection is impossible.

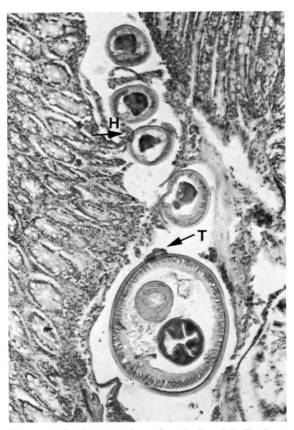

Figures 2.5. Cross section of a single adult *Trichuris trichiura* in the large intestine. Note the variation in the diameter between the tail (*arrow T*) and the head regions (*arrow H*). ×160.

References

1. Morgagni GB: Epistolarum anatomicarum duodeviginti ad scripta pertinentium celeberrimi viri Antonii Marie Valsalvae pars altera. Epistola Anatomica XIV. Apud Franciscum Pitheri, Venice, 1740
2. Roederer JG: Nachrichten von der Trichuriden, der Societät der Wissenschaften in Göttingen. Göttingische Anzeigen von gelehrten Sachen: Unter der Aufsicht der Königliche Gesellschaft der Wissenschaften. Part 25, 1761, pp 243–245
3. Pike EH: Bionomics, blood and Cr.[51] Investigations of *Trichuris muris* and studies with two related species. Doctoral dissertation, Columbia University, 1963, pp 1–207
4. Bown HW: The whipworm of man. Seminar (Merck, Sharpe and Dohme) 16:19–22, 1954
5. Belding D: Textbook of Parasitology. Meredith, New York, 1965, pp 397–398
6. Brown HW: Studies on the rate of development and viability of the eggs of *Ascaris lumbricoides* and *Trichuris trichiura* under field conditions. Parasitol 14:1–15, 1927
   Gilman RH, Chong YH, Davis C, et al.: The adverse consequences of heavy Trichuris infection. Trans Roy Soc Trop Med Hyg 77:432–438, 1983
8. Maqbool S, Lawrence D, Katz M: Treatment of trichuriasis with a new drug, mebendazole. J Pediatr 86:463–465, 1975

3. *Ascaris lumbricoides* (Linnaeus 1758)

Ascaris lumbricoides, which lives in the upper part of the small intestine, is often referred to as the giant intestinal worm because it can grow to a length of more than 30 cm. It has a worldwide distribution and is thought to affect some 1 billion people.[1] Although its eggs fare best in warm, moist soil they are highly resistant to a variety of environmental conditions and can survive even in the sub-arctic regions.[2] There are no reservoir hosts.

Historical Information

In 1683, Edward Tyson described the anatomy of *A. lumbricoides,* then known as *Lumbricus teres.*[3] Linnaeus gave it its current name on the basis of its remarkable similarity to the earthworm, *Lumbricus terrestrias,* which he also named. The life cycle was accurately described by Brayton Ransom and Winthrop Foster in 1917.[4]

In a remarkable series of experiments with himself and his younger brother as subjects, Shimesu Koino, in 1922, described the clinical spectrum of disease induced by this nematode.[5] Although in this experiment *Ascaris suum,* the ascarid of pigs, failed to complete its life cycle in man, it is now known that in some cases this infection in man can result in the development of adult worms.[6] In addition, he proved that a pneumonia-like syndrome developed during the early phase of the infection and that it was caused by third-stage larvae migrating through the lungs, on their way to the stomach. Koino, who swallowed 2000 *A. lumbricoides* eggs, became seriously ill, but fortunately did not suffer permanent disability. His younger brother, given 500 larvae of *A. suum,* did not experience as severe a disease.

Life Cycle

The adult worms (Fig. 3.1) live in the lumen of the upper small intestine, where they consume predigested food. On the average, each female produces 200,000 eggs per day.

The worms maintain themselves in the lumen of the small intestine by assuming an S-shaped configuration and pressing their cuticular surfaces against the columnar epithelium of the intestine and continually moving against the peristalsis. The worms secrete antitrypsins and as a result compete successfully for proteins that the host ingests.

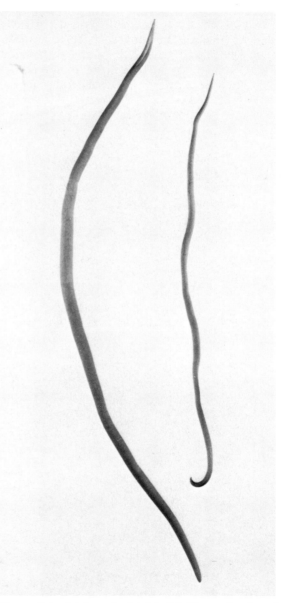

Figure 3.1. Adult male (*right*) (15–31 cm long) and female (*left*) (20–35 cm long) *Ascaris lumbricoides.* Note the hook-like tail of the male. ×0.50.

The eggs (Fig. 3.2) the worm lays are fertilized but nonembryonated. They become incorporated into the fecal mass in the large intestine.

Embryonation of the fertilized eggs takes place in the soil. If the eggs are deposited in the soil directly, the embryonation is completed within 2–4 weeks, depending on the ambient temperature and moisture. The eggs need not reach the soil directly; they can survive for several months before beginning embryonation.[7] The infective embryonated egg must be swallowed for the life cycle to be completed. Hatching of the larvae is stimulated in the small intestine by the combined action of bile salts and alkalinity of the enteric juice. The second-stage larvae then penetrate the

lumen of the intestine and enter the lamina propria, where they move further into a capillary and are carried passively to the liver (Fig. 3.3). From there they migrate to the heart through the inferior vena cava. On reaching the lung through the pulmonary circulation, the now third-stage larvae lodge in alveolar capillaries and break out into the alveolar spaces (Fig. 3.4). Rarely, the

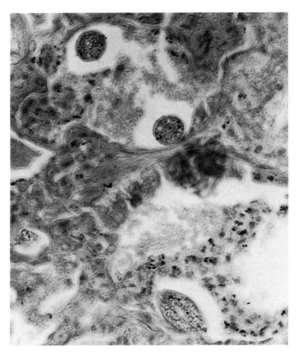

Figure 3.4. Larvae of *Ascaris lumbricoides* in lung. ×400.

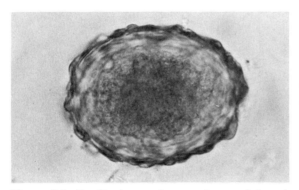

Figure 3.2. Fertilized, unembryonated egg of *Ascaris lumbricoides*. The outer coating (i.e., cortical layer) is characteristically irregular. ×700.

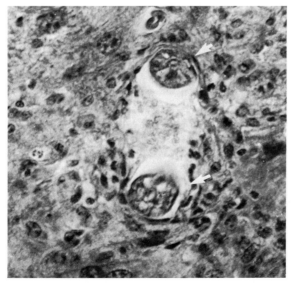

Figure 3.3. Larvae (*arrows*) of *Ascaris lumbricoides* in liver. ×360.

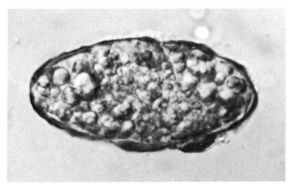

Figure 3.5. The unfertilized egg of *Ascaris lumbricoides* is characterized by a thin inner shell and disorganized yoke material. Usually, the cortical layer is also missing. Unfertilized eggs are characteristic of infections in which only a few female worms are present. ×700.

Ascaris lumbricoides

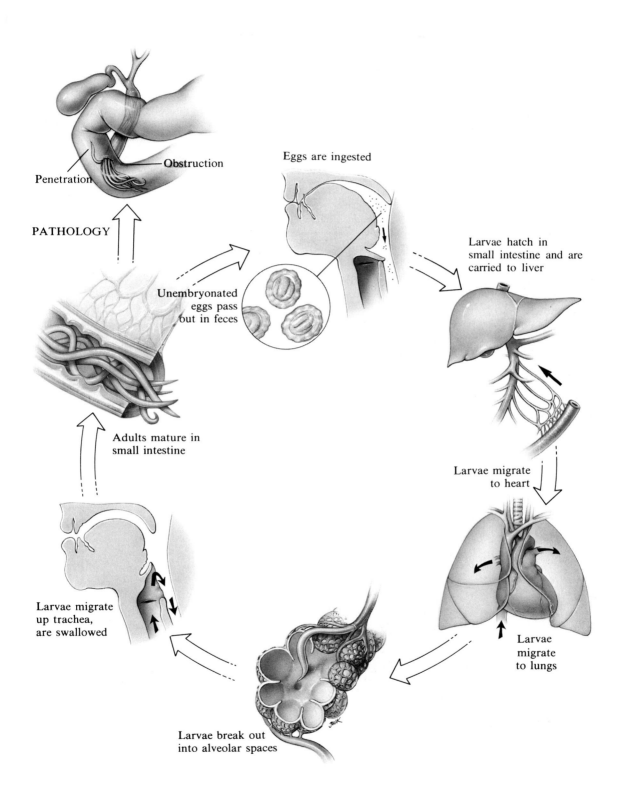

PATHOLOGY

Penetration — Obstruction

Eggs are ingested

Unembryonated
eggs pass
out in feces

Larvae hatch in
small intestine and are
carried to liver

Adults mature in
small intestine

Larvae migrate
to heart

Larvae migrate
up trachea,
are swallowed

Larvae
migrate
to lungs

Larvae break out
into alveolar spaces

immature worms leave the capillaries and wander about in the parenchymal tissues of the liver.

The larvae migrate actively up the bronchi into the trachea, across the epiglottis, and are then swallowed, finally reaching the lumen of the small intestine. There, after two more molts, the worms mature to adulthood. Occasionally, egg production may precede mating. When this occurs, infertile eggs (Fig. 3.5) are passed by the worm. Worms reach sexual maturity within 6 weeks after the final molt and cease growing.

Pathogenesis

As the Koinos showed, most intense host reactions occur during the migratory phase of infection. Ascaris antigens released during the molting of the larvae cause inflammation associated with eosinophilic infiltration of the tissues, peripheral eosinophilia, and an antibody response leading to an increase in the serum IgG levels. Specific antibodies of the IgG class form the basis of complement fixation and precipitin tests. The secretory IgA responses have not been well studied.

Ascaris may affect nutrition of infected children, especially those already in a state of marginal adequate nutrition.[8] It has been hypothesized that this results from secretion of antitrypsin factors by the worms. Moreover, it has been suggested that ascaris induces malabsorption of fats and carbohydrates. However, the data supporting these hypotheses are weak and the significance of such malabsorption in well-nourished children is doubtful.

The adult worms in the intestine cause few symptoms, although when they are numerous their sheer bulk may cause fullness and even obstruction. Through aberrant migration they may perforate the intestine, penetrate the liver (Fig.

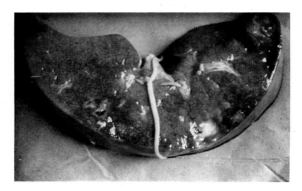

Figure 3.6. Fatal case of ascariasis caused by aberrant migration of adult worms into the liver.

3.6), obstruct the biliary tract, or cause peritonitis.

Clinical Disease

The intensity of the systemic response to the migratory phase of ascaris is related directly to the number of larvae migrating simultaneously. If the infection is light and only a few larvae traverse the tissues, the host response is negligible and clinically inapparent. If the infection is heavy, after ingestion of hundreds or more eggs, the patient experiences intense pneumonitis, enlargement of the liver, and generalized toxicity that may last up to 2 weeks.

In the intestinal phase of the disease, the worms may become entangled and form a bolus obstructing the lumen. This is a rare consequence of ascaris infection, with an incidence of approximately two cases per 1000 infected children per year.[9] If intestinal blockage is recognized early, it may be managed medically; if this fails, surgical intervention is mandatory.

Less frequent complications are perforations of the intestine, blockage of the bile duct, and other aberrant migrations of the adult worm. Certain irritants, such as tetrachlorethylene (which had been used in therapy of certain hookworm infections) and fever tend to stimulate migration of the adult worms.

The majority of people with moderate infections are rarely symptomatic. Most commonly, such individuals become aware of the infection through casual examination of the stools for another reason, because of passage of an adult worm in the stool, or by regurgitation of it during an episode of vomiting.

Diagnosis

Specific diagnosis of *A. lumbricoides* infection cannot be made on the basis of signs or symptoms during the migratory or intestinal phases of the infection. The clinical suspicion of infection with intestinal helminths is the usual reason for request of a stool examination.

Eggs of ascaris are quite characteristic (Fig. 3.2) and are easily recognized. If only few eggs are present, they may be missed but can be readily found if the stool specimen is concentrated by any of several standard techniques (see Methods, Appendix I). Usually, so many eggs are passed each day by individual female worms that the likelihood of finding them, even in light

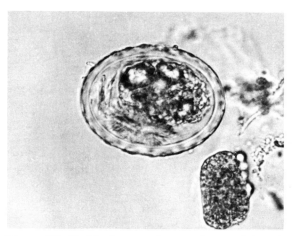

Figure 3.7. Fertilized, nonembryonated egg of *Ascaris lumbricoides* which lacks the cortical layer. This type of egg is rarely seen. ×700.

infections, is quite high. The presence of infertile ascaris eggs (Fig. 3.5) is still diagnostically important, because the presence of even a single female worm could have serious consequences if she were to migrate. Infrequently, defective eggs without mammilations are seen (Fig. 3.7); they can be difficult to recognize.

Treatment

There is no specific treatment for the migratory phase of the worm, and if the infection is heavy and the patient quite ill, symptomatic therapy with corticosteroids may be advised. There has been very little experience with the management of this phase of the disease because its diagnosis is almost impossible. The presence of adult worms in the intestine is readily treated with a single dose of pyrantel pamoate.[10] An alternative drug, mebendazole,[11] is as effective, but must be administered over a period of 3 days, which is a disadvantage.

In cases of intestinal obstruction, piperazine citrate can be used because it paralyzes the myoneural junction and relaxes the worms, which can then be expelled.

Prevention and Control

This parasite is prominent in temperate and tropical zones, but has highest prevalence in warm countries where sanitation is deficient. In some parts of Africa, 95% of the population is infected in parts of Central and South America, 45%. In the United States, the infection is most prevalent in southern communities, and in surveys conducted largely, or predominantly, among children, 20%-67% infection rates were noted.[9] There is no differential susceptibility according to sex or race. Although persons of all ages are susceptible, the infection predominates among young children because they are most likely to be exposed to contaminated soil.

Areas of the world with moist and loose soil are especially contaminated. The eggs can be destroyed by exposure to direct sunlight for 12 h and are quickly killed by temperatures in excess of 40°C. Exposure to cold, however, does not affect the eggs. They have been known to survive the ordinary freezing temperatures of winter months in the temperate zones. The eggs are also resistant to chemical disinfectants and have survived treatment of sewage.[7]

References

1. Crompton DWT: The prevalence of ascariasis. Parasit Today 4:162–169, 1988
2. Embil JA, Pereira CH, White FH, et al.: Prevalence of *Ascaris lumbricoides* infection in a small Nova Scotian community. Am J Trop Med Hyg 33:595–598, 1984
3. Tyson E: *Lumbricus teres,* or some anatomical observations on the roundworm bred on the human bodies. Philos Trans 13:153–161, 1683
4. Ransom BH, Foster WD: Life history of *Ascaris lumbricoides* and related forms. J Agr Res 11:395–398, 1917
5. Koino S: Experimental infections on human body with Ascarides. Jpn Med World 2:317–320, 1922
6. Davies NJ, Goldsmid JM: Intestinal obstruction due to *Ascaris suum* infection. Trans R Soc Trop Med Hyg 72:107, 1978
7. Bryan FD: Diseases transmitted by foods contaminated by waste water. J Food Prot 40:45–56, 1977
8. Stephenson LS, Crompton DWT, Latham MC, et al.: Relationships between ascaris infection and growth of malnourished preschool children in Kenya. Am J Clin Nutr 33:1165–1172, 1980
9. Blumenthal DS, Schultz MG: Incidence of intestinal obstruction in children infected with *Ascaris lumbricoides.* Am J Trop Med Hyg 24:801–805, 1975
10. Aubry ML, Cowell P, Davey MJ, et al.: Aspects of the phamacology of a new anthelmintic, pyrantel. Br J Pharmacol 38:332–344, 1970
11. Chevarria AP, Schwartzwelder JC, Villarejos VM, et al.: Mebendazole, an effective broad spectrum anthelminthic. Am J Trop Med Hyg 22:592–595, 1973

4. The Hookworms: *Necator americanus* (Stiles 1902) and *Ancylostoma duodenale* (Dubini 1843)

Two major species of hookworm infect man: *Necator americanus* (the New World hookworm) and *Ancylostoma duodenale* (the Old World hookworm). Adults of both species inhabit the small intestine and feed upon villi.

The distribution of the two species was thought at one time to be discrete and nonoverlapping; however, both species have been shown to occupy at least some of the same regions of Africa, South America, and Asia. A third species, *A. ceylanicum,* is found mainly in cats, but has occasionally been described in man. *A. braziliensis,* whose definitive host is cat, and *A. caninum,* whose definitive host is dog, cause in man aberrant infection of skin (see Chapter 11).

Accurate data regarding prevalence are difficult to obtain, but a conservative estimate, based on a survey reported in 1947,[1] suggests that there are at present some 700 million infections in the world.

There are no known reservoir hosts for *A. duodenale* or *N. americanus*.

Historical Information

Hookworm disease is widespread in the tropics. It had been common in the United States in the past, found primarily in the rural South, and in Puerto Rico. Because hookworm disease was thought to be a major obstacle to the economic development of the affected areas, John D. Rockefeller Jr. established, in 1909, the Rockefeller Sanitary Commission (which later became the Rockefeller Foundation) for the sole purpose of eliminating hookworm from the United States and Puerto Rico. Stiles, who described *N. americanus* in 1902, was largely responsible for convincing Rockefeller to establish the Commission.[2] The prevalence of hookworm infections in the United States and Puerto Rico has been much reduced, but this resulted less from any planned intervention than from the general improvement in socio-economic conditions.

Dubini, in 1843, first reported human infection with *A. duodenale*.[3] Most of its clinical and epidemiological features were identified during epidemics that occurred in association with the building of the St. Gotthard Tunnel through the Alps in Switzerland.

Life Cycle

The adult worms live in the small intestine, where they feed on the mucosal villi (Fig. 4.1).

Morphologically, each species can be differentiated on the basis of the mouth parts of the adults. *A. duodenale* possesses cutting teeth (Fig. 4.2) whereas *N. americanus* has rounded cutting plates (Fig. 4.3). Moreover, their body sizes differ (Table 4.1).

The adult males are differentiated from the females by the presence of a copulatory bursa (Fig. 4–4).

The life cycles of these worms are identical. The female passes eggs into the lumen of the small intestine. *A. duodenale* produces about 28,000 and *N. americanus* 10,000 eggs per day.

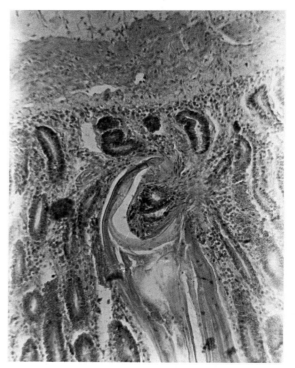

Figure 4.1. Cross section of an adult *Ancylostoma duodenale* engulfing a portion of villus. ×80.

Necator americanus

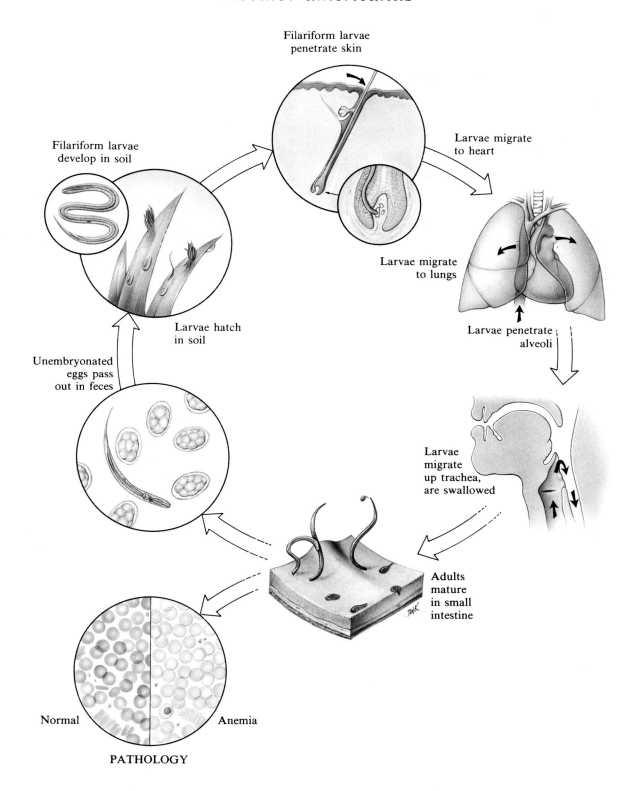

Filariform larvae penetrate skin

Filariform larvae develop in soil

Larvae migrate to heart

Larvae migrate to lungs

Larvae hatch in soil

Larvae penetrate alveoli

Unembryonated eggs pass out in feces

Larvae migrate up trachea, are swallowed

Adults mature in small intestine

Normal

Anemia

PATHOLOGY

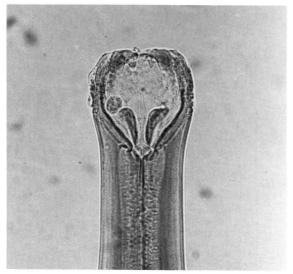

Figured 4.2. Head of adult *Ancylostoma duodenale*. Note teeth (*arrow T*) in upper region of oral cavity (*OC*). ×70.

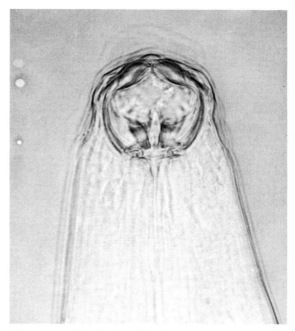

Figure 4.3. Head of adult *Necator americanus*. Note cutting plates. ×100.

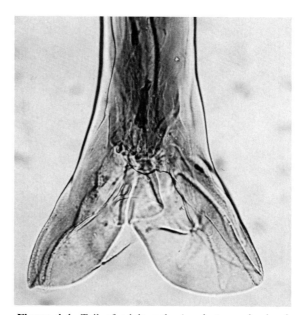

Figure 4.4. Tail of adult male *Ancylostoma duodenale*. The bursa is used to hold onto the female during copulation. ×100.

The eggs (Fig. 4.5A) begin to embryonate immediately after they are passed, reaching the four- (Fig. 4.5B) or the eight-cell stage (Fig. 4.5C) by the time they are deposited outside the body. In warm, moist, sandy, or loamy soil the eggs develop further until the first-stage (rhabditiform) larvae (Fig. 4.6A and B) hatch within 48 h of deposition in the soil. After feeding on debris in the immediate surroundings, the larvae grow and molt twice, and are transformed into the infective third-stage (filariform) larvae (Fig. 4.7A and B).

The filariform larvae do not consume food. They seek out the highest point in their environment (e.g., the tops of grass blades, small rocks, etc.) where they can come into direct contact with human skin. In endemic areas it is common for many third-stage larvae to aggregate on dewy grass, increasing the chances for multiple infections of the same host.

On contact with the skin, the filariform larvae actively penetrate the subcutaneous tissues, usually through a hair follicle (Fig. 4.8) or an

Table 4.1.

Sex	Species	Average Length	Average Width
♂	*A. duodenale*	10 mm	0.45 mm
♀	*A. duodenale*	12 mm	0.60 mm
♂	*N. americanus*	7 mm	0.30 mm
♀	*N. americanus*	10 mm	0.35 mm

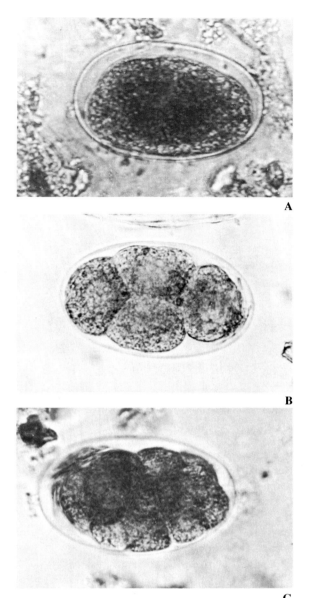

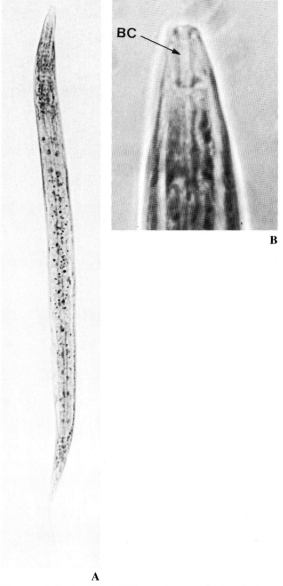

Figure 4.5. A. Hoodworm egg. No cell division has occurred within the embryo. **B.** Hookworm egg in the four-cell stage of embryonation. **C.** Hookworm egg in the eight-cell stage of embryonation. **A, B,** and **C,** ×630.

Figure 4.6. A. Rhabditiform larva of *Ancylostoma duodenale*. **B.** This stage has an elongated buccal cavity (*BC*), and can be distinguished from the same stage of *Strongyloides stercoralis* by this anatomic feature (see Fig. 5.1). **A,** ×150; **B,** ×1500.

abraided area. Once in the subcutaneous tissue, the larvae enter capillaries and are carried passively through the bloodstream to the capillaries of the lungs. The larvae, now fourth-stage worms, break out of the alveolar capillaries and complete the migratory phase of the life cycle by crawling up the bronchi and trachea, over the epiglottis, and into the pharynx. They are then

swallowed and proceed into the stomach. This portion of the life cycle (i.e., the parenteral phase) closely parallels that of *A. lumbricoides* (see Chapter 3) and *Strongyloides stercoralis* (see Chapter 5). One last molt takes place in the small intestine, resulting in the emergence of an adult worm.

Forty days later, following maturation and

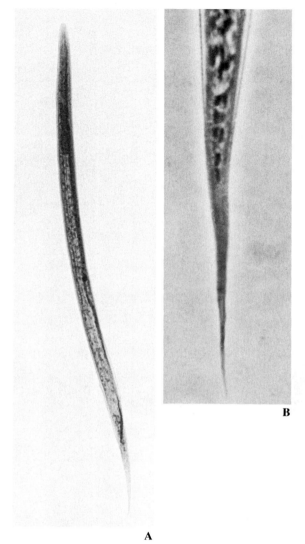

A

Figure 4.7. A and **B.** The third-stage filariform larva (i.e., the infective stage) has a pointed tail, in contrast to the same stage of *Strongyloides stercoralis,* which has a notched tail (see Fig. 5.3B). **A,** ×400; **B,** ×1600.

B

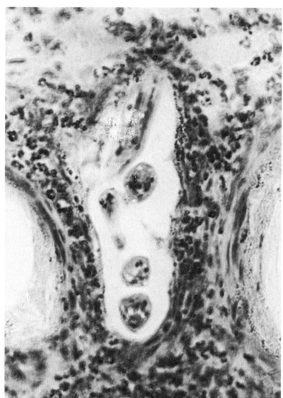

Figure 4.8. Hookworm larvae in skin. ×630.

copulation, the female worms begin laying eggs and thus complete the life cycle. Adult worms live an average of 5 years in the case of *A. duodenale,* and 4 years in the case of *N. americanus.*[5] The maximum recorded survival is 15 years.[6]

In endemic areas, where reinfections are continual, the development of some filariform larvae is interrupted and they remain dormant within bundles of skeletal muscles. After the adult worms are lost from the host's small intestine (i.e., as the result of either immune expulsion or chemotherapy), these larvae resume their development and complete the life cycle.[4] It is thought that the immune mechanisms of the host are responsible for blocking the development of the worms. As the immunity wanes, following loss of the adults from the intestine, the block is removed. This mechanism could be responsible for the reported "drug failures."

Pathogenesis

The adult worms derive their nourishment from eating villous tissue. They also suck blood directly from the site of attachment to the intestinal mucosa. They accomplish this by a pump-like action of their muscular esophageal bulb. The worms secrete an anticoagulant, which facilitates bleeding. Hence blood loss continues even after the worms have moved to a new location. *A. duodenale* adult is responsible for loss of 0.1–0.2 ml of blood per day, and *N. americanus* for 0.01–0.02 ml of blood per day.[7]

The precise role of the ingested blood is not understood. It remains unaltered by passage through the gut tract of the worm, except that the red cells emerging are somewhat depleted of oxygen. It is possible that the adult hookworms require red cells of the host to maintain aerobic existence.

Repeated exposure to the filariform larvae may cause hypersensitization. Thus, individuals respond to a reinfection with an inflammatory reaction, which results in death of many of the larvae.

Clinical Disease

Penetration of the skin by the filariform larvae may be asymptomatic in previously uninfected individuals. However, those experiencing repeated infections develop itching, known as "ground itch," or "dew itch." This may be a protective mechanism against infection. There is evidence suggesting acquired resistance to reinfection. Individuals living in endemic areas are less likely to be infected than people who have recently entered those areas.

In heavily infected individuals (i.e., 500–1000 worms), there can be symptoms of pneumonia during the migratory phase in the developmental cycle of these worms. The parenteral stages induce an intense circulating eosinophilia. It is made up, predominantly, of hypodense activated eosinophils.[8] The intestinal phase can be symptomatic—epigastric pain being the most common complaint—even in lightly infected well-nourished individuals.[9] Those subsisting on marginal diets who are heavily infected (especially young children) usually become anemic and, in addition, more hypoproteinemic because of some loss of serum proteins. In patients who are hypoproteinemic, that deficiency can be corrected by diet alone. Anemia is also correctable by an adequate intake of iron. However, because both of the above conditions are more commonly seen in impoverished areas, the rapid elimination of the intestinal infection by drug treatment is usually the most practical approach.

Diagnosis

Diagnosis is established by the identification of characteristic eggs (Fig. 4.5) in the stool. No distinction can be made among eggs of any of the hookworm species. Differentiation depends on the examination of adult worms. It is possible to base an informed guess about the infecting species on epidemiologic information regarding the area where the infection was acquired.

Treatment

All adult hookworms are susceptible to treatment with a single dose of pyrantel pamoate.[10] Likewise mebendazole,[11] administered over a period of 3 days, is effective, but has the disadvantage of multiple dose requirement. Although *A. duodenale* is more susceptible to mebendazole than to pyrantel pamoate and, in controlled circumstances, mebendazole may be considered the appropriate drug, if there is any doubt about compliance, treatment with pyrantel pamoate is the better choice. A single dose of tetrachloroethylene[12] is quite effective, but again more so for necator than for ancylostoma. Tetrachloroethylene is a relatively safe drug, but does produce troublesome side effects and therefore is not recommended.

Prevention and Control

Hookworms are most prevalent in the tropical and subtropical zones, but are also found in certain temperate zones in isolated areas. *N. americanus* prevails in the Western Hemisphere, most of Africa, southern Asia, Indonesia, parts of Australia, and some islands in the South Pacific. *A. duodenale* is seen predominantly in the Mediterranean region, northern Asia, and the west coast of South America. In areas where one species of hookworm predominates, the other is usually also found, in smaller numbers. Moist, shady, sandy, or loamy soil favors persistence of these worms. Larvae can survive in such soils for up to 6 weeks but do not live long in clay, dry, hard packed soils, or where temperatures are freezing, or are higher than 45°C.[13]

Sanitary disposal of human feces is the single most effective control measure in preventing the spread of infection with the hookworms. The Rockefeller Sanitary Commission discovered that hookworm larvae could not migrate very far in soil. The introduction of pit privies, with 2 m deep and 0.5 m wide holes, was sufficient to contain the larvae.

In addition, education of the public regarding

the mode of transmission of the infection led to the regular wearing of shoes, which reduced further the chances of exposure to the larvae. Poverty, however, often precludes buying shoes by many people. The use of human feces as fertilizer is still a time-honored and economically profitable practice in many countries, one that puts at risk large segments of the population.

References

1. Stoll NR: This wormy world. J Parasitol 33:1–18, 1947
2. Stiles CW: A new species of hookworm (*Uncinaria americana*) parasitic in man. Am Med 3:777–778, 1902
3. Dubini A: Nuovo verme intestinale umano *Ancylostoma duodenale*, constitutente un sesto genere dei nematoidei proprii dell'uomo. Ann Univ di Med Milano 106:5–13, 1843
4. Schad GA, Chowdhury AB, Dean CG, et al.: Arrested development in human hookworm infections: An adaptation to a seasonally unfavorable external environment. Science 180:502–504, 1973
5. Kendrick JF: The length of life and rate of loss of hookworm, *Acylostoma duodenale* and *Necator americanus*. Am J Trop Med 14:363–379, 1934
6. Palmer ED: Course of egg output over a 15 year period in a case of experimentally induced necatoriasis americanus. Am J Trop Med Hyg 4:756–757, 1955
7. Roche M, Layrisse M: The nature and causes of "hookworm anemia." Am J Trop Med Hyg 15:1031–1102, 1966
8. White CJ, Maxwell CJ, Gallin JI: Changes in the structural and functional properties of human eosinophils during experimental hookworm infection. J Infect Dis 159:778–783, 1986
9. Maxwell CJ, Hussain R, Nutman TB, et al.: The clinical and immunologic responses of normal human volunteers to low dose hookworm (*Necator americanus*) infection. Am J Trop Med Hyg 37:126–134, 1987
10. Blumenthal DS, Schultz MG: Incidence of intestinal obstruction in children infected with *Ascaris lumbricoides*. Am J Trop Med Hyg 28:801–805, 1975
11. Aubry ML, Cowell P, Davey MJ, et al.: Aspects of the pharmacology of a new anthelmintic, pyrantel. Br J Pharmacol 38:332–344, 1970
12. Lamson PD, Brown HW, Ward CB: Anthelmintics, some therapeutic and practical considerations of their use. JAMA 99:292–295, 1932
13. Kobayashi A, Suzuki N, Yasuda I, et al.: The resistance of hookworm eggs to lower temperatures. Japn J Parasitol 8:637, 1959.

5. *Strongyloides stercoralis* (Bavay 1876)

Strongyloides stercoralis is an intestinal nematode found throughout the tropical and subtropical world. It is also present in certain temperate zones as a zoonotic and, occasionally, human infection. Dogs and nonhuman primates can harbor strongyloides, and outbreaks of this infection among animal handlers have occurred.[1] *S. stercoralis* can exist in a nonparasitic, free-living state in the soil. Thus there are many potential sources of human infection with this pathogen.

Under special conditions strongyloides can maintain infection without passing into the soil. It is the only nematode parasite of man that can reproduce within the host and thus becomes a chronic infection lasting many years.[2,3]

The number of infected people in the world at present has been estimated as 100—200 million.

Historical Information

S. stercoralis and its relationship to disease were first described by Bavay[4] and Normand[5] in 1876 while they were working together in Toulon, France. Their patients were French army personnel, newly arrived from Cochin, Indochina, hence the common term for the strongyloidal enteritis, "Cochin China Diarrhea." Bavay was able to recover from the stools of these patients numerous larvae of a nematode not previously described. He named it *Anguillula stercoralis*.

Strongyloides stercoralis

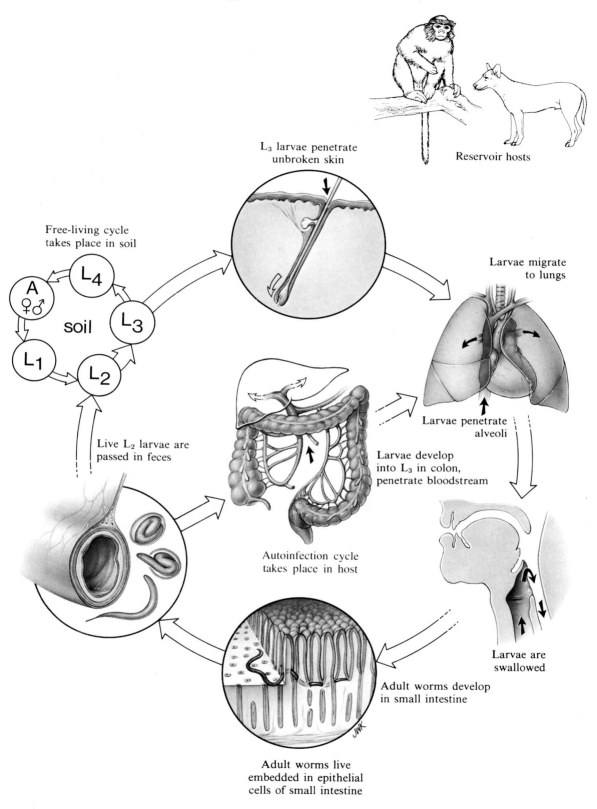

Reservoir hosts

L_3 larvae penetrate
unbroken skin

Free-living cycle
takes place in soil

A
♀♂

soil

L₄

L₃

L₂

L₁

Larvae migrate
to lungs

Larvae penetrate
alveoli

Larvae develop
into L_3 in colon,
penetrate bloodstream

Live L_2 larvae are
passed in feces

Autoinfection cycle
takes place in host

Larvae are
swallowed

Adult worms develop
in small intestine

Adult worms live
embedded in epithelial
cells of small intestine

Pathology of strongyloidiasis was described by Askanazy[6] and the life cycle of the worm by Fullerborn,[7] who in 1914 initiated experimental infections in dogs and discovered that the infective larvae can penetrate unbroken skin.

Autoinfection with *S. stercoralis* was studied first in 1928 by Nishigoii,[8] who found that infected dogs made constipated with morphine and bismuth subnitrate passed infective third-stage larvae, rather than the noninfective second-stage larvae. In addition, he noted that the number of larvae passed by these animals continued to increase as long as their constipation was maintained. These studies preceded the clinical description of the situation now known to occur in man.

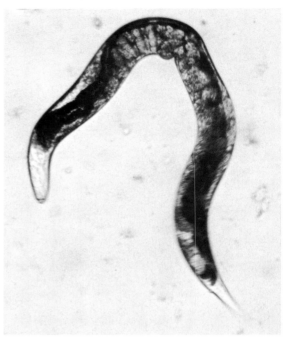

Figure 5.2. Free-living adult female of *Strongyloides stercoralis*. ×260.

Life Cycle

Strongyloides stercoralis has a free-living phase and a parasitic phase of its life cycle.

Free-Living Phase

The second-stage rhabditiform larvae (Fig. 5.1A and B) must be deposited in warm, moist, sandy, or loamy soil for the next developmental phase of the cycle to take place. If they molt twice in the soil, they become free-living adult worms (Fig. 5.2.). Unlike the parasitic phase, the free-living phase contains worms of both sexes. They copulate and the female then produces embryonated eggs, which are deposited in the soil where larvae hatch and repeat the pattern of molting, becoming adults within 3–5 days. When conditions become unfavorable for the continuation of the free-living phase, the surviving infective third-stage larvae (Fig. 5.3A and B) can then penetrate the skin of the host, and begin parasitic infection. Penetration takes place usually through a hair follicle, but may also occur through abraided skin. Once in the host, the larvae are carried passively through the bloodstream and eventually break out into the alveolar space. From there,

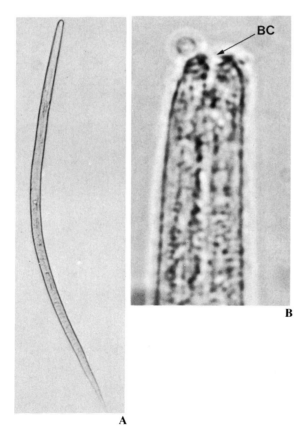

Figure 5.1. A. Rhabditiform larva of *Strongyloides stercoralis*. **B.** Note the short buccal cavity (*arrow BC*) that distinguishes this larva from that of the rhabditiform larva of hookworm (see Fig. 4.6A). **A,** ×150; **B,** ×1500.

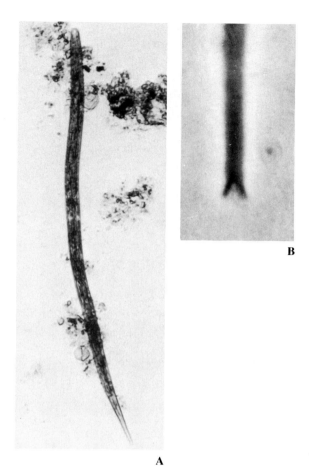

A

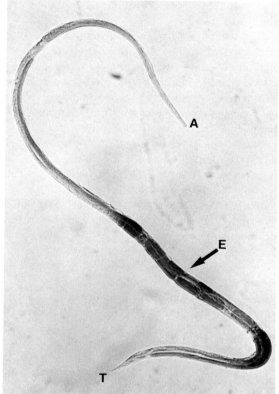

Figure 5.4. Parasitic female *Strongyloides stercoralis*. *A*, Anterior end; *E*, eggs; *T*, tail. ×210.

Figure 5.3. A. Infective third-stage larva (filariform) of *Strongyloides stercoralis* can be distinguished from the filariform larva of hookworm (see Fig. 4.7A and B) by the notched tail (**B**). **A**, ×350; **B**, ×1000.

they actively crawl up the respiratory tree, pass through the trachea into the pharynx, go over the epiglottis, and are swallowed. The larvae undergo a final molt in the small intestine and become parasitic females (Fig. 5.4).

Parasitic Phase
The adult parasitic female is about 2 mm long and 0.04 mm wide and lives within columnar epithelial cells of the small intestine (Fig. 5.5). There is no information concerning its nutritional requirements. In the parasitic phase, reproduction is protandrous, a process that includes early maturation of the male gonad and production of sperm, followed by involution of the male gonad and development of a female gonad; this in turn

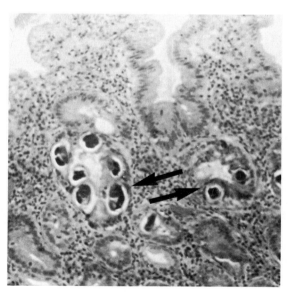

Figure 5.5. Adults (*arrows*) of *Strongyloides stercoralis* in situ in the small intestine. ×150. (Courtesy of Dr. T. Brasitus)

is followed by self-fertilization. There is no parasitic male.

The embryonated eggs hatch rapidly into first-stage larvae, which emerge into the lumen of the small intestine and proceed into the colon. They molt there once, becoming second-stage rhabditiform larvae. Ordinarily, the rhabditiform larvae are deposited in the soil with feces. However, if there is a delay in their deposition in the soil, the larvae molt into third-stage filariform larvae within the lumen of the colon, burrow into the mucosa, and enter the circulation directly. This aspect of the parasitic phase of the life cycle is known as autoinfection. It represents an infrequent event that does not result in a noticeable increase in numbers of adult worms in the small intestine. In the usual form of infection, the larvae from the soil penetrate the skin of the host and follow a pattern of migration identical to that of hookworm larvae, finally differentiating into adult females in the small intestine. They begin

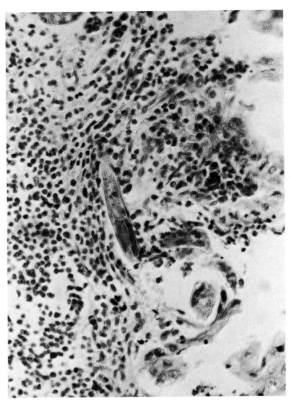

Figure 5.7. Larvae of *Strongyloides stercoralis* in stomach of the patient in Fig. 5.6. ×200.

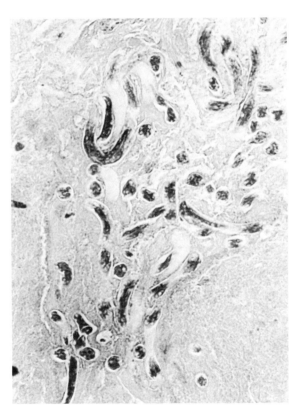

Figure 5.6. Larvae of *Strongyloides stercoralis* in small intestine of a patient who died of an overwhelming infection. ×150.

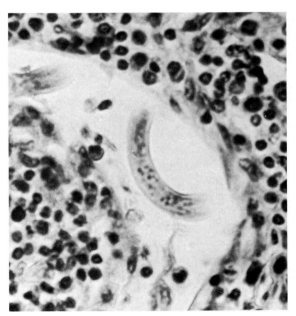

Figure 5.8. Larvae of *Strongyloides stercoralis* in a lymph node of the patient in Fig. 5.6. ×200.

egg production within 25–30 days after the initial infection.

In immunocompromised hosts,[9] many infective larvae develop within the colon, making it possible to increase the numbers of adult worms in the small intestine. This exaggeration of autoinfection is known as hyperinfection and represents the most serious and often fatal consequence of infection with *S. stercoralis*.

Pathogenesis

In small numbers, the parasitic females cause little or no damage to the mucosa of the small intestine, but they do induce a local inflammatory reaction. The kinins provoking the mixed granulocyte response have not been identified, but it is likely that they are induced by antigens of the worm, because in states of immunodeficiency inflammation is less intense or absent and hyperinfection often develops.

In experimental studies, T cell function appears to be necessary for the development of resistance to infection.[10] However, in man the mechanism of this protection is not understood.[11]

Diarrhea, often severe, is related to heavy infection with *S. stercoralis* and has been attributed to malabsorption, the evidence for which is indirect.

In cases of auto- or hyperinfection, penetrating larvae often carry enteric microorganisms, which may cause local infection or sepsis. Larvae can be found throughout the body at this time (Figs. 5.6–5.8). In immunosuppressed individuals with strongyloidiasis, bacterial infections are common causes of death.[12]

Clinical Disease

The characteristic clinical disease presents itself as a watery, mucous diarrhea, the degree of which varies with the intensity of the infection. States of alternating diarrhea and constipation have been described. Malabsorption syndrome has also been reported.[13]

During the migratory phase of the infection, there can be symptoms resembling those described for ascariasis and hookworm disease (e.g., pneumonitis). This phase is associated with circulating eosinophilia. The above symptoms are exaggerated if hyperinfection is superimposed upon an already chronic infection.

In the immunocompromised individuals, such as those suffering from debilitating diseases, or those undergoing chemotherapy as treatment of a malignancy or in preparation for organ transplantation, massive invasion by strongyloides larvae due to hyperinfection can occur and can lead to death. In such situations it is mandatory to treat promptly, but most important, it is crucial to make the diagnosis as early as possible, preferably in advance of immunosuppression.

Diagnosis

The diagnosis depends on microscopic examination of the stool. It can be difficult if only a single, casual stool specimen is examined, because often the number of rhabditiform larvae (Fig. 5.1) is small. It is necessary to examine a large quantity of stool (e.g., a 24-h sample) and to use a sedimentation method (see Appendix I).

Even when sedimentation techniques are used, low-grade infections are usually missed, and therefore a rigorous search must be carried out before a patient can be declared free of the infection. Discovery of strongyloides is made more likely by examination of duodenal fluid, mucosal biopsy, or application of the string test.[14]

Immunological tests are based on the ELISA method. They are both specific and sensitive,[15] but their availability is limited. Individuals who test positive should be treated.

Treatment

The drug of choice is thiabendazole. Cure rates of nearly 100% have been achieved. This drug is detoxified in the liver and therefore can reach undesirably high blood levels in patients with liver disease. Unfortunately, no guidelines to reduction of the dose have been clinically determined. For hyperinfection, thiabendazole therapy is extended to 5 days. Other benzimidazoles (e.g. cambendazole[16]) are also effective.

Prevention and Control

Dogs and certain primates, notably chimpanzees, are naturally infected with *S. stercoralis*. Whether these animals form an important reservoir of human disease is undetermined. As already mentioned, a small outbreak of human strongyloidiasis that may have originated in dogs has been described.[1]

Custodial institutions are foci of infection, which are most intense among mentally retarded patients.

References

1. Georgi JR, Sprinkle CL: A case of human strongyloidosis apparently contracted from asymptomatic colony dogs. Am J Trop Med Hyg 23:899–901, 1974

2. Pelleteir LL, Gabre-Kidan T: Chronic strongyloidiasis in Vietnam Veterans. Am J Med 78:139–140, 1985

3. Genta RM, Weesner R, Douce RW, et al.: Strongyloidiasis in US veterans of the Vietnam and other wars. JAMA 258:49–52, 1987

4. Bavay A: Sur l'anguillule stercorale. C R Acad Sci (Paris) 83:694–696, 1876

5. Normand LA: Sur la maladie dite diarrhie de Cochinchine. C R Hebd Sean Acad Sci 83:316–318, 1876

6. Askanazy M: Über Art und Zweck der Invasion der Anguillula intestinalis in die Darmwand. Centr Bakt Parasitol Infekt Abtiebung I Originale. 27:569–578, 1900

7. Fullerborn F: Untersuchungen über den Infektionsweg bei Strongyloides und Ankylostomum und die Biologie diesen Parasiten. Arch Schiffs Trop 18:26–80, 1914

8. Nishigoii M: On various factors influencing the development of Strongyloides stercoralis and autoinfection. Taiwan Sgakkai Zassi 27:1–56, 1928

9. Shekamer JH, Neva FA, Finn DR: Persistent strongyloidiasis in an immunodeficient patient. Am J Trop Med Hyg. 31:746–751, 1982

10. Olson CE, Schiller EL: Strongyloides ratti infections in rats. I. Immunopathology. Am J Trop Med Hyg 27:521–526, 1978

11. Neva FA: Biology and immunology of human strongyloidiasis. J Infect Dis 153:397–406, 1986

12. Cuni LJ, Rosner F, Chawla SK: Fatal strongyloidiasis in immunosuppressed patients. NY State J Med 77:2109–2113, 1977

13. Milner PF, Irvine RA, Burton CL, et al.: Intestinal malabsorption in Strongyloides stercoralis infestation. Gut 6:574–581, 1965

14. Robert-Thomson IC, Mitchell GF: Giardiasis in mice. I. Prolonged infections in certain mouse strains and hypothymic (nude) mice. Gastroenterology 75:42–46, 1978

15. Sato Y, Takara M, Otsuru M: Detection of antibodies in strongyloidiasis by enzyme-linked immunosorbent assay. Trans Roy Soc Trop Med Hyg 79:51–55, 1985

16. Bicalho SA, Leao OJ, Pena, Q Jr: Cambendazole in the treatment of human strongyloidiasis. Am J Trop Med Hyg 32:1181–1183, 1983

6. *Trichinella spiralis* (Railliet 1896)

Trichinella spiralis is capable of infecting all mammals. The disease it causes is referred to as trichinellosis.

Some 10 to 15 million people in North America are infected with *T. spiralis*.[1] In Europe and in Asia, its prevalence is also high. There have been recent epidemics in Japan and China.[2] In fact, the infection has been diagnosed in most parts of the world. Puerto Rico and Australia are among the exceptions.

Historical Information

Credit is usually given to Sir Richard Owen for being the first to describe, in 1835, the larva of *T. spiralis*, which he observed in a vertebrate muscle.[3] However, it was Sir James Paget, then a first-year medical student, who, while watching an autopsy, obtained a piece of the diaphragm in which he and Owen first saw the worms. Unfortunately, Owen chose not to share with Paget glory of the discovery, and promptly read a short report on the morphology of the nematode to the Zoological Society of London. Had Paget not written a letter to his brother the day after the event, describing the finding, history would to this date be giving Owen credit for the discovery.

The main features of the life cycle of *T. spiralis* were reported in 1859 by Virchow[4] and Leuckart.[5] The first clinical case of trichinellosis was described by Friedriech in 1862[6] and the first fatality was reported by Zenker in 1860.[7]

Life Cycle

The host consumes larvae encysted in a striated skeletal muscle. The larvae are liberated by the action of digestive enzymes and are transported

Trichinella spiralis

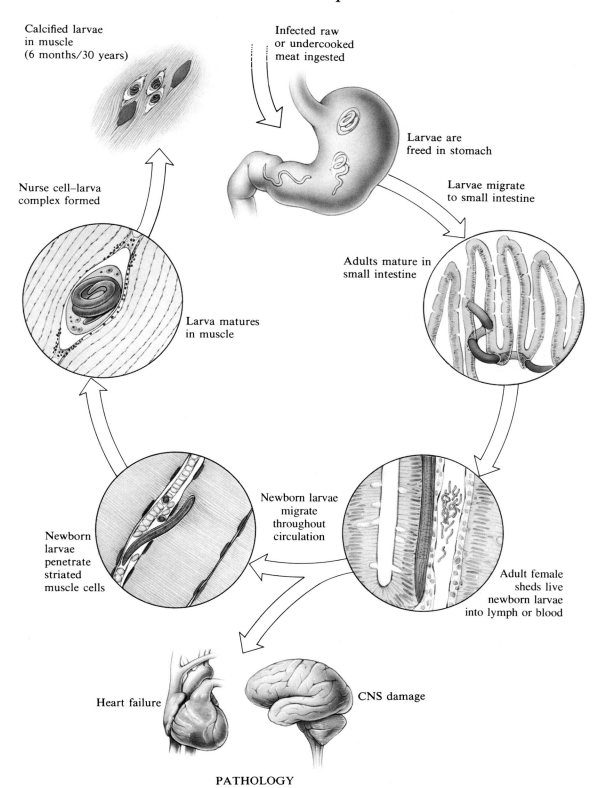

Calcified larvae
in muscle
(6 months/30 years)

Infected raw
or undercooked
meat ingested

Larvae are
freed in stomach

Larvae migrate
to small intestine

Nurse cell–larva
complex formed

Adults mature in
small intestine

Larva matures
in muscle

Newborn larvae
migrate
throughout
circulation

Newborn
larvae
penetrate
striated
muscle cells

Adult female
sheds live
newborn larvae
into lymph or blood

Heart failure

CNS damage

PATHOLOGY

passively by peristalsis to the upper two-thirds of the small intestine. There they penetrate the columnar epithelium (Fig. 6.1) at the base of the villus[8] and, after undergoing four molts during a 30-h period, become adult worms. The female is 3 mm in length (Fig. 6.2) and the male 1.5 mm (Figs. 6.3A and B). Five days after copulation, the female begins to deposit live larvae (Fig. 6.4), which are 0.08 mm long. The female continues producing larvae for 5–10 days, giving birth to some 1000 of them.

Most of the newborn larvae migrate into the lamina propria and then either into the mesenteric lymphatics or directly into the bloodstream. All larvae eventually end up in general circulation and become distributed throughout the body. They are capable of emerging from the capillaries and penetrating any cell. Most cells die as the result of invasion by the larvae, but skeletal muscle fibers are an exception (Fig. 6.5). Not only do they remain alive after invasion by the larvae, but also they are capable of supporting further growth and development of the larvae. Twenty days after penetration, the larvae have so altered their intramuscular environment that they have become "encysted." In fact, the term "cyst" is a misnomer, because in this case it is a modified, but active, muscle cell. It was named the Nurse cell[9] (Fig. 6.6) because it brings nutrients to the larva.[10]

Larvae that have penetrated tissues other than striated muscle fail to induce Nurse cell formation and either reenter the capillaries or become surrounded by granulomas and eventually die. Lar-

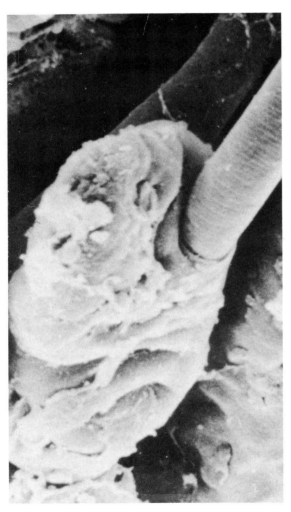

Figure 6.1. Scanning electron micrograph of an infective larva of *Trichinella spiralis* entering its intramulticellular niche in the columnar epithelium of the small intestine. ×5300. (Courtesy of Dr. M. Sukhdeo)

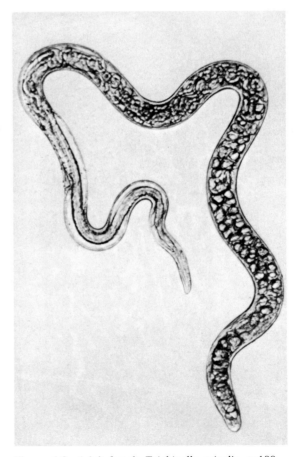

Figure 6.2. Adult female *Trichinella spiralis*. ×100.

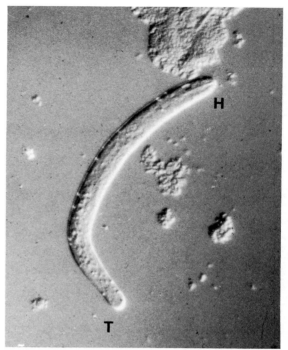

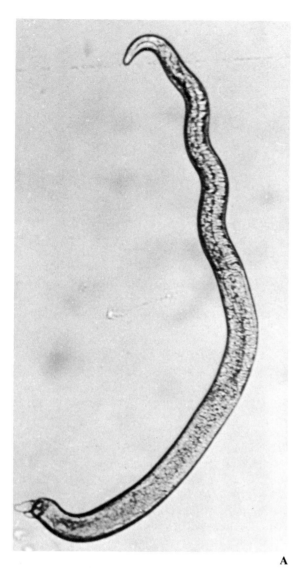

Figure 6.4. Newborn larva of *Trichinella spiralis*. This stage of the infection induces most of the pathologic changes associated with clinical trichinellosis. *H*, head; *T*, tail. × 1,000.

vae in Nurse cells can survive for years, but eventually become calcified and die. This may occur as early as 2 months or as late as 31 years after the infection.

The enteral phase of the infection in the small intestine can last for 2–3 weeks, but eventually the adult worms are expelled by the protective immune responses of the host. Although the mechanism of this expulsion is not completely understood, it is thought that antibodies play a central role.[11]

Pathogenesis

Enteral Stages
The enteral (intestinal) stages include larval stages 1 through 4 and the immature and reproductive adult stages. During the several-week period of

◀**Figure 6.3. A.** Adult male *Trichinella spiralis*. **B.** Copulatory papillae of the male *Trichinella spiralis* as seen under the scanning electron microscope. **A,** × 125; **B,** × 4,500.

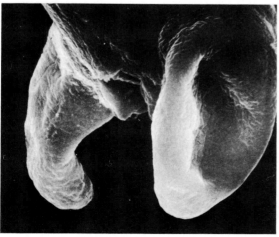

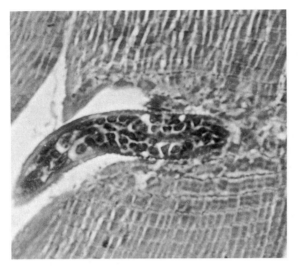

Figure 6.5. Newborn larva penetrating a skeletal muscle cell. × 1,700.

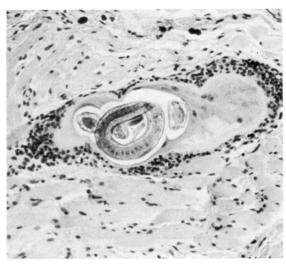

Figure 6.7. Intense inflammatory response around the Nurse cell–larva complex. This early lesion consists largely of neutrophils, eosinophils, and macrophages. × 140.

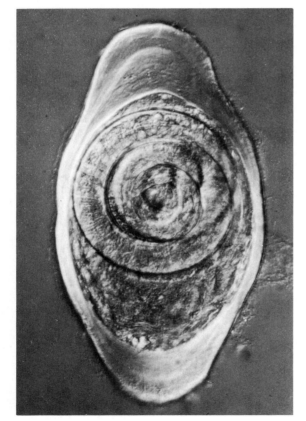

Figure 6.6. Nurse cell–infective larva complex of *Trichinella spiralis*. This biological unit is derived from a skeletal muscle cell and is anatomically independent of the surrounding host tissue. × 220.

the enteral infection, much damage can occur in the intestine.

When the larval stages are developing in the columnar epithelium, there is associated enteritis. As the worms begin to shed newborn larvae, 5–21 days after infection, the inflammation consisting of infiltration by eosinophils, neutrophils, and lymphocytes becomes intensified. The larvae penetrate the mesenteric lymphatics and capillaries. The precise mechanism of this process is not known. It is of interest that this stage of the infection is associated with bacteremia due to enteric flora, and cases of death due to sepsis have been reported.

Ultimately, the host expels the adult worms by immune defense mechanisms.

Parenteral Stages

As larvae penetrate various cells, they cause damage. This is most problematic to the host when it involves the heart and central nervous system. The myocarditis is transient and rarely consequential, because the larvae exit from the myocardium soon after penetration. However, in the central nervous system, they tend to wander, causing damage before either leaving the tissue by reentering the bloodstream or being trapped and killed within a granuloma. Much of the inflammation in the brain is initiated by petechial hemorrhages.

Following their entry into the skeletal muscle fibers, the larvae induce a progressive infiltration by the inflammatory cells (Fig. 6.7). Edema and myositis develop about 14 days following the penetration of muscle fibers.

Petechial hemorrhages noted in the conjunctivae and under the nail beds are also associated with penetration by the larvae.

Clinical Disease

Trichinellosis can mimic many clinical syndromes and, as a consequence, is often misdiagnosed. However, there are certain clues, even early in the disease, that should alert the physician to consideration of this diagnosis.

Classically, a patient has fever and myalgia, periorbital edema, petechial hemorrhages, seen most clearly in the subungual skin, but also observed in the conjunctivae and mucous membranes. Tenderness of muscles can be readily elicited. Laboratory studies reveal moderately elevated WBC (12–15,000/mm) and eosinophilia, ranging from 5% to 50%. History of eating insufficiently cooked pork, or meat that passed for something other than pork, 2 weeks or so earlier and history of a "gastroenteritis" or "flu-like illness" that followed the ingestion of the suspect meat by 2 or 3 days gives a clue to the diagnosis. As the infection progresses, larvae penetrating a variety of tissues can give rise to symptoms and signs mimicking different diseases, such as viral encephalidities and cardiomyopathies.

Diagnosis

Once the diagnosis is suspected, the approach to its establishment is relatively straightforward. One can review the history with the patient to bring out facts that may have been missed in the initial inquiry. Most important are details of consumption of meat during the preceding 1–5 weeks. It is especially important to determine what pork or pork products the patient consumed, and also to take into account any consumption of ground meats that may have been sold as, for example, beef, but in reality were pork. Homemade pork sausages and similar products usually escape proper inspection and therefore can be sources of trichinellosis. Epidemiological information about a similar disease, however mild, in people who shared the suspect meal can be very helpful in arriving at the diagnosis. Wild mammals can also be sources of infection. Outbreaks of trichinellosis have been traced to the consumption of flesh of grizzly bear, black bear, raccoon, and fox.

Patients with moderate to severe disease begin to show eosinophilia (5–10%) on about the 12th day after infection; it reaches 30–50% in two to two and a half weeks. It is probable that the eosinophilia is due to the presence of adult worms in the small intestine,[12] because it is not induced by the migrating larvae, as had previously been supposed.

Immunological tests begin to show positive results within 2 weeks. Counterimmunoelectrophoresis (CIE) and ELISA can detect antibodies in some patients even as early as 12 days after infection.[13] The bentonite flocculation test becomes positive about 3 weeks after the infection. Both remain positive for at least 2–3 months after the patient has recovered.

The definitive diagnosis of trichinellosis can be made only by finding larvae in a biopsy specimen obtained from a skeletal muscle (Fig. 6.8). The deltoids and gastrocnemii are the best muscles for this purpose.[14]

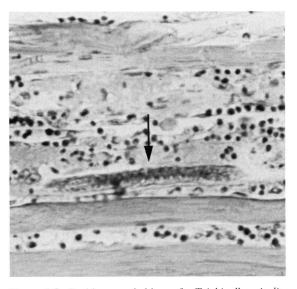

Figure 6.8. Positive muscle biopsy for *Trichinella spiralis*. The larva (*arrow*) is young (probably 6–8 days old) and has not yet begun to coil up in its Nurse cell. × 400. (Courtesy of Dr. H. Zaiman)

Proper handling of the tissue at biopsy is crucial to the success of the test. Although some of it should be processed in the routine fashion for histopathological studies, a part must be provided fresh and uncut for a direct microscopic examination. It is carried out by squashing the fresh tissue between two microscope slides and examining it under low power and reduced light, to observe the larvae. Although the larvae are characteristically coiled in a long standing infection, in the early phase of the infection they may still be straight, parallel to the muscle fibers. A cube of a few millimeters of tissue is usually sufficient to make the diagnosis in all but lightly infected individuals. If larvae are more than 12 days old, they can be released from the tissue by digestion with pepsin-HC1 mixture and concentrated by centrifugation. This improves the chances of microscopic identification.

Adult worms may be present in the stool, but are difficult to detect because they are few in number and tend to be degenerated.

Treatment

Once the diagnosis is made, there is little that the physician can offer in the way of therapy. The most important reason for establishment of this diagnosis is that it relieves the concern about more serious and consequential diseases.

If the patient is toxic, he should be treated symptomatically with antipyretics and analgesics (aspirin, acetaminophen). More seriously ill patients may require therapy with one of the oral corticosteroids (e.g., prednisone) for several days. No currently available drug can alter the course of the infection, once the migratory phase has begun. Thiabendazole can affect the adult worms,[15] but not the migratory newborn larvae. Unfortunately, trichinellosis is seldom suspected during the early phase of the disease, and therefore the use of this drug is not practical.

Prevention and Control

Prevention may be readily accomplished by thorough cooking of pork at 58.5°C for 10 min or by freezing it at −20°C for 3 days. The majority (90-95%) of infections with T. spiralis in the United States result from the eating of undercooked or raw pork obtained from commercial sources.[1] In addition, outbreaks of the disease have been traced to ground beef that had been adulterated with pork scraps. Finally, sporadic epidemics have been caused by the ingestion of undercooked meat of bears and other wild animals.

Only 80–100 cases are reported each year to the Centers for Disease Control, whereas more than 200,000 new infections are estimated to occur each year. The apparent low incidence may be accounted for by the relatively mild symptoms of some infections, in which the diagnosis is missed, and by the subclinical course of most.

It is usually impossible to trace a supply of pork to its source, because the origin of individual pigs is not identifiable after the animals are sold at auctions. Large numbers of people raise their own pigs for private consumption and do not take the recommended precautions of cooking refuse that is used to feed the pigs. Besides the uncooked garbage that contains infected meat scraps, there are other sources of infection for pigs, such as consumption of infected rats and other small animals, and cannibalism of dead infected pigs. Singularly raised pigs represent a major source of trichinellosis in the United States.

United States federal law requires that all refuse destined for the pig farms be cooked to avoid certain viral infections, such as vesicular exanthema, foot and mouth disease, and hog cholera, but it is difficult to enforce this law. Moreover, the United States, in contrast, for example, with Germany, does not require microscopic examination of pork for T. spiralis.

Thorough cooking or freezing of pork will destroy the infective larvae and prevent infection. However, certain wild animals, such as bears and raccoons, have substances in their muscles that prevent ice crystals from forming, thus permitting the survival of larvae. Hence, their flesh must be cooked to destroy the larvae.

References

1. Kim CW: Epidemiology II. Geographic distribution and prevalance. in: Trichinella and Trichinosis (Campbell WC, ed.) Plenum Press, New York and London, 1983, pp 445–500
2. Au ACS, Ko RC, Simon JW, et al.: Study of acute trichinosis in Gurkas: specificity and sensitivity of enzyme linked immunosorbent assays for IgM and IgE antibodies to trichinella larval anti-

gens in diagnosis. Trans Roy Soc Trop Med Hyg 77:412–415, 1983

3. Owen R: Description of a microscopic entozoan infesting the muscles of the human body. Trans Zool Soc 1:315–324, 1835

4. Virchow R: Recherche sur le development du *Trichina spiralis*. C R Acad Sci 49:660–662, 1860

5. Leuckart R: Untersuchungen über *Trichina Spiralis*. Zugleich ein Beitrag zur Kenntnis der Wurmkrankheiten. Winter, Leipzig

6. Friedriech N: Ein Beitrag zur Pathologie der Trichinenkrankheit beim Menschen. Virchows Arch Path Anat 25:399–413, 1862

7. Zenker FA: Über die Trichinen-Krankheit des Menschen. Virchows Arch Path Anat 18:561–572, 1860

8. Wright K: *Trichinella spiralis:* An intracellular parasite in the intestinal phase. J Parasitol 65:441–445, 1979

9. Purkerson M, Despommier DD: Fine structure of the muscle phase of *Trichinella spiralis* in the mouse. In (Kim C, ed): Trichinellosis. New York, Intext Educational Publishers, 1974, pp 7–23

10. Stewart GL, Read CP: Desoxyribonucleic acid metabolism in mouse trichinosis. J Parasitol 59:164–167, 1973

11. Despommier DD: The Immunobiology of *Trichinella spiralis* in: Immune Responses in Parasitic Infections: Immunology, Immunopathology, and Immunoprophylaxis Vol. 1 Nematodes. Soulsby EJL, ed. CRC Press, Inc. Boca Raton, Florida, 1987, pp 43–60

12. Despommier DD, Weisbroth S, Fass C: Circulating eosinophils and trichinosis in the rat: The stage responsible for induction during infection. J Parasitol 60: 280–284, 1974

13. Despommier DD, Müller M, Jenks B, et al.: Immunodiagnosis of human trichinosis using counterelectrophoresis and agar gel diffusion techniques. Am J Trop Med Hyg 23:41–44, 1974

14. Despommier DD: Trichinellosis. in: Immunodiagnosis of Parasitic Diseases. Vol 1. Helminthic Diseases. Schantz PM and Walls KW eds. Academic Press, Inc., Orlando, 1987 pp 43–60

15. Campbell WC, Cuckler AC: Comparative studies on the chemotherapy of experimental trichinosis in mice. Z Tropenmed Parasitol 18:408–417, 1967

16. Zimmerman WJ: The current status of trichinellosis in the United States. In: Trichinellosis (Kim C ed.). New York, Intext Educational Publishers, 1974, pp 609–614

7. *Wuchereria bancrofti* (Cobbold 1877)

Wuchereria bancrofti is a thread-like nematode, whose adults live within lymphatic vessels. The worms are ovoviviparous; their larvae are called microfilariae. Approximately 400 million people are at present infected with this filarial worm.[1]

There are apparently three forms of *W. bancrofti*, one of which is more widely distributed in the tropics and is primarily spread by culicine mosquitoes; the other two, spread mainly by anopheline mosquitoes, are most commonly seen in Africa, Southeast Asia, South America, and the island of Timor in New Guinea. A diurnal *W. bancrofti* exists in the South Pacific area, which has day-biting mosquitoes of the *Aedes* sp. as its primary vector. There are no animal reservoir hosts for this parasite.

Historical Information

The microfilariae of *W. bancrofti* were first described by Demarquay[2] in 1863 and the adult worms in 1877 by Bancroft[3] in Australia and by Lewis[4] in India. Manson,[5] also in 1877, completed the description of the cycle by showing that mosquitoes acted as intermediate hosts for the parasite. For two decades Manson persisted in his belief that infection occurred when individuals drank water containing larvae released from dead or dying mosquitoes. He eventually accepted the concept that the larvae were transmitted by the bite of the mosquito. Nevertheless, filariasis may be a water-borne disease under some circumstances, because experimental infections can be induced by the oral route.[6]

Life Cycle

Adult worms (Figs. 7.1 and 7.2) occupy the lumen of lymphatic vessels (Fig. 7.3), and have been found at all sites within the lymphatic circulation. The female is approximately 8 cm by 300 μm; the male 4 cm by 100 μm. The microfilariae (Fig. 7.4 A and B and 12.1A), the first-stage larvae, find their way from the lym-

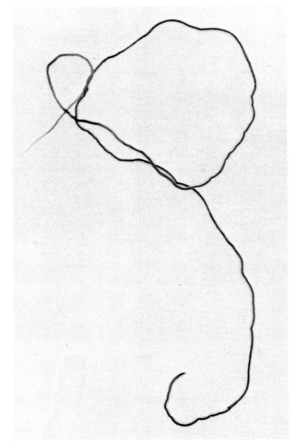

Figure 7.1. Adult female *Wuchereria bancrofti.* ×4.

phatic circulation into the bloodstream. They measure approximately 270 μm by 9 μm and are ensheathed. Their nuclei do not extend to the tip of the tail. In most endemic areas of the world, microfilariae are present in large numbers in the peripheral blood only during the night, but in a few regions they have a diurnal cycle. During the time of low peripheral microfilariaemia, the microfilariae aggregate in the capillaries of the lungs. Nocturnal periodicity can be a result of the microfilariae's penchant for low oxygen tension.[7] Experiments in which sleep habits of infected volunteers were reversed also reversed the periodicity of microfilariae. The diurnal periodicity pattern has not been satisfactorily explained. A less frequently occurring subperiodic filariasis caused by *W. bancrofti* occurs in certain regions of the world.

Microfilariae, which live for about 1½ years, must be ingested by a mosquito to continue the life cycle.

A large number of mosquito species transmit *W. bancrofti;* the most important include *Culex pipiens quinquefasciatus, Culex pipiens pipiens, Anopheles gambiae,* and *A. polynesiensis* (see Chapter 38). In all cases, it is the female insect that acquires the larvae with her blood meal.

Ingested microfilariae penetrate the stomach wall of the mosquito and migrate into the thoracic flight muscles. There they undergo three molts and develop into third-stage larvae (Fig. 7.5), becoming infective after 10–20 days of morphogenesis in the insect muscle tissue.

The infective larvae migrate from the muscles to the biting mouth parts (Fig. 7.6) and during consumption of a subsequent blood meal are deposited onto the skin adjacent to the bite wound. When the mosquito withdraws her mouth parts from the epidermis, the larvae crawl into the

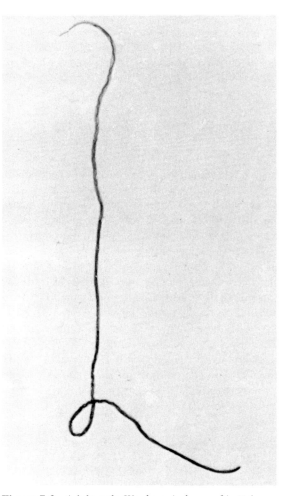

Figure 7.2. Adult male *Wuchereria bancrofti.* ×4.

Wuchereria bancrofti

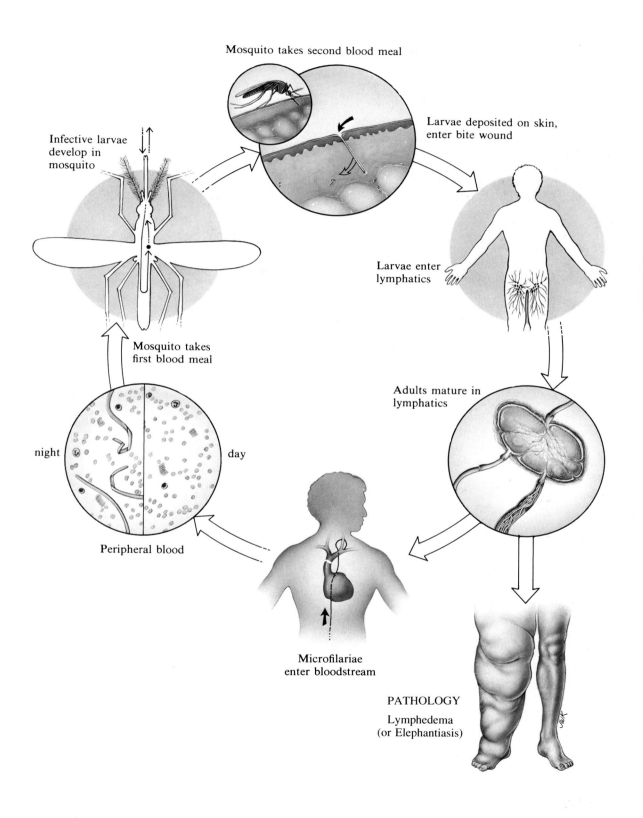

Mosquito takes second blood meal

Larvae deposited on skin, enter bite wound

Infective larvae develop in mosquito

Larvae enter lymphatics

Mosquito takes first blood meal

Adults mature in lymphatics

night   day

Peripheral blood

Microfilariae enter bloodstream

PATHOLOGY

Lymphedema (or Elephantiasis)

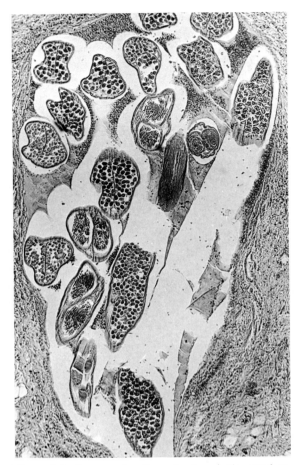

Figure 7.3. Cross section through a lymphatic vessel occupied by adult *Wuchereria bancrofti*. Various stages of microfilarial embryogenesis are seen in the sections of worm. × 54.

open wound and migrate through the subcutaneous tissues to the lymphatic vessels. The worms develop into mature adults in about 1 year and, soon after copulation, begin shedding microfilariae. The longevity of adult worms, measured by the continued production of micorfilariae, is estimated at 5–8 years, but infections lasting 40 years have been reported.[8]

Pathogenesis

Secreted metabolic products of the adult worms (i.e., various peptides, proteins, etc.) induce immunological reactions causing alterations of the walls of the lymphatics. As a direct result of hypersensitization, the walls thicken and become distended, but the drainage of lymph remains largely unaffected. Neither the microfilariae nor their metabolic products cause any overt pathological changes. When the adult worms die, the sudden release of antigenic material from the disintegrating worms exacerbates the inflammatory response in the wall of the lymphatic vessel. Following an intense lymphocytic infiltration, the lumen of the vessel eventually closes, and the remnants of the adult worms calcify (Fig. 7.7). The blockage of lymphatic circulation continues in heavily infected individuals until most major lymph channels are occluded, causing lymphedema in the affected region of the body. In addition, hypertrophy of smooth muscle tissue occurs in the area immediately surrounding the site of involvement.

As already implied, the process of lymphatic blockage is a protracted one and results from repeated infections. Consequently, people visiting endemic areas for short periods of time usually do not develop lymphedema, even as they often have microfilariaemia.

Clinical Disease

Usually, clinical disease begins with the inflammatory process, i.e., lymphangitis, dermatitis, and cellulitis, which are all associated with fever. After several days, the lymph nodes draining the involved areas become enlarged and tender. The skin becomes doughy and exhibits some degree of pitting, but is rather firm. As the inflammatory reaction continues, the area becomes firmer still and pitting disappears. There is substantial encroachment on the subcutaneous tissue and consequent loss of elasticity of the overlying skin. Characteristically, and in contradistinction to cellulitis caused by some bacteria, filarial cellulitis shows no demarcation line between the affected and the healthy skin. In Bancroftian filariasis the legs are more likely to be involved than the upper extremities and the lower portions of the legs more involved than the upper ones. The scrotum is frequently affected and may become gigantic, weighing up to 10 kg; much larger scrotums have been described in rare cases.

Diagnosis

Definitive diagnosis is based on the demonstration of the characteristic microfilariae in the blood (Fig. 7.4). This can be achieved by examination of a blood smear stained by Giemsa solution. In

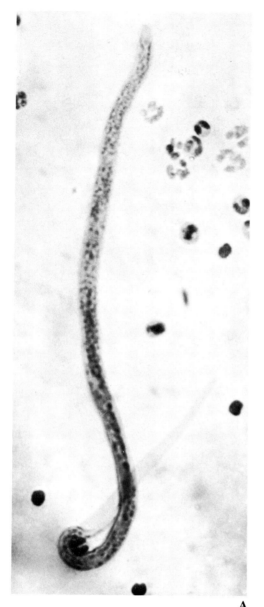

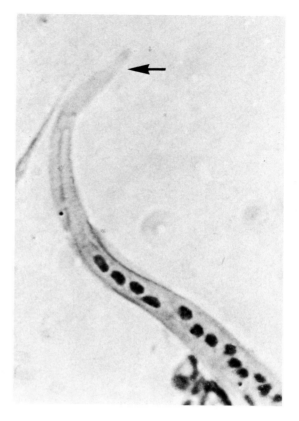

A

Figure 7.4. A. Microfilaria of *Wuchereria bancrofti*. **B.** Tail of the microfilaria of *Wuchereria bancrofti*. Note that the nuclei do not extend to the tip of the tail and the sheath (*arrow*) extends beyond the tip of the tail (see Figure 12.1). **A,** ×650; **B,** ×1,600.

the case of light infection, 1 ml of blood is preserved in 9 ml of 1% formalin and then concentrated by centrifugation (Knott test). The pellet contains red cell ghosts and microfilariae. Stained smears of the pellet are then examined microscopically. Another technique for concentration depends on filtration of 10 ml of heparinized blood through a filter with a pore size of 10 μm, which permits the red cells to pass through. The filter containing only white cells and microfilariae is then stained and examined.

Because of the periodicity, it is best to draw blood during the customary hours of sleep. It is possible, however, to provoke migration of microfilariae at other times by administration of 100 mg of diethylcarbamazine to an adult, and collecting blood 45 min to 1 h subsequently.

Immunological tests for the diagnosis of *Wuchereria bancrofti* infection have been developed, although they are not yet widely available. They are based both on the measurements of the host's antibody response to the antigens of the

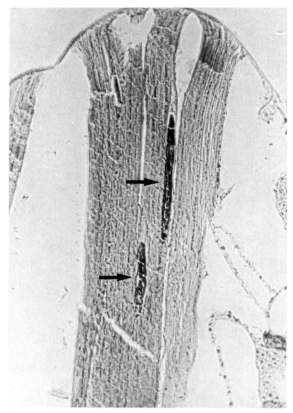

Figure 7.5. Larvae (*arrows*) of *Wuchereria bancrofti* in the flight wing muscles of a mosquito. × 150.

worm[9], and on the detection by monoclonal antibodies of circulating worm antigens[10].

Treatment

Therapy is inadequate and is effective only in eradication of the microfilariae. Administration of diethylcarbamazine for 10–30 days is the current recommended treatment. This therapy can be associated with fever, probably resulting from the disintegration of a few of the adult worms, occasional nausea and vomiting, and fleeting skin rashes. Ivermectin, a drug effective in therapy of onchocerciasis, has the capacity to kill the microfilariae of *W. bancrofti*. It has an advantage over diethylcarbamazine in that only one dose of it is required. However there have been insufficient clinical trials to recommend it as a drug of choice. Moreover, by causing release of the antigens from the dying parasites, it can cause side effects similar to those of diethylcarbamazine.

Treatment of lymphedema is symptomatic, but in certain affected areas, such as the scrotum,

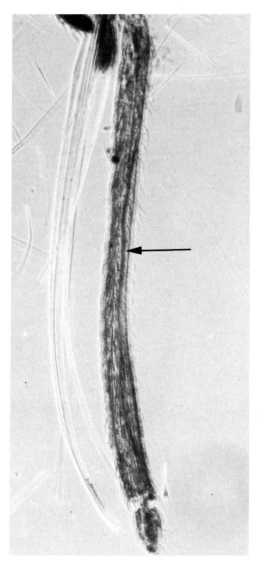

Figure 7.6. Infective larva (*arrow*) of *Wuchereria bancrofti* lying within the biting mouth parts of a mosquito. × 76.

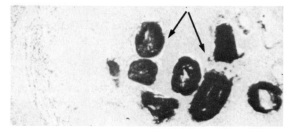

Figure 7.7. Calcified, dead adults of *Wuchereria bancrofti* (*arrows*) within an occluded lymphatic vessel. Extensive fibrosis surrounds the dead worms. × 25.

surgical excision and exteriorization of the testes to restore fertility may be required. However, even after surgery, the affected area invariably becomes edematous once again.

Prevention and Control

Prevention depends primarily on the control of the mosquito vectors and has had limited success because the mosquitoes develop resistance to the insecticides. The increased urbanization of vast areas of tropical Asia has resulted in the concomitant rise in the prevalence of both Bancroftian and Malayian varieties of filariasis carried by mosquitoes that breed in non-sylvatic habitats. Mass treatment with ivermectin may become useful in the control of Bancroftian filariasis by reducing the load of microfilariae in the treated person. This would make transmission less likely.

References

1. Nelson GS: Filariasis. N Engl J Med 300: 1136–1139, 1979
2. Demarquay M: Note sur une tumeur des bourses contenant un liquide laiteux (galactocele de Vidal) et refermant des petits etres vermiformes que l'on peut considerer comme des helminthes hematoides a l'etat d'embryon. Gaz Med Paris 18:665–667, 1863
3. Cobbold TS: Discovery of the adult representative of microscopic filariae. Lancet 2:70–71, 1877
4. Lewis T: *Filaria sanguinis hominis* (mature form), found in a blood-clot in naevoid elephantiasis of the scrotum. Lancet 2:453–455, 1877
5. Manson P: Further observations on *Filaria sanguinis hominis*. Medical Reports China Imperial Maritime Customs, Shanghai, no. 14, 1878, pp 1–26
6. Gwadz RW, Chernin E: Oral transmission of *Brugia pahangi* to jirds *(Meriones unguiculatus)*. Nature 238:524–525, 1972
7. Hawking F, Pattanayak S, Sharma HL: The periodicity of microfilariae. XI. The effect of body temperature and other stimuli upon the cycles of *Wuchereria bancrofti*, *Brugia malayi*, *B. ceylonensis* and *Dirofilaria repens*. Trans Soc Trop Med Hyg 60:497–513, 1966
8. Carme B, Laigret J: Longevity of *Wuchereria bancrofti var. pacifica* and mosquito infection acquired from a patient with low parasitemia. Am J Trop Med Hyg 28:53–55, 1979
9. Dissanoyake S, Ismail MM: Immunodiagnosis of Bancroftian filariasis. in: Filariasis (Evered D and Clark S, eds). Ciba Foundation Symposium 127. John Wiley and Sons, Chichester, New York, 1987, pp 203–224
10. Weil GJ, Jain DC, Santhanam S, et al.: A monoclonal antibody-based enzyme immunoassay for detecting parasite antigenemia in Bancroftian filariasis. J Infect Dis 156:350–355, 1987

8. *Onchocerca volvulus* (Leuckart 1893)

Onchocerca volvulus is a filarial nematode living in the subcutaneous tissues. Man is its only host. The vector of *O. volvulus* is the blackfly *Simulium* sp. (see Chapter 38). *O. volvulus* is prevalent in Africa, and in Central and South America where it is the major cause of blindness, often affecting more than 50% of the inhabitants of towns and villages in endemic areas. The breeding habitat of the blackfly is rivers and streams; hence the common term "river blindness" has been applied to onchocerciasis. Approximately 17 million people throughout the world are infected, with over 330,000 cases of blindness.

Historical Information

Onchocercal infection was first described in Africa by Leuckart. He recounted his discovery of the parasite to Manson, who, in turn, published the full description in 1893, giving Leuckart credit.[1]

Earlier, O'Neill[2] observed the microfilariae of this filarial nematode in the skin of a patient from West Africa. Clinical onchocerciasis in Latin America was not reported until 1917, when Robles[3] found ocular disease associated with the presence of nodules on the forehead of a small boy. He dissected the nodule, and found that it contained the adult worms. Later he described the worm, the pathology of the disease, and epidemiology of the infection. Moreover, he suspected that the blackfly was the vector, which was proved by Blacklock[4] in 1927.

Life Cycle

The adult female measures about 40 cm in length and 300 μm in width; the male 30 mm by 150

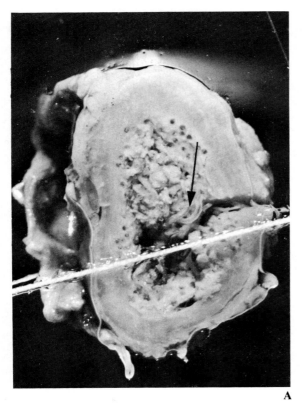
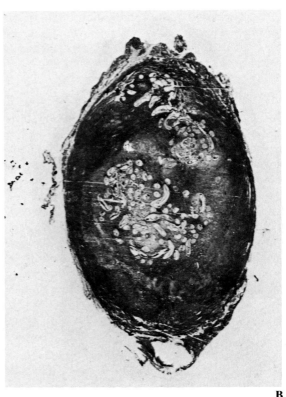

A   B

Figure 8.1. A. Bisected whole nodule removed from the head of a patient infected with *Onchocerca volvulus.* Adult worms can be seen in various sections throughout the center portion of the nodule (*arrow*). The specimen is suspended by a piece of string for purposes of orientation. **B.** Cross section of a nodule containing adults of *Onchocerca volvulus.* **A,** ×2; **B,** ×2.

μm. Both sexes, entwined about each other, live embedded in subcutaneous fibrous nodules, which vary in size depending on the number of adult worms in them (Fig. 8.1A and B). Microfilariae are produced within the nodules, but leave these sites and wander through the subcutaneous tissues.

The blackfly (Fig. 8.2) acquires the larvae in the process of taking a blood meal. The immature worms penetrate the insect's hemocoele and then muscle fibers of the flight wing bundles in the thorax. After 6–8 days of development, during which the larvae molt twice, the now infective larvae migrate out of the muscles into the cavity of the proboscis and are deposited on human skin when the fly bites. The larvae enter the bite wound after the fly has withdrawn its biting mouth parts, and take up residence in subcutaneous tissues, where they complete their development and mate. The adults produce hundreds of thousands of microfilariae (Figs. 8.3 and 12.1B) during their life span of 8–10 years. The growth and molting of the worms in the subcutaneous tissues induce formation of the fibrous nodules (Fig. 8.4).

Pathogenesis

The degree of infection varies directly with the intensity and frequency of exposure to the bite of the vector. The disease results from a severe inflammatory reaction elicited by the foreign protein of the worms. There is no evidence that live microfilariae cause *any* reaction, but dead ones induce inflammation that becomes more severe the longer the infection has persisted within the host. This has an important implication in consideration of the therapy.

The lesions primarily involve the skin and the eyes. Although some reports have suggested that

Onchocerca volvulus

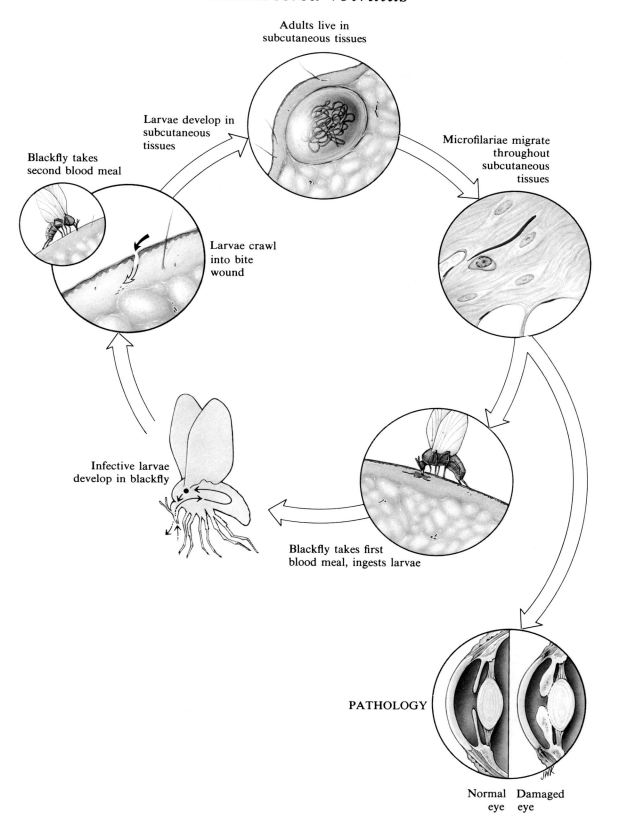

Adults live in
subcutaneous tissues

Larvae develop in
subcutaneous
tissues

Blackfly takes
second blood meal

Larvae crawl
into bite
wound

Microfilariae migrate
throughout
subcutaneous
tissues

Infective larvae
develop in blackfly

Blackfly takes first
blood meal, ingests larvae

PATHOLOGY

Normal
eye

Damaged
eye

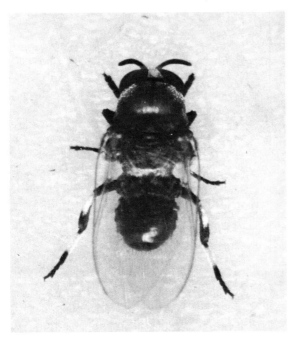

Figure 8.2. Female blackfly, *Simulium damnosum*, vector of *Onchocerca volvulus*. ×22. (Courtesy of Armed Forces Institute of Pathology, Neg. no. 72-4519E)

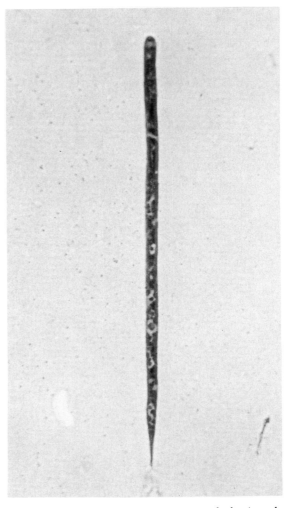

Figure 8.3. Microfilaria of *Onchocerca volvulus* (see also Fig. 12.1B). ×240.

lymphadenopathy, particularly in the inguinal region, may be due to onchocercal infections, this is probably incorrect because these studies failed to eliminate the strong possibility of concomitant infections with those filariae that are known to cause lymphedema (viz. Wuchereria and Brugia; see Chapter 7).

Nodules in the subcutaneous tissues vary in size from barely noticeable to those the size of a lemon. The numbers of nodules also vary from an occasional one to several hundreds, occupying virtually every bit of subcutaneous tissue. Those areas in which peripheral lymphatics converge (e.g., the occiput, suboccipital areas, intercostal spaces, the axilla, and iliac crests) have the highest predilection to nodules. The body regions most affected differ in different geographic locales. In Africa, for example, the nodules predominate in the lower part of the body, whereas in Central America they tend to be found more often in the upper portions of the body. This is related to the biting habits of the vector insects and the styles of clothing worn by the inhabitants of each endemic area. The eye lesions develop as a result of the invasion by microfilariae of the optic nerve and the retina, wherein an inflamma-

tory reaction leading to atrophy develops. Eye lesions are common in geographic areas where nodules tend to be concentrated in the upper part of the body. Nothing is known concerning the nature of either the irritants released by the adults, which induce nodule formation, or those associated with the microfilariae, which elicit the inflammatory responses described above.

Clinical Disease

Skin Lesions

Mild infections produce no symptoms at all, but moderate to severe infections produce correspondingly more serious and more numerous

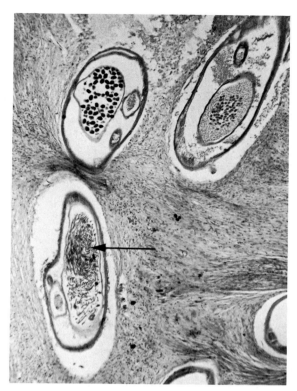

Figure 8.4. Section through a nodule containing adults of *Onchocerca volvulus*. Note presence of microfilariae (*arrow*) in uterus of female. ×54.

symptoms. The involvement of the skin is heralded by an intense itching reaction, associated with a rash consisting of numerous small circular, elevated papules, 1–3 mm in diameter. On white skin these papules are reddish in color, but on black skin they tend to be dark brown. The involved areas eventually become endematous and thickened, giving rise to the characteristic appearance resembling orange skin ("peau d'orange"). Later the skin becomes even thicker and is lichenified, before it becomes atrophic and loses its elasticity, giving rise to a condition called presbyderma.

This severe involvement of the skin is more common in Africa than in Central America, but Central American children who are infected may have facial lesions, reddish in color and described as "erisipela de la costa."

Eye Lesions
Eye lesions involve all parts of the eye. Initially, there may be conjunctivitis, a reaction analogous to the dermatitis in response to dead microfilar-

iae, and associated with irritation, lacrimation, and photophobia. Examination of the cornea at this time will reveal punctate lesions of keratitis. Slit-lamp examination will reveal motile or dead microfilariae in the conjunctiva. A long-standing infection will produce sclerosis and vascularization. The anterior chamber is also invaded and microfilariae can be seen there with a slit lamp. Finally there may be iritis, iridocyclitis, and secondary glaucoma, which is the main cause of blindness. Invasion of the posterior segment of the eye causes optic neuritis, or at least papillitis; the choroid and the retina are also involved. Inguinal lymphadenopathy, often leading to scrotal enlargement, has been attributed to onchocercal infection.[5]

Diagnosis

Diagnosis is made by examination of a piece of skin (2–5 mm^2) cut from the affected part of the body; in Africa the specimen should be obtained from the lower part and in Central America, from the upper. The skin should be cleansed, elevated with a needle, and snipped with a sharp knife blade; next, a preferably bloodless piece should be examined directly in saline solution to note motile microfilariae. A representative sample of this skin can be weighed and the number of microfilariae per milligram of tissue calculated as an index of the intensity of infection. In addition, the piece of skin can be pressed against a dry microscope slide and the impression stained with Giemsa solution and examined for presence of microfilariae (Fig. 8.5). Section of a subcutaneous nodule will also reveal microfilariae.

Serological tests have not yet been perfected to provide an accurate diagnosis. The Mazzotti test consists of observation of the clinical reaction to a test dose of diethylcarbamazine. Positive response results in an exacerbation of the skin itch or induction of itching of the skin or rash in patients who were previously free of it.

Treatment

Ivermectin, given as a single dose, is the drug of choice recently approved by the U.S. F.D.A. for use in this infection. It affects a wider variety of invertebrates, including most filarial parasites, by either interfering with the presynaptic release of gamma amino benzoic acid or interfering with

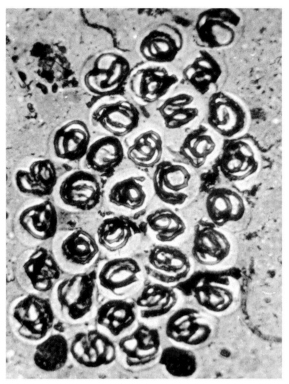

Figure 8.5. Impression smear from a nodule showing numerous coiled microfilariae of *Onchocerca volvulus*. ×240.

neurotransmission in the parasite. Ivermectin has a high therapeutic index and is effective in microgram amounts.[6].

Surgical removal of the nodules acts as prophylaxis of intense involvement of the eyes.

Prevention and Control

Distribution of onchocerciasis follows that of the vector. Blackflies breed in fast running water of mountainous streams in regions of Africa and South and Central America.

Blackflies have a fairly long flight range. As a result, onchocerciasis can be found several miles from the nearest endemic breeding site. Since much of the coffee of the world is grown on mountainous hillsides, the prevalence of onchocerciasis among workers on coffee plantations is high.

The first step in control of the disease should be directed toward infected populations through the use of surgery (i.e., removal of nodules) and drug therapy against the microfilariae.

The second step should be an attempt to reduce the vector population in the larval stages of development by the use of DDT and other insecticides in streams and rivers. However, since all species of insects in the treated rivers are affected by DDT, severe, adverse effects on food chains and food webs may result. Moreover, because the dose of DDT added into the rivers and streams cannot be precisely controlled, resistance of blackflies to DDT has developed.

Recently a multidisciplinary program was initiated by the World Health Organization in the Volta River basin, in West Africa, which serves as a model for control programs of onchocerciasis in other regions.[7] This program incorporates elements of vector control, chemotherapy with ivermectin, and surveillance. It still lacks immunological or molecular biological methods for precise diagnosis, which would be of immense value to the surveillance.

References

1. Manson P: *Filaria volvuloxus* In Davidson AH: Hygiene and Diseases of Warm Climates. London, Y.J. Pentland, 1893, p. 1016
2. O'Neill J: On the presence of a filaria in "craw-craw." Lancet 1:265–266, 1875
3. Robles R: Enfermidad nueva en Guatemala. La Juventud Medica 17:97–115, 1917
4. Blacklock DB: The insect transmission of *Onchocerca volvulus* (Leuckart 1893). The cause of worm nodules in man in Africa. Br Med J 1:129–133, 1927
5. Connor 'DH, Morrison NE, Kerdel-Vegas F, et al.: Onchocercal dermatitis, lymphadenitis, and elephatiasis in the Ubangi territory. Hum Pathol 1:553, 1970
6. Rew RS, Fetterer RH: Mode of action of antinematodal drugs. In: Chemotherapy of Parasitic Diseases (Campbell WC, Rew RS, eds). Plenum Press. New York and London, 1986, pp 321–337.
7. Taylor HR: Global priorities in the control of onchocerciasis. Rev Infect Dis 7:844–846, 1985

9. *Loa loa* (Cobbold 1864)

Loa loa, the filarial worm causing loaiasis, is limited to Africa, where it infects some 20 million people. The adult worms live in subcutaneous tissues. Their main vectors are dipteran flies of the genus Chrysops; there are no reservoir hosts.

Historical Information

Argyll-Robertson[1] provided the first accurate and complete description of the worm and the clinical presentation of the infection in 1895. The woman from whom he removed two adult worms (one of each sex) had lived in West Africa in Old Calabar. Swellings in her arms accompanied her infection and were described in detail by Argyll-Robertson. Today, these inflammatory lesions are still referred to as Calabar swellings.

Flies of two species, *Chrysops dimidiata* and *C. silacae,* were found by Leiper[2] to be the proper vectors of *L. loa.*

Life Cycle

The adult females are about 0.5 mm wide and 60 mm long (Fig. 9.1); the males, 0.4 mm by 32 mm. The adult worms wander throughout the subcutaneous tissues, where the female deposits microfilariae. The microfilariae (Figs. 9.2A and B, and 12.1A) penetrate capillaries and enter the bloodstream, where they remain until they are ingested in a blood meal by a mango fly, *Chrysops* spp.

The larvae penetrate the stomach of the fly and come to rest inside a structure known as the fat body. From 8–10 days later, the infective third-stage larvae move into the cavity of the biting mouth parts, and are released into the bite wound as the fly feeds. The larvae, in the subcutaneous tissues of the host, molt to adults within 1–4 years, mate, and the females begin depositing microfilariae.

The nutritional requirements of *L. loa* are unknown.

Pathogenesis

Neither the adult worms in the subcutaneous tissues of the host nor the microfilariae in the

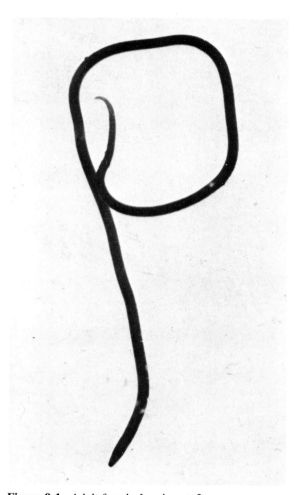

Figure 9.1. Adult female *Loa loa.* ×2.

bloodstream cause any pathological changes. However, in time, the infected person becomes hypersensitive to the secretions of the adult worms. This immunological reaction expresses itself in swelling of tissues traversed by the worm, the Calabar swellings.

Clinical Disease

The hot, erythematous Calabar swellings occurring on the extremities and in the periorbital tissues may be quite painful, but last only a few days. More disturbing to the patient is the occasional passage of an adult worm across the subconjunctival space. On rare occasions, adult par-

Loa loa

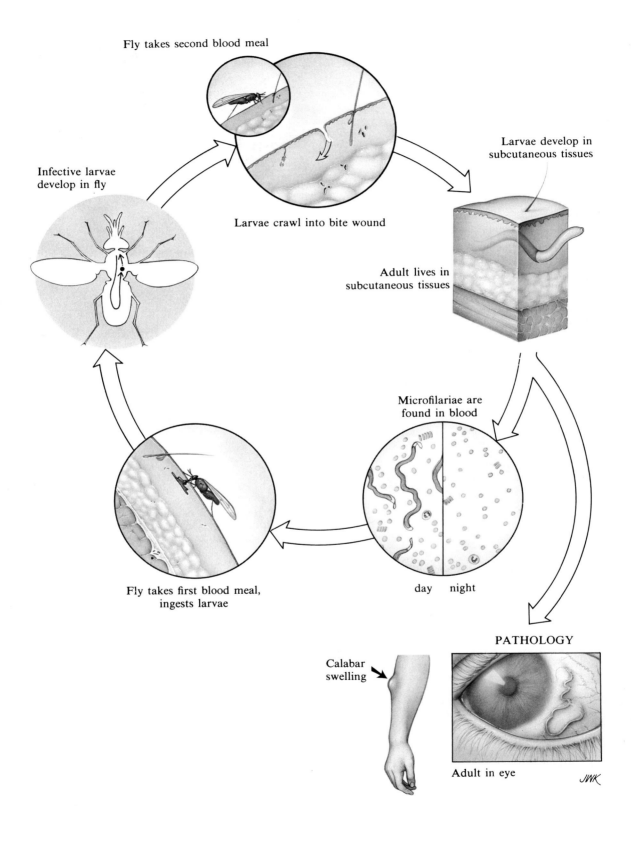

Fly takes second blood meal

Larvae crawl into bite wound

Infective larvae
develop in fly

Larvae develop in
subcutaneous tissues

Adult lives in
subcutaneous tissues

Microfilariae are
found in blood

Fly takes first blood meal,
ingests larvae

day   night

PATHOLOGY

Calabar
swelling

Adult in eye

JWK

asites have been found in the cerebrospinal fluid, in association with meningoencephalitis.

Diagnosis

Diagnosis is made by finding the microfilariae in a thin blood smear stained with either Giemsa or Wright's solution (Fig. 9.2A and B). It is also possible to recover an adult worm from the sub-

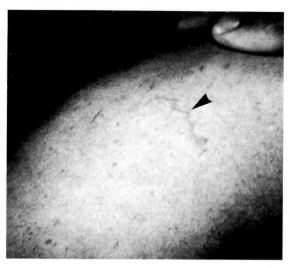

Figure 9.3. Adult *Loa loa* in the subcutaneous tissues (*arrow*) of a patient. (Courtesy of Dr. C. Panosian)

conjunctival space and various subcutaneous tissues (Fig. 9.3). There are no reliable serological tests.

Treatment

Diethylcarbamazine kills the microfilariae, but not the adult worms. An allergic inflammatory response may follow death of the microfilariae and may have to be treated with corticosteroids. Adult worms in the eye must be removed surgically.

Prevention and Control

Spraying mango groves with insecticides, particularly DDT, remains an effective method of controlling populations of the vector. Dieldrin applied to breeding sites kills the larvae.

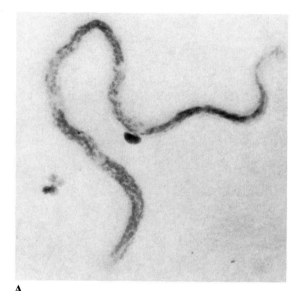

A

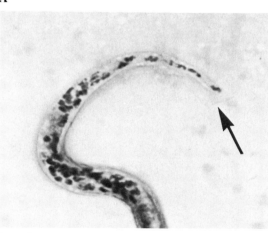

B

Figure 9.2. A. Microfilaria of *Loa loa*. **B.** Tail of the microfilaria of *Loa loa* has nuclei that extend to the tip. A sheath (*arrow*) is also present (see also Fig. 12.1A). **A,** ×600; **B,** ×1,300.

References

1. Argyll-Robertson DMCL: Case of *Filaria loa* in which the parasite was removed from under the conjunctiva. Trans Ophthalmol Soc UK 15:137–167, 1895

2. Leiper RT: Report of the helminthologist for the half year ending 30 April, 1913. Report Adv Commis Trop Dis Res Fund, 1913–1914

10. *Dracunculus medinensis* (Linnaeus 1758)

Dracunculus medinensis, commonly known as the Guinea Fire Worm, causes infection throughout Central Africa, the Middle East, India, and to a lesser extent, South America. Estimates of prevalence suggest that the number of infected individuals is nearly 50 million.[1]

This parasite affects the skin and subcutaneous tissues and causes a relatively benign infection. Nevertheless, because of secondary bacterial infections of the skin lesions, and the high prevalence of this nematode, *D. medinensis* ranks as one of the most important infections in the developing world. It has a number of reservoir hosts, including dogs, monkeys, horses, cattle, raccoons, and foxes, but none of these are thought to aid in the spread of human disease caused by this worm.

Historical Information

Infection with *D. medinensis* has been known for thousands of years, because its clinical presentation is so conspicuous and therapy so dramatic. The latter, which involves gradual mechanical extraction by pulling the head out and then winding the worm on a stick, until it is fully extracted, is still used by traditional healers (Fig. 10.3B).

Bastian[2] provided the first formal description of the anatomy of *D. medinensis* in 1863. Seven years later, Fedchenko[3] reported a partial outline of its life cycle in which he recognized a crustacean, cyclops, as the intermediate host. Finally, Turkhud[4] in India in 1914 pieced together all of the crucial steps in the life cycle and fulfilled the

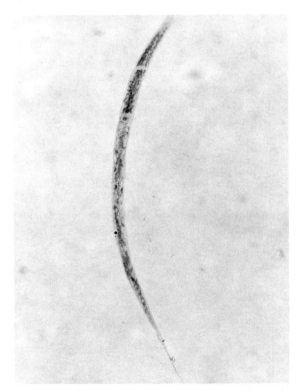

Figure 10.1. The first stage larva of *Dracunculus medinensis.* × 170.

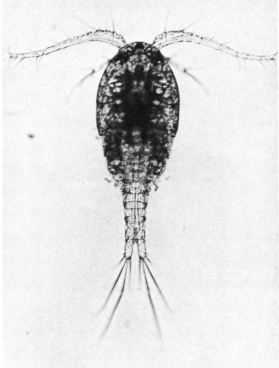

Figure 10.2. Copepod intermediate host for *Dracunculus medinensis.* × 100.

Dracunculus medinensis

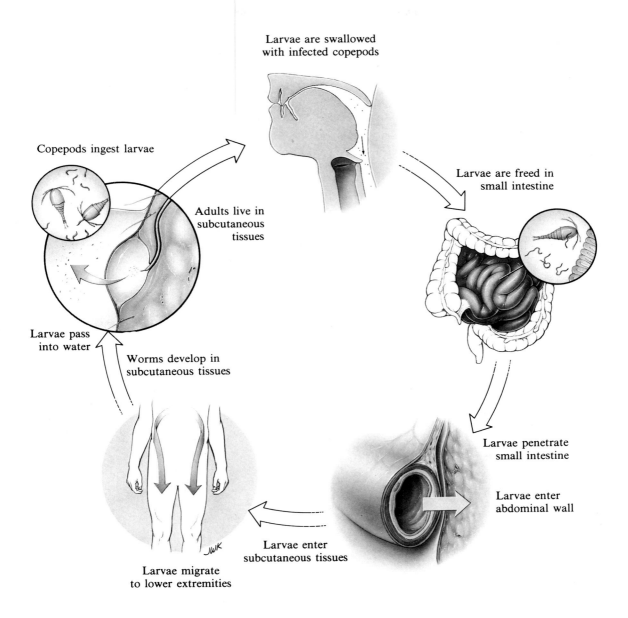

Larvae are swallowed
with infected copepods

Copepods ingest larvae

Larvae are freed in
small intestine

Adults live in
subcutaneous
tissues

Larvae pass
into water

Worms develop in
subcutaneous tissues

Larvae penetrate
small intestine

Larvae enter
abdominal wall

Larvae migrate
to lower extremities

Larvae enter
subcutaneous tissues

JWK

requirements of Koch's postulates for this infection in human volunteers.

Life Cycle

The female worm (Fig. 10.3A) is long and thin, often measuring more than 100 cm by 1.5 mm. The dimunitive male measures approximately 40 mm by 0.4 mm. The adult worms live in the subcutaneous tissues, usually in the lower extremities. Members of both sexes have acutely curved tails, which serve to anchor the worms in the tissues. Few male worms have ever been recovered from the infected individuals. The female induces a vesicular, ulcerated, lesion in the skin of the host surrounding her oral cavity. When the ulcer comes in contact with fresh water, the worm undergoes a uterine prolapse, which releases motile larvae (Fig. 10.1) into the oral cavity and then into the water. The larvae are ingested by copepods (Fig. 10.2) of the genera Cyclops, Mesocyclops, and Thermocyclops. They quickly enter the hemocoel of the crustacean and develop within 2–3 weeks into the infective third-stage larvae. The copepods, in turn, are swallowed by man, usually in drinking water, and are digested in the small intestine, releasing the infective larvae. The larvae penetrate the wall of the small intestine and migrate within the connective tissues for as long as a year, during which time they molt two more times and mature to adult worms. Gravid female worms migrate through the subcutaneous tissues into the extremities or the trunk, where they cause indurated papules that vesiculate and eventually become ulcerated (Fig. 10.3B) When the ulcer comes in contact with water, the life cycle has been completed.

Pathogenesis

There is no host response to the migration of the worm during its maturation process. If the worm does not complete its migration and dies, it may either disintegrate or become calcified. At the conclusion of a successful migration, the worm secretes a toxin, which causes local inflammation and the eventual formation of an ulcer. These ulcers tend to occur most frequently on the lower portions of the body, such as the legs and feet,

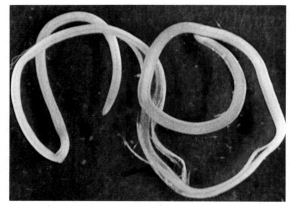

A

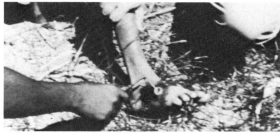

B

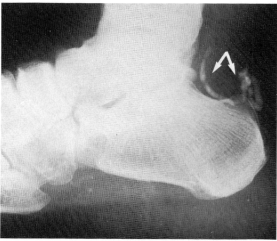

C

Figure 10.3. A. Adult ♀ *Dracunculus medinensis.* ×2 **B.** Removal of adult *Dracunculus medinensis* from the foot of an infected individual. Note the large ulcer from which the worm is being extracted. **C.** Radiogram of a calcified adult *Dracunculus medinensis (arrows)* in the foot of a patient from Ghana. (**A.** Courtesy of Dr. M. Klebs; **B.** Courtesy of Dr. J. Breman; **C.** Courtesy of Drs. R. Schlaeger and L.D. Carmichael)

but are also found on the upper extremities and the trunk.

Patients can become sensitized to secretions of the worm with the consequent allergic reactions of urticaria and pruritis. Anaphylactic reactions have also been reported. The ulcers can become secondarily infected.

Clinical Disease

Multiple blisters and ulcers are the only cutaneous manifestations of this infection. Allergic reactions usually occur in advance of the rupture of the blister, or in association with attempts to remove a worm. Although dracunculiasis is not a fatal disease, it causes substantial disability in nearly half of the affected individuals. Secondary bacterial infections occur with cellulitis spreading along the track of the worm. Rarely ankylosing of joints, arthritis, or contractures of tendons develops and leads to permanent disability.[5]

Diagnosis

The diagnosis depends on finding the head of the adult worm in the skin lesion and identifying the larvae that are released upon exposure to fresh water. Radiograms (Fig. 10.3C) may reveal calcifications corresponding to the adult worms in the subcutaneous tissues.

There are no serological tests for this infection.

Treatment

The time-honored therapy involves winding the worm gradually on a matchstick until it is totally extracted. Surgical excision of the worms has been effective, but may exaggerate the allergic reactions. The currently available drugs, niridazole and metronidazole, render the older treatments obsolete. Niridazole is the drug of choice.

Prevention and Control

This infection has been completely eliminated in some areas where pumps were installed to supply drinking water. Spread of the infection is facilitated by the step-in open wells prevalent throughout India and the Middle East. The strategy outlined by Hopkins and Foege[6] serves to point up that water sanitation would eliminate *D. medinensis*.

References

1. Muller R: Guinea worm disease: epidemiology, control, and treatment. Bull WHO 57:683,689. 1979
2. Bastian HC: On the structure and the nature of *Dracunculus,* or Guinea worm. Trans Linn Soc 24:101–134, 1863
3. Fedchenko AP: Concerning the structure and reproduction of the Guinea worm (*Filaria medinensis, L.*) Izv Imper Obsch Liubit Estes Anthrop Ethnog 8:71–81, 1870
4. Turkhud DA: Report of the Bombay bacteriological laboratory for the year 1913. Report presented by Maj. W. Glen Liston. Bombay, Government Central Press, 1914, pp 14–16
5. Ilegbodu VA, Oladele KO, Wise RA, *et al.*: Impact of Guinea worm disease on children in Nigeria. Am J Trop Med Hyg 35:962–964, 1986.
6. Hopkins DR, Foege WH: Guinea worm disease. (Letter to the Editor.) Science 212:495, 1981

11. Aberrant Nematode Infections

Many nematodes whose definitive hosts are various animals other than man can infect man, but are incapable of maturing to adult parasites in the human body and thus completing their life cycles. Two important human diseases, cutaneous larva migrans (CLM) and visceral larva migrans (VLM), are a result of such aberrant infections with larval nematodes. The pathogens causing CLM and VLM and the clinical manifestations of these diseases are listed in Tables 11.1 and 11.2. Although the number of nematodes causing aberrant human infections is large, this chapter will emphasize only the most important of these agents.

Cutaneous Larva Migrans

Cutaneous larva migrans (Table 11.1) is caused by infection with larvae of the dog and cat hookworms, which have worldwide distribution.

Third-stage larvae of *Ancylostoma caninum*

Table 11.1. Cutaneous Larva Migrans

Organism	Predominant Location in Body	Major Pathological Consequences	Diagnosis	Treatment
Ancylostoma caninum	Subcutaneous tissues	Urticaria, serpiginous lesion	Biopsy	Topical thiabendazole
Ancylostoma braziliensis	Subcutaneous tissues	Urticaria, serpiginous lesion	Biopsy	Topical thiabendazole
Dirofilaria conjunctivae	Palpebral conjuctivae, subcutaneous tissues	Abscess formation	Biopsy	Surgical removal
Dirofilaria repens	Subcutaneous tissues	Fibrotic, painless nodule formation	Biopsy	Surgical removal
Anatrichosoma cutaneum	Subcutaneous tissues	Serpiginous lesions	Biopsy	Surgical removal
Rhabditis niellyi	Skin	Papule, urticaria	Biopsy	Surgical removal
Lagochilascasris minor	Subcutaneous tissues around head and neck	Abscess formation	Biopsy	Surgical removal
Gnathostoma spinigerum	Subcutaneous tissues	Abscess formation	Biopsy, ELISA	Surgical removal
Thelazia callipaeda	Conjunctival sac, corneal conjunctiva	Paralysis of lower eyelid muscles, ectropion, fibrotic scarring	Ophthalmoscopic examination of conjunctiva	Surgical removal

(Fig. 11.1) and *A. braziliensis* can penetrate unbroken skin and wander throughout the subcutaneous tissues. The larvae can survive in sandy soil for several days. Within the human skin, they live for about 10 days.

The infected person develops an inflammatory reaction associated with intense itching in the affected areas, provoked by the secretions of the larvae, which consist largely of proteolytic enzymes. The serpigenous lesions, known as "creeping eruption" (Fig. 11.2), develop after an incubation period of 1 week. Secondary bacterial infections, caused by scratching, are common.

Topical application of thiabendazole to the affected areas kills the larvae.[1] Ethyl chloride spray relieves symptoms quickly, but for only a short time.

Visceral Larva Migrans

Aberrant migration of larvae through the viscera (Table 11.2) is a far more serious condition than the aberrant infection of the skin.

Toxocara canis (Johnston 1916) and *Toxocara cati* (Brumpt 1927)

Human infection with *Toxocara* spp. was recognized in 1950 by Wilder,[2] who discovered a larva within a retinal granuloma of a child. In 1952, Beaver and colleagues[3] described a series of children who had eosinophilia and suffered severe multisystem disease caused by *T. canis* and *T. cati* larvae.

Both *Toxocara* spp. have a life cycle in their

Table 11.2. Visceral Larva Migrans

Organism	Predominant Location in Body	Major Pathological Consequences	Diagnosis	Treatment
Toxocara cati *Toxocara canis*	Viscera, eye	Blindness	ELISA or RIA	Corticosteroids, thiabendazole
Angiostrongylus cantonensis	Meninges	Meningoencephalitis	CSF examination	Corticosteroids
Angiostrongylus costaricensis	Mesenteric arterioles	Peritonitis	Biopsy	Corticosteroids
Anisakis sp.	Stomach wall	Granuloma	Biopsy	Surgical removal
Baylisascaris procyonis	Brain and other tissues	Granuloma	Biopsy	None
Phocanema sp.	Stomach wall	Granuloma	Biopsy	Surgical removal
Terranova sp.	Stomach wall	Granuloma	Biopsy	Surgical removal
Oesophagostomum stephanostomum var. *thomasi*	Small and large intestinal wall	Granuloma	Biopsy	Surgical removal
Oesophagostamum bifurcum	Large intestinal wall	Granuloma	Biopsy	Surgical removal
Gnathostoma spinigerum	Striated muscles, subcutaneous tissues, brain, small intestinal wall	Abscess, meningo-encephalitis	Biopsy, ELISA	Surgical removal
Dirofilaria immitis	Lung, heart	Granuloma in lung	Biopsy	Surgical removal

respective hosts resembling that of ascaris in man. The adults of toxocara are smaller than those of ascaris (Fig. 11.3). They resemble the human parasite with respect to nutritional requirements and physiological behavior. In man the life cycle of toxocara is initiated by ingestion of embryonated eggs (Fig. 11.4A and B). After the larvae hatch, the third-stage larvae wander through the body, invading all organs. Unlike larvae of ascaris, larvae of toxocara do not break out of the capillaries in the alveolar spaces in the lungs, but pass through and eventually reach the systemic circulation. The degree of damage varies with the tissues invaded, the eye being the most seriously affected organ. Ultimately, the larvae die and provoke granuloma formation. Epidemiological evidence suggests that ocular disease tends to occur in the absence of systemic involvement and vice versa. This has led Glickman and

Schantz to propose that the two manifestations of this infection be reclassified as ocular larva migrans and visceral larva migrans.[4] Thus, there may be strains of *T. canis* with specific tropisms.

Larvae of *T. canis* secrete proteolytic enzymes, which facilitate movement through the tissues. Host response to the infection is an intense eosinophilic inflammation. The host develops both immediate and delayed types of hypersensitivity, which are responsible, in part, for the damage caused by the larvae. When a larva dies its concentrated proteins stimulate formation of granulomas (Fig. 11.5A). In the retina, such a granuloma grossly resembles retinoblastoma (Fig. 11.5B). As a result of this resemblance, in some cases an unnecessary enucleation was carried out. In many other cases, the granuloma itself was responsible for the loss of sight.

Toxocariasis is mainly a disease of young

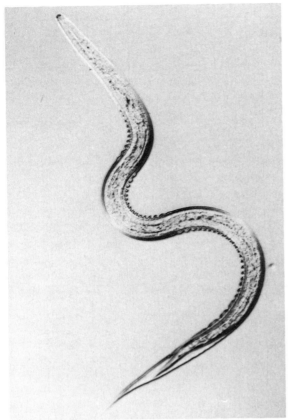

Figure 11.1. Filariform (third-stage) larva of *Ancylostoma caninum*, which induces creeping eruption after penetrating the skin. ×224.

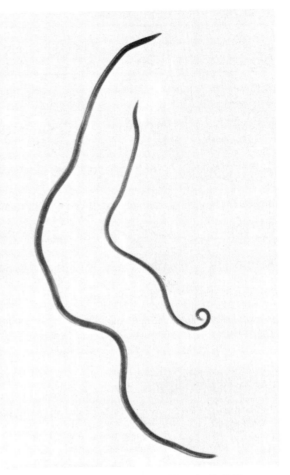

Figure 11.3. Adult male (*right*) and female (*left*) *Toxocara canis*. ×1.7.

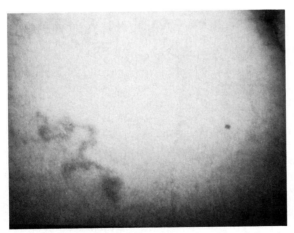

Figure 11.2. Serpiginous lesion on the skin of the abdomen of a patient with creeping eruption due to the L₃ larva of *Ancylostoma*. The patient acquired this infection by sunbathing on a public beach on which dogs and other animals were allowed to roam. (Courtesy of·Dr. R. Armstrong)

children.[5] It presents with fever, enlargement of the liver and the spleen, lower respiratory symptoms (particularly bronchospasm, resembling asthma), eosinophilia, sometimes approaching 70%, and hypergammaglobulinemia of both IgM and IgG classes. Myocarditis, nephritis, and involvement of the central nervous system have been described.

The most serious consequence of the infection is invasion of the retina. The degree of impairment of visual acuity depends on the specific area involved, but blindness is common (Fig. 11.6). Later effects of the eye infection are iridocyclitis, endophthalmitis, and detachment of the retina. Secondary glaucoma can follow.

Any pediatric-age patient with an unexplained febrile illness and eosinophilia should be suspected of VLM. Hepatosplenomegaly and evi-

Toxocara canis

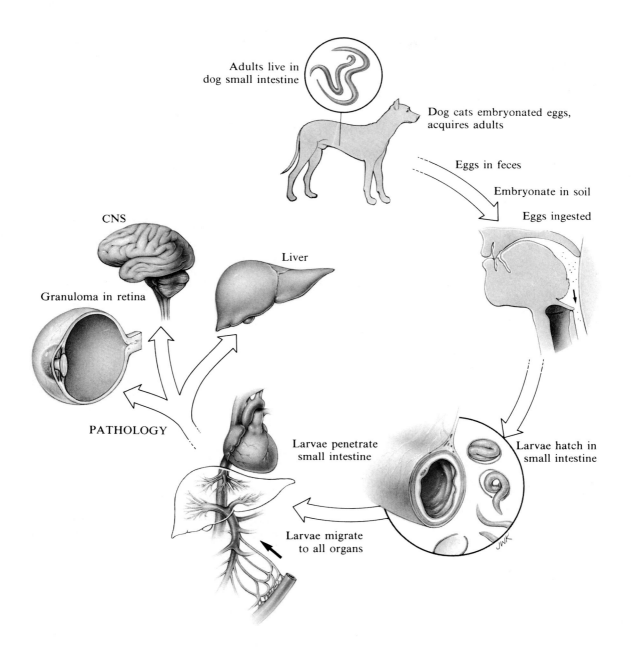

Adults live in dog small intestine

Dog cats embryonated eggs, acquires adults

Eggs in feces

Embryonate in soil

Eggs ingested

CNS

Liver

Granuloma in retina

PATHOLOGY

Larvae penetrate small intestine

Larvae hatch in small intestine

Larvae migrate to all organs

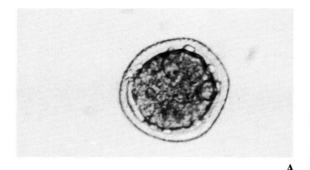

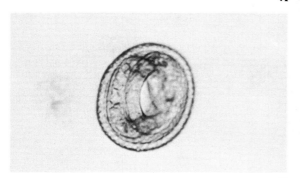

Figure 11.4. Fertilized unembryonated (**A**) and embryonated (**B**) eggs of *Toxocara canis.* × 430.

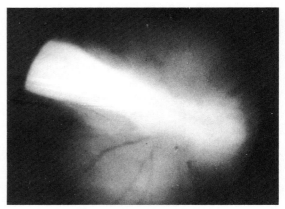

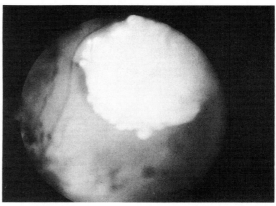

Figure 11.5. Ophthalmoscopic view of granuloma due to *Toxocara canis* (**A**), resembling an early stage of retinoblastoma (**B**). (**A** and **B:** Courtesy of Dr. B. Haik)

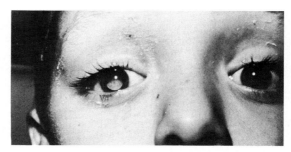

Figure 11.6. Leukocoria due to ocular infection with the larva of *Toxocara canis.* (Courtesy of Dr. Z. Pollard)

dence of multisystem disease and history of pica make the diagnosis of VLM more likely.

Diagnostic tests for *Toxocara* spp. are primarily immunologic.[6] The precipitin test is subject to cross-reactions with common antigens of the larvae and blood group substance A. The enzyme-linked immunosorbent assay (ELISA) test, which employs antigens secreted by the second-stage larva, has sufficient specificity to be the best indirect test in the diagnosis of this infection. About 80% of those infected are positive in this test.[7]

Other indicators include hypergammaglobulinemia and an elevation of the isohemoagglutin titers. Thus, a constellation of clinical disease described above, a history of pica, eosinophilia, and positivity of the immunological tests mentioned strongly point to the diagnosis. Liver biopsy may reveal a granuloma surrounding a larva, but success of sampling is fortuitous.

There is no specific treatment. Although claims have been made for effectiveness of thiabendazole and diethylcarbamazine, no definitive evidence of beneficial effects of these drugs has been established. Symptomatic treatment, including administration of corticosteroids, has been helpful in suppressing the intense manifestations of the infection. Most children improve within 1 to 3 months, regardless of treatment.

The worms are common parasites of pets; young puppies often harbor them, because the infection can be acquired transplacentally. Children with pica are at the greatest risk of ingesting embryonated eggs from the soil.

Treatment of dogs and strict control of their excreta are the only measures for control of this disease. A raccoon ascarid *Baylisascaris procyonis* has caused two reported fatal infections in children. Death was caused by meningoencephalitis, but virtually all organs were involved and contained granulomas. It is a particularly severe form of visceral larva migrans, whose prevalence is unknown.[8,9]

Angiostrongylus cantonensis (Chen 1935) and *Angiostrongylus costaricensis* (Morera and Cespedes) 1971)

A. cantonensis is a larval infection of man throughout Southeast Asia, Micronesia, Hawaii, and the Philippines. The definitive host is the rat, whose infection is more widely distributed, being found in all countries bordering on the Indian Ocean and South Pacific.[10] *A. costaricensis* is restricted to Costa Rica, Mexico, Venezuela and El Salvador.[11]

The adult female *A. cantonensis* is 400 μm long and 28 μm in diameter; the male measures 350 μm by 22 μm. The worms live and lay eggs in the pulmonary arteries of the wild rats (Fig. 11.7). The eggs are carried through the bloodstream to the lung capillaries, where they break out into the alveolar spaces. There they hatch and the larvae actively migrate up the respiratory tree, across the epiglottis, and are swallowed.

The larvae pass out with the feces, incubate in the soil, and are consumed by a wide variety of molluscs and crustaceans. Wild rats become in-fected by ingesting these intermediate hosts.

The infective third-stage larvae (Fig. 11.8) are released in the rat's stomach, penetrate the wall of the small intestine, and migrate with the bloodstream to the capillaries of the brain. In the brain, they undergo further development, and transform into adults (Fig. 11.9). The mature worms finally migrate from the brain to the pulmonary arteries, where they copulate, and thus complete the life cycle.

In contrast, adults of *A. costaricensis* live in the mesenteric arteries of wild rats and are infective only for one type of invertebrate, the slug. Otherwise, their life cycle is identical to that of *A. cantonensis*.

Human infection is acquired through ingestion of an undercooked or raw infected intermediate host. In man, the pattern of infection varies with the species of the two nematodes.

In the case of *A. cantonensis*, the third-stage

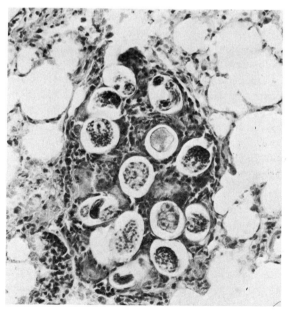

Figure 11.7. Larvae of *Angiostrongylus cantonensis* in the lung of a rat. ×200.

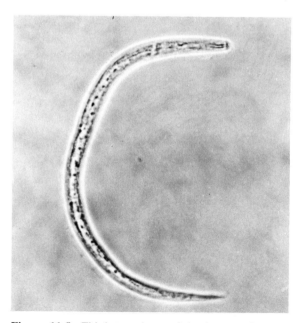

Figure 11.8. Third-stage larva of *Angiostrongylus cantonensis*. ×280.

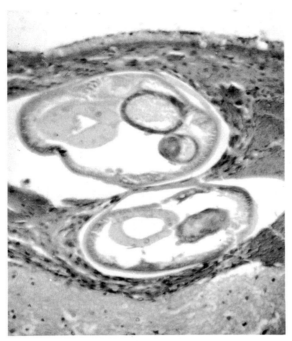

Figure 11.9. Adult worms of *Angiostrongylus cantonensis* in the cross-section of an infected rat. × 100.

larvae migrate to the capillaries of the meninges. There they induce an eosinophilic inflammatory response, resulting in a meningoencephalitis. The larvae never complete their life cycle and eventually die within eosinophilic granulomata that surround them.

Larvae of *A. costaricensis* lodge in the mesenteric arterioles and cause arteritis, thrombosis, and small infarcts. The consequence is necrotic ulceration, followed by the development of peritonitis, and formation of fistulas. Infection in the human host has rarely led to the development of adult worms.

Patients infected with larvae of *A. cantonensis* usually experience headaches and meningismus. In addition, they may show focal findings of central nervous system involvement, such as parasthesiae (in about one-half of the cases), and

cranial nerve palsies (in about one-quarter). The infection is associated with eosinophilia in the cerebrospinal fluid (CSF) and blood. The vast majority of patients recover within 3 weeks with no apparent residual abnormalities.

Patients infected with *A. costaricensis* usually exhibit right iliac fossa pain, may have fever, and always present with peripheral eosinophilia. In advanced disease, there are palpable abdominal masses representing eosinophilic granulomas.

There is no specific diagnostic test for either parasite. The disease must therefore be suspected on the basis of the clinical presentation, history of residence in endemic areas, and presence of peripheral eosinophilia. In the case of infection with *A. cantonensis,* eosinophilia in the CSF suggests the diagnosis.

There is no evidence that any treatment affects the outcome, although claim has been made that thiabendazole shortens the duration of symptoms. This may be due to the antiinflammatory properties of the drug, rather than its antihelminthic activity. In cases of severe discomfort and an intense inflammatory reaction, corticosteroids are recommended.

Disease caused by *A. cantonensis*[12] occurs in Southeast Asia, the Philippine Islands, Taiwan, and the North and South Pacific islands. Human infection was first described in Taiwan when larvae of the parasite were isolated from the CSF of a child. Infected rodents, but not human cases, have also been reported from East Africa. A survey of wharf rats in New Orleans revealed a high rate of infection; several years prior to that study none had been detected.[13]

Acquisition of human infection depends on the locale and the nutritional habits of specific populations. A case in Hawaii resulted from ingestion of a raw slug, for traditional medicinal purpose. In Tahiti, epidemics have resulted from consumption of raw freshwater prawns (i.e., shrimp-like crustaceans), and elsewhere other invertebrates either consumed directly or in vegetation have been the causes of infections.

Gnathostoma spinigerum (Owen 1838)

Gnathostoma spinigerum is a parasite whose definitive hosts are a variety of mammals and the intermediate hosts are, first, copepods of the genus Cyclops, and, second, birds, fish, snakes,

and frogs. Females measure 25–54 mm in length; the males 11–25 mm. In the definitive host, the adults live coiled in the wall of the small intestine. Eggs, released with feces, hatch in the water and released larvae are ingested by the cyclops. Man ingesting the second intermediate host becomes infected and, in the process of larval migration, may develop eosinophilic meningitis. The disease is self-limited and there is no known treatment.

Anisakiasis

Anisakiasis[14] refers to infection with a number of species of marine nematodes belonging to the genera *Anisakis, Phocanema, Terranova,* and *Contracoecum,* which infect sea mammals, particularly dolphins, whales, sea lions, and seals. In these hosts, the anisakiid adults, which are distantly related to ascariids (see Chapter 3), live in the lumen of the intestinal tract. These worms, as first-stage larvae, infect a wide variety of crustaceans. As second-, third-, or fourth-stage larvae, they infect a number of fish species.

When man ingests raw or undercooked saltwater fish and, with it, the larval form of the worm, the larva burrows into the wall of the stomach or the small intestine and dies within a few days. The dead organism provokes granuloma reaction characterized by eosinophilic infiltration. The initial stages of the infection may be asymptomatic; the later stages are often associated with vague upper abdominal pain. Radiographic diagnosis can suggest a tumor, which has sometimes been thought to be carcinoma of the stomach. Definitive diagnosis can be made only by gastroscopy and biopsy or by surgical excision. Treatment requires removal of the larva.

References

1. Whitting DA: The successful treatment of creeping eruption with topical thiabendazole. S Afr Med J 50:253–255, 1976
2. Wilder HC: Nematode endophthalmitis. Trans Am Acad Ophthalmol Otolaryngol 55:99–104, 1950
3. Beaver PC, Snyde CH, Carrera GM, et al.: Chronic eosinophilia due to visceral larva migrans. Pediatrics 9:7–19, 1952
4. Glickman LT, Schantz PM: Epidemiology and pathogenesis of zoonotic toxocariasis. Epidemiol Rev 10:143–148, 1982
5. Worley G, Green JA, Frothingham TE, *et al.: Toxocara canis* infection: clinical and epidemiological associations with seropositivity in kindergarten children. J Infect Dis 149:591–597, 1984
6. Cypess RH, Karol MH, Zidian JL, et al.: Larva-specific antibody in patients with visceral larva migrans. J Infect Dis 135:633–640, 1977
7. Glickman LT, Schantz PM, Dombroske R, et al.: Evaluation of serodiagnostic tests for visceral larva migrans. Am J Trop Med Hyg 27:492–498, 1978
8. Huff DS, Neafie RC, Binder MJ *et al.:* Case 4. The first fatal *Baylisascaris* infection in humans: an infant with eosinophilic meningoencephalitis. Pediatric Pathology 3:345–352, 1984
9. Fox AS, Kazacos KR, Gould NS, *et al.:* Fatal eosinophilic meningoencephalitis and visceral larva migrans caused by the racoon ascarid *Baylisascaris procyonis.* N Engl J Med 312:1619–1624, 1985
10. Cross JH (ed): Studies on angiostrongyliasis in eastern Asia and Australia. NAMRU-2-SP-44, 1–164, 1979
11. Morera P: Life history and redescription of *Angiostrongylus costaricensis* (Morera and Cespedes, 1971). Am J Trop Med Hyg 22:613–621, 1973
12. Cheng CW, Chen ER: Clinical observation on 30 cases of eosinophilic meningitis and meningoencephalitis. J Formosan Med Assoc 75:586–587, 1975
13. Campbell B G, Little MD: The finding of *Angiostrongylus cantonensis* in rats in New Orleans. Am J Trop Med Hyg 38:568–573, 1988
14. Jackson GJ: The ''new disease'' status of human anisakiasis and North American cases: A review. J Milk Food Technol 38:769–773, 1975

12. Nematode Infections of Minor Medical Importance

Several nematode infections of high prevalence warrant mention, although the clinical manifestations they cause are of minor importance. Table 12.1 lists their geographic distribution, major pathological effects, mode of infection, method of diagnosis, and therapy. A brief description of those preceded by an asterisk is given in the text that follows.

Table 12.1. Nematode Infections of High Prevalence

Parasite	Geographic Distribution	Major Pathological Consequences	Mode of Infection	Diagnosis	Therapy
*Capillaria hepatica**	Worldwide	Necrotic lesions in liver	Oral route	Biopsy	None
*Capillaria philippinensis**	The Philippines	Malabsorption syndrome, diarrhea	Oral route	Stool examination for larvae and eggs	Thiabendazole
Dioctophyma renale	North and South America, China	Complete destruction of kidney	Oral route	Urine examination for eggs	Surgical removal of the worm
*Dipetalonema perstans**	Central and South America, Africa	None	Bite of infected midge	Blood smear or Knott test for microfilariae	None
*Dipetalonema streptocerca**	Africa	Pruritic dermatitis	Bite of infected midge	Impression smear of skin snip for microfilariae	Diethylcarbamazine
*Mansonella ozzardi**	Central and South America, the Caribbean	None	Bite of infected midge	Blood smear or Knott test for microfilariae	None
Syngamus laryngeus	South America, the Caribbean, the Philippines	Asthma, hemoptysis	Unknown	Sputnum or stool examination for eggs	None
Ternides deminutus	Africa	Iron-deficiency anemia	Unknown	Stool examination for eggs	Not established
Trichostrongylus spp.	Worldwide	Anemia	Oral route	Stool examination for eggs	Thiabendazole

*These parasites are discussed in the text.

Mansonella ozzardi (Manson 1897)

This filarial infection is found throughout South and Central America and the Caribbean islands. It is transmitted by the bite of an infected midge (see Chapter 38). The adult worms inhabit the visceral adipose tissue of the host. The microfilariae (Fig. 12.1A) can be found in the blood. As far as is known, this infection does not induce any disease. Diagnosis depends on finding the microfilariae on a stained blood smear or by the Knott test (see Appendix III).

Dipetalonema perstans (Manson 1891)

This filarial worm is found in Africa and in South and Central America. It is transmitted from person to person by the biting midges. The adults live free in the abdominal or pericardial cavity,

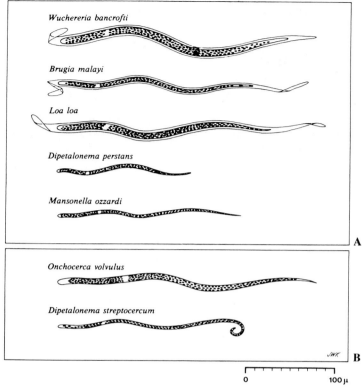

Figure 12.1. A. Microfilariae that are found in blood. The microfilariae of *W. bancrofti*, *B. malayi* and *L. loa* are sheathed, whereas those of *D. perstans* and *M. ozzardi* are not. **B.** Microfilariae that are found within the subcutaneous tissues. Neither of these microfilariae has a sheath.

where they produce microfilariae, which circulate in the blood. There is no known associated disease. The infection is discovered by the examination of the stained blood smear (Fig. 12.1A) or by the Knott test.

Dipetalonema streptocerca (Macfie and Corson 1922)

Infections with *Dipetalonema streptocerca* are widely distributed throughout Central Africa. The adult worms live in the subcutaneous tissues, as do the microfilariae. The infection is transmitted by the biting midges. The only clinical manifestation of this infection is a pruritic dermatitis. Diagnosis is made by finding microfilariae (Fig. 12.1B) in specimens of skin or impression smears made from them. The microfilariae must be differentiated from those of *O. volvulus*. Therapy with diethylcarbamazine may exacerbate the pruritis, in which case it may be necessary to prescribe corticosteroids.

Capillaria hepatica (Bancroft 1893)

Capillaria hepatica is a parasite of rodents, particularly the rat. Adult worms live and lay eggs in the liver parenchyma within a syncytium (Fig. 12.2). After the host dies, the eggs embryonate within 2 to 6 weeks and are then infective for another host. The infective eggs (Fig. 12.3) are ingested and hatch in the small intestine. The exact route of infection after the egg hatches is

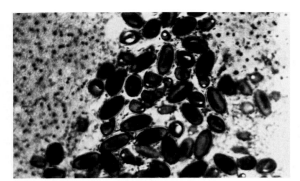

Figure 12.2. Egg of *Capillaria hepatica*

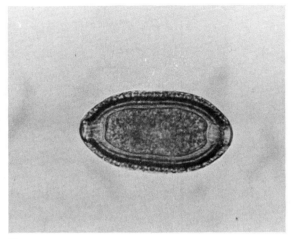

Figure 12.3. Isolated egg of *Capillaria hepatica*

still unknown. Eventually, the larvae mature and reach the liver. After mating, they begin to lay eggs and thus complete the life cycle. The liver serves as the source of nourishment for the adult worms. If enough worms are present, the host may suffer liver failure and die. Man rarely becomes infected by ingesting the eggs. Too few clinical cases of this infection have been recorded to determine what constitues a lethal dose. Diagnosis requires liver biopsy. Often the disease is unsuspected and discovered only at autopsy. No treatment has been developed.[1]

Capillaria philippinensis (Chitwood, Valesquez, and Salazar 1968)

Infection with *Capillaria philippinensis* occurs mainly in the Philippines, where some 1000 cases and 100 deaths have been documented in the northern provinces,[2] and is less frequent in Thailand.

The adult worms resemble those of *Trichinella spiralis* (see Chapter 6) both in size and biology. They live in the columnar epithelium of the small intestine, and deposit living larvae there. These larvae are infectious within the host and in this respect mimic the autoinfectious cycle of *Strongyloides stercoralis* (see Chapter 5). There is no evidence, however, that the host of *C. philippinensis* is immunosuppressed. As the infection progresses, the host begins to pass in his stools first embryonated and then unembryonated eggs.

C. philippinensis is probably a parasite of birds that feed upon fish and crustaceans, the intermediate hosts for this nematode. Man becomes infected by eating raw or undercooked infected fish or shrimp. In the Philippines, ingestion of "jumping salad," which consists of vegetables and a variety of live aquatic animals including shrimp, is thought to be a common source of this infection.

Clinical disease is a rampant diarrhea,[3] quickly followed by malabsorption of fats and carbohydrates. Prolonged infection leads to electrolyte imbalance, and occasionally death. It is estimated that the mortality rate approaches 10% in some endemic areas. Diagnosis depends on finding eggs or living larvae in the feces. Treatment is administration of mebendazole or thiabendazole.[4]

References

1. McQuown AL: *Capillaria hepatica;* reported genuine and spurious cases. Am J Trop Med 30:761–767, 1950

2. Watten RH, Beckner WM, Cross JH, et al.: Clinical studies of *Capillaria philippinensis*. Trans Roy Soc Trop Med Hyg 66:828–832, 1970

3. Cross JH, Banzon TC, Murrell KD, et al.: A new epidemic diarrheal disease, caused by a nematode, *Capillaria philippinenesis*. Indust Trop Health 7:124–131, 1970

4. Singson CN, Banzon TC, Cross JH: Mebendazole in the treatment of intestinal capillariasis. Am J Trop Med Hyg 24:932–934, 1975

II
The Cestodes

Introduction

The class Cestoidea belongs to the phylum Platyhelminthes and includes parasitic tapeworms. Tapeworms have flat, segmented bodies consisting of a head, known as scolex and a series of segments, known as proglottids. The adults of this class are all parasitic and live in the intestinal lumen of a large number of vertebrate hosts, including man and other mammals.

Anatomy and Physiology

Anatomically, the adult tapeworm is constituted of a head, or scolex, and a segmented portion, or strobila, comprised of individual proglottids.

Scolex

The scolex is the only point of attachment between the host and the parasite. It may be equipped with suckers, hooks, or grooves, which aid in the attachment. The scolex contains ganglia.

The neck region of the scolex, which is metabolically very active, is the site at which new proglottids form.

Proglottids

The outer surface of adult tapeworms consists of a tegument whose structure and function are related to feeding. It is covered by evenly spaced microvilli, underneath which lie mitochondria, pinocytic vesicles, and related structures. The tapeworms, which lack a digestive system, must obtain all of their nutrients by actively transporting them across their teguments. While each proglottid is able to absorb various small molecular weight nutrients, its precise metabolic requirements have yet to be fully defined.

The high levels of ATPase in the tegument are related to active transport, but may also help the worm resist digestion by the mammalian host. Inhibitors of tapeworm ATPase, such as niclosamide, cause disintegration of adult tapeworms.

There are two layers of muscles in each proglottid, a longitudinal one and a transverse, enabling the proglottid to move. The worms are innervated by a pair of lateral nerves, with perpendicular commissures branching out into the parenchyma of each segment. Although each segment is anatomically independent, all are connected by a common nervous system that emanates from a set of cerebral ganglia in the scolex.

Excretion or osmoregulation is associated with a lateral pair of excretory tubules.

Each proglottid possesses both male and female sex organs, but self-mating within a segment is unusual. Typically, sperm are transferred between adjacent mature proglottids of the worm.

13. *Taenia saginata* (Goeze 1782)

The beef tapeworm, *Taenia saginata*, is one of the longest human parasites, capable of growing to 10 m. It lives in the upper half of the small intestine.

The geographic distribution of *T. saginata* reflects cattle husbandry in areas where human excreta are not disposed of in a sanitary manner. Hence, large areas of Africa, portions of Mexico and Argentina, and, to a lesser extent, middle Europe are endemic foci. It is infrequently acquired in the United States; most clinical cases are imported.

Historical Information

Tapeworms had been known for many years before Tyson,[1] in 1683, formally described several species, which he recovered from dogs. In 1656, Plater, a Swiss physician, wrote about the distinctions between *Taenia* sp. and *Diphyllobothrium latum* (which was then called *Lumbricus latus*).[2] The first report of *T. saginata* came from Andry,[3] in 1700, but he failed to recognize the individuality of each proglottid, nor did he distinguish this worm from other similar tapeworms. Thus, Goeze must be credited with the first correct description of the worm, for in 1782, he published his treatise on helminthology in which he presented the first recognizable classification of *T. saginata* and *T. solium* adult worms.[4] Von Siebold, in 1850, speculated that "bladder worms" (i.e., cysticerci) could develop into adult tapeworms,[5] which was the correct supposition; unfortunately, he also offered the alternate hypothesis that these were nothing more than degenerated adults.

Leuckart, in 1863, showed experimentally that the proglottids of *T. saginata*, when fed to young calfs, developed into cysticerci in the animal's muscles.[6] Oliver, in 1870, discovered that following ingestion of the "bladder worms" man developed adult *T. saginata*.[7] He further suggested in the same report that thorough cooking of the infected meat would prevent infection with the adult tapeworms.

Life Cycle

Most infected individuals harbor only one adult worm (Fig. 13.1). It is attached to the mucosal surface of the small intestine with the aid of four suckers located on the scolex (Fig. 13.2). No hooks or other organelles of attachment are present on *T. saginata*. The developing proglottids extend down the small intestine, sometimes reaching the jejunum.

The most distal proglottids (Fig. 13.3) are gravid (i.e., contain infective eggs) and tend to break off from the rest of the worm. The egg-laden segments then actively migrate through the large intestine, rectum, and anus to the outside. Some eggs are usually expressed from the proglottid as it exits the body and are deposited on the perianal skin. Large ribbons of gravid proglottids may also be passed with the feces.

If the gravid segments come to rest in grazing areas, they may become ingested by the cattle, the proglottids are then digested, and the eggs (Fig. 13.4) released.

The hexacanth (i.e., six-hooked) larva, the oncosphere, (Fig. 13.5) hatches from its egg, actively penetrates the small intestine, and migrates by the hematogenous route to all organ systems. Most oncospheres lodge in the skeletal muscles, where they encyst in the fascial tissues and develop into cysticerci, the stage infective for man.

The adult tapeworm is acquired by consumption of raw or undercooked beef containing the infective cysticerci. The cysticercus, released from its surrounding muscle tissue by digestion in the small intestine, everts its scolex and attaches to the mucosa, where it develops to a fully grown tapeworm within 3 months.

Eggs of *T. saginata*, ingested by man, do not result in an infection.

Pathogenesis

Although this large tapeworm occupies a substantial proportion of the lumen of the small intestine, it is flexible and relatively fragile. Therefore, it does not obstruct. There are no host responses against the worm and therefore no tissue reactions.

Clinical Disease

Most infected individuals are asymptomatic, but those in whom the worm has become very large

Taenia saginata

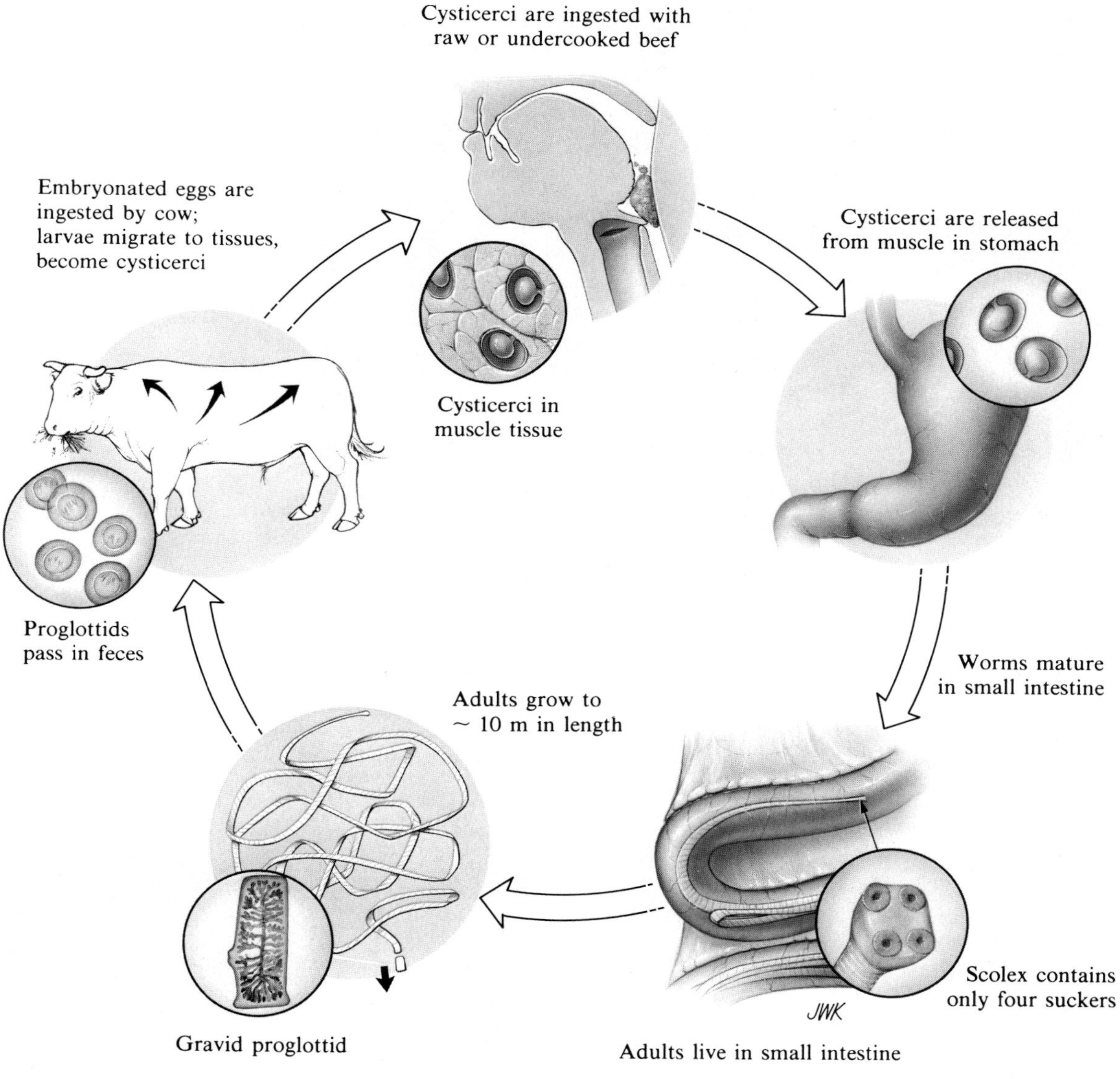

Cysticerci are ingested with
raw or undercooked beef

Embryonated eggs are
ingested by cow;
larvae migrate to tissues,
become cysticerci

Cysticerci in
muscle tissue

Cysticerci are released
from muscle in stomach

Proglottids
pass in feces

Worms mature
in small intestine

Adults grow to
~ 10 m in length

Gravid proglottid

Scolex contains
only four suckers

Adults live in small intestine

JWK

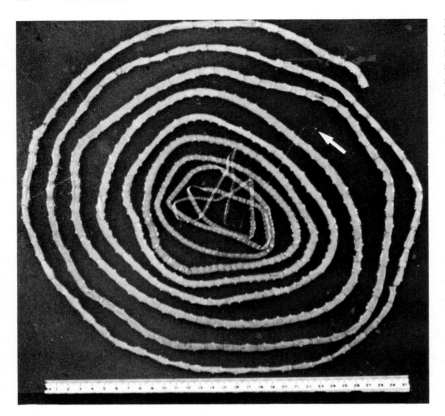

Figure 13.1. The adult of *Taenia saginata*. The *arrow* indicates the position of the scolex. The entire worm measures over 5.4 m in length. (Courtesy of Mr. U. Martin)

may feel epigastric fullness. Rarely an infected individual will experience postprandial nausea and vomiting. The patient becomes aware of the infection by noting proglottids in the stool. Occasionally, a proglottid may emerge from the anus and crawl down the thigh; this produces a tickling sensation. Frequently, proglottids pass from the patient during periods of sleep, and are found in bedding or clothing the following morning. In other instances, the patient may pass a large segment of the worm, either during defecation or spontaneously.

Diagnosis

Definitive diagnosis depends on identification of the proglottids passed by the patient. Gravid proglottids should be fixed in 10% formaldehyde solution and the uterine branches injected with India ink. Twelve or more uterine branches on one side are characteristic of gravid *T. saginata* (Fig. 13.3). Eggs in the stool can be identified only as *Taenia* sp., because the eggs of all tapeworms in the taeneid group look alike. The

eggs may adhere to the perianal skin and it is possible to detect them on transparent plastic adhesive tape in the manner described for detection of pinworm infections (see Chapter 1).

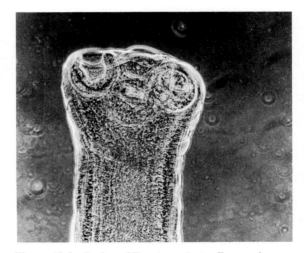

Figure 13.2. Scolex of *Taenia saginata*. Four suckers on the scolex attach the worm to the small intestine. No hooks are present. ×50.

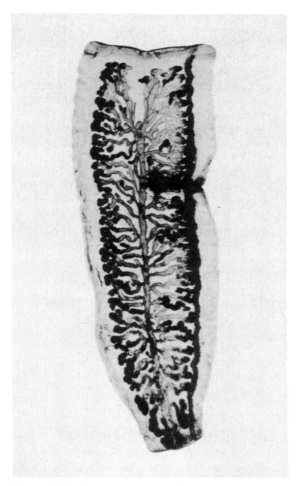

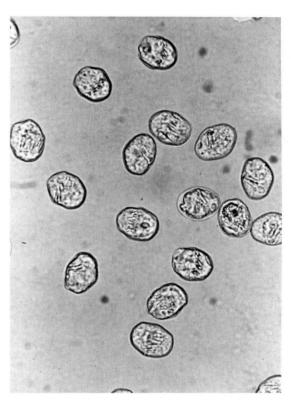

Figure 13.5. Oncospheres of *Taenia saginata* (Courtesy of Dr. M. Rickard.) ×700.

Figure 13.3. Gravid proglottid of *Taenia saginata*. This segment contains more than 15 lateral uterine branches per side. This differentiates it from *Taenia solium*, which has fewer than 10 branches per side (cf. Fig. 14.3). ×2.

Treatment

The drug of choice is niclosamide[8] usually effective in a single dose administration.[9] The consequence of this drug's action is damage, to the point of dissolution of the worm. Hence, a search for the scolex, a time-honored procedure in the older therapy with quinacrine, is not warranted.

Prevention and Control

The most effective method to prevent tapeworm infection in the community is protection of cattle from coming in contact with human excrement. In some areas of the world, this has been very difficult to achieve because human feces are widely used as fertilizer. On an individual basis, the infection is fully preventable by thorough cooking of beef. Inspection of beef readily identifies taeniasis, but it is not carried out thoroughly or at all in many endemic areas.

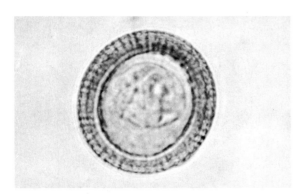

Figure 13.4. Egg of *Taenia saginata*. This egg cannot be differentiated from any other member of the taeniid family (e.g., *T. solium*, *Echinococcus granulosus*, or *E. multilocularis*). ×1000.

References

1. Tyson E: *Lumbricus latus*, or a discourse read before the Royal Society, of the joynted worm, wherein great many mistakes of former writers concerning it, are remarked; its natural history from more exact information is attempted; and the whole urged, as a difficulty against doctrine of univocal generation. Philos Trans 13:113–144, 1683
2. Plater F: Praxeos medicae opus. Basel, 1656
3. Andry N: De la generation des vers dans le corps de l'homme. Paris, 1700
4. Goeze JAE: Versuch einer Naturgeschichte der Eingeweiderwurmer Thierischer Körper. Blankenburg, P. A. Pape, 1782
5. von Siebold CTE: Über den Generationswechsel der Cestoden nebst einer Revision der Gattung Tetrarhynchus. Ztschr Wissensch Zool 2:198–253, 1850
6. Leuckart R: Die menschlichen Parasiten und die von ihnen herruhenden Krankheiten. Ein Hand- und Lehrbuch für Naturforscher und Ärzte. Leipzig, C. E. Wintersche Verlagshandlung, 1863
7. Oliver JH: The importance of feeding of cattle and the thorough cooking of the meat, as the best preservatives against tapeworms. Seventh Annual Rep of the Sanitary Commissioner (1870) with the Government of India, Calcutta. 1871, pp 82–83
8. Keeling JED: The chemotherapy of cestode infections. Adv Chemother 3:109–152, 1968
9. Vermund SH, MacLeod S, and Goldstein RG: Taeniasis unresponsive to a single dose of niclosamide: Case report of persistent infection with *Taenia saginata* and a review of therapy. Rev Infect Dis 8:423–426, 1986

14. *Taenia solium* (Linnaeus 1758)

Taenia solium is distributed throughout the world and coincides with the raising of pigs, especially in the areas where human feces are used as fertilizer. In parts of Southeast Asia, Micronesia, the Philippines, Mexico, South America (particularly Ecuador), and eastern Europe, the infection is endemic. *T. solium* is a large tapeworm, more than 6 m in length. It lives attached to the wall of the small intestine. Although presence of the adult tapeworm in the intestine usually does not result in any clinical disease, infection with the larval form, referred to as cysticercosis (see Chapter 16), can be a serious, even fatal disease.

Historical Information

Long before the adult of *T. solium* was described by Goeze[1] in 1782, Aristotle wrote about the cysticercus stage of the worm in the muscles of pigs. However, there is no evidence that he understood the relationship between the larval infection in the pig and the adult infection in man. Cysticercosis in pigs was formally described by Hartman in 1688.[2] Küchenmeister, in 1855, transmitted the infection to a man who was a condemned murderer, by secretly contaminating his food with cysticerci that Küchenmeister recovered from meat he had purchased at a local restaurant. At autopsy 120 h later, the small intestine of the prisoner was shown to contain immature adults of *T. solium*.

Life Cycle

Morphologically, the adult of *T. solium* closely resembles adult *T. saginata*. However, its scolex possesses, besides the four sucker discs, two rows of hooks, which it uses as an additional attachment mechanism (Fig. 14.1).

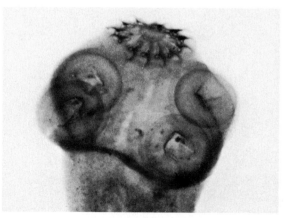

Figure 14.1. Scolex of *Taenia solium*. The scolex possesses four suckers and two rows of hooks by which it attaches to the small intestine. × 33.

Taenia solium

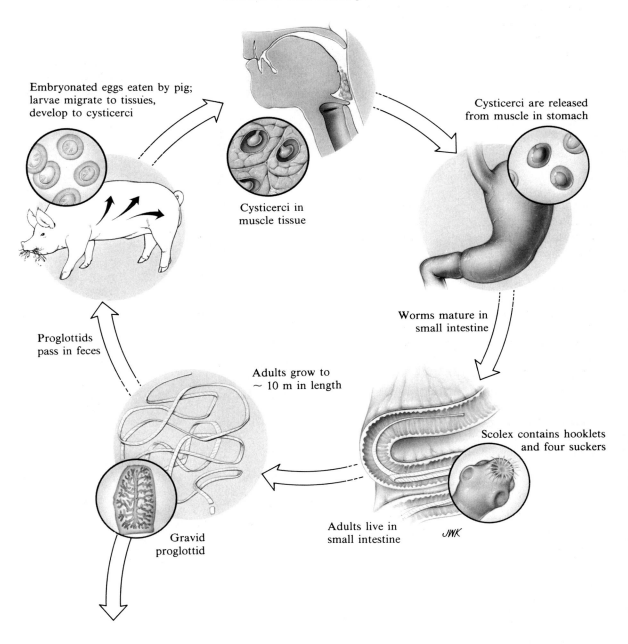

Cysticerci are ingested
with raw or undercooked pork

Embryonated eggs eaten by pig;
larvae migrate to tissues,
develop to cysticerci

Cysticerci in
muscle tissue

Cysticerci are released
from muscle in stomach

Worms mature in
small intestine

Proglottids
pass in feces

Adults grow to
~ 10 m in length

Scolex contains hooklets
and four suckers

Gravid
proglottid

Adults live in
small intestine

JWK

Man becomes infected with *T. solium* by ingesting raw or undercooked pork that harbors the larval (i.e., cysticercus) stage of the worm (Fig. 14.2A and B). From this point on, the life cycle follows the pattern of the life cycle of *T. saginata* (see Chapter 13).

In addition to infection with the ingested cysticercus, man can also become infected with the eggs of this parasite. If man swallows eggs of *T. solium*, they will hatch and go on to produce a larval infection, or cysticercosis (see Chapter 16).

Pathogenesis

The adult parasite induces no host reaction.

Clinical Disease

Unlike *T. saginata*, which is much larger, *T. solium* does not usually give rise to symptoms of epigastric fullness. The patients are asymptomatic and become aware of the infection only when they discover the proglottids in their stools or on the perianal skin.

Diagnosis

Diagnosis is established by the identification of the gravid proglottids. These segments should be fixed in 10% formaldehyde solution and injected with India ink to reveal the uterine branches, which are 5–10 in number on each side (Fig. 14.3). Eggs present on the patient's perineum can be identified by application of transparent adhesive tape, which is then examined under a microscope (see Chapter 13). Presence of eggs (Fig. 13.4) confirms the diagnosis of infection with a taenia, but does not identify its species, because eggs of all taeniae are morphologically alike. It must be remembered that unfixed proglottids and eggs of *T. solium* are infectious for man, and the examiner must exercise appropriate caution to prevent self-infection.

Treatment

The drug of choice is Niclosamide.[3] No purgatives should be used,[4] because purging increases the risk of regurgitation of the eggs into the stomach and initiation of an aberrant infection leading to cysticercosis.[5]

A

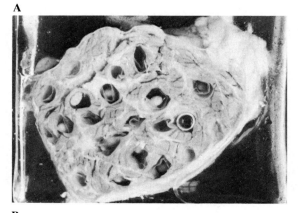

B

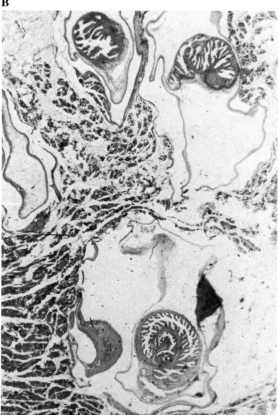

Figure 14.2. A. A piece of pork infected with the cysticercus stage of *T. solium* ("measly pork"). **B.** Section through a piece of pork infected with cysticerci. × 10.

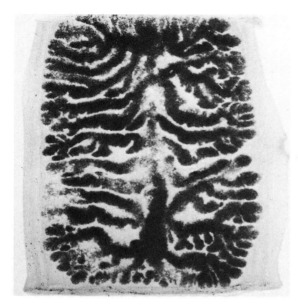

Figure 14.3. Gravid proglottid of *Taenia solium*. The lateral uterine branches number fewer than 10 on each side. This identifies the source of the proglottid as *T. solium*. ×7.5.

Prevention and Control

The infection is totally preventable by protection of the feed from contamination by human feces. Individual infection is prevented by thorough cooking of pork or by freezing it at −10°C for at least 5 days.

References

1. Goeze JAE: Versuch einer Naturgeschichte der Eingewiderwurmer Thierischer Körper. Blankenburg, P. A. Pape, 1782
2. Hartman PJ: Miscellanea curiosa sive ephemeridium medico-physicarum Germanicarum Academiae Imperialis Leopoldineae naturae curiosorum decuriae II. Observatio 34. Nürnberg, Literis Joonnis Ernesti Adelbuneri, 1688, pp 58–59
3. Keeling JED: The chemotherapy of cestode infections. Adv Chemother 3:109–152, 1968
4. The medical letter, 26:32 (footnote 30), 1984
5. Richards F. Jr., Schantz PM: Treatment of *Taenia solium* infections. Lancet June 1:1264–1265, 1985

15. *Diphyllobothrium latum* (Linnaeus 1758)

Diphyllobothrium latum, which can grow to more than 10 m in length, is the longest of the tapeworms that parasitize human small intestine. Like other tapeworms of man, this parasite does little harm. Its location in the upper part of the small intestine, which is rich in nutrients, and its feeding mechanisms are similar to those of the other tapeworms. However, in addition, it has a unique affinity for vitamin B_{12}.

D. latum infection is common throughout Scandinavia, Switzerland, Hungary, the Great Lakes region of the United States, and western U.S.S.R.

Historical Information

D. latum was first accurately reported as a human infection by Plater,[1] in 1609, and later classified taxonomically by Linneaus in 1758. However, its complex life cycle was defined only in 1917 by Janicki.[2]

Life Cycle

The adult worm resides in the small intestine, loosely attached to the villous surface by its scolex (Fig. 15.1). The scolex, 3 mm long, has two lateral grooves, or bothria, which it uses to create suction between itself and the host tissues. It has no hooks or suckers.

D. latum is nourished through its tegumental surface by active transport mechanisms, absorbing small-molecular-weight nutrients obtained in the ingested foodstuffs.

Each proglottid (Fig. 15.2) is greater in width than length and contains both sets of sex organs. Therefore, self-mating is the rule, with each proglottid fertilizing the eggs in the adjacent one.

As the fertilized proglottids become gravid, eggs are shed from the centrally located uterine pore directly into the lumen of the intestine. They also can break off from the strobila and disintegrate in the small intestine. The eggs (Fig. 15.3A) pass out of the host with the feces and

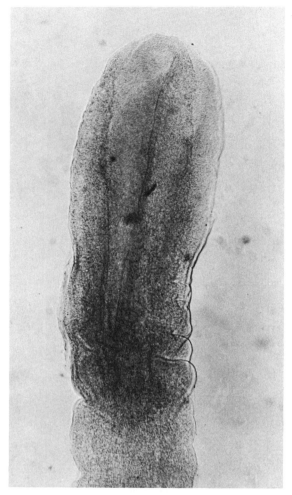

Figure 15.1. Scolex of *Diphyllobothrium latum*. The groove on the scolex extends down its entire length and attaches this tapeworm to the small intestine. × 120.

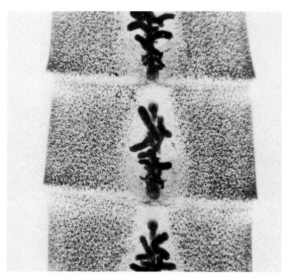

Figure 15.2. Mature proglottids of *Diphyllobothrium latum*. The segments are greater in width than in length, hence the common name "broad" fish tapeworm. × 12.

must be deposited in fresh water if the life cycle is to continue.

The eggs, measuring 70 μm × 45 μm, must incubate for 9–12 days in water prior to hatching (Fig. 15.3B). The ciliated coracidium (Fig. 15.4) emerges from the egg and immediately begins to swim. Free-living coracidia survive for 3–4 days before exhausting their food reserves. Some coracidia are ingested by microscopic crustacea, such as *Cyclops* sp. and *Diaptomus* sp., which are the first intermediate hosts for *D. latum*. The coracidium burrows into the crustacean's body cavity and develops into the procercoid larva (Fig. 15.5).

When the infected crustacea are consumed by small freshwater fish, particularly various species of minnows, the released procercoid larva penetrates the wall of the small intestine of the fish and takes up residence in the muscles. It then transforms into the pleurocercoid larva (Fig. 15.6), the infective stage for man.

Infected minnows eaten by large predator species of fish, such as members of the perch and pike families, transfer the larvae to the larger fish. The pleurocercoid larva is capable of infecting the predator species, but it remains biologically unchanged.

When an undercooked or raw infected fish is ingested by man, the pleurocercoid larva passes to the small intestine, where it develops into the adult worm, becoming a fully formed strobila within 3 months (Fig. 15.7).

Most carnivores can harbor *D. latum*, and dog, bear, cat, fox, martin, mink, and other mammals serve as reservoir hosts for this parasite.

Pathogenesis

Vitamin B$_{12}$ deficiency in *D. latum* infection results from absorption of this vitamin by the worm. The full picture of megaloblastic anemia is indistinguishable from that due to other causes. The reason for the relative infrequency of mega-

Diphyllobothrium latum

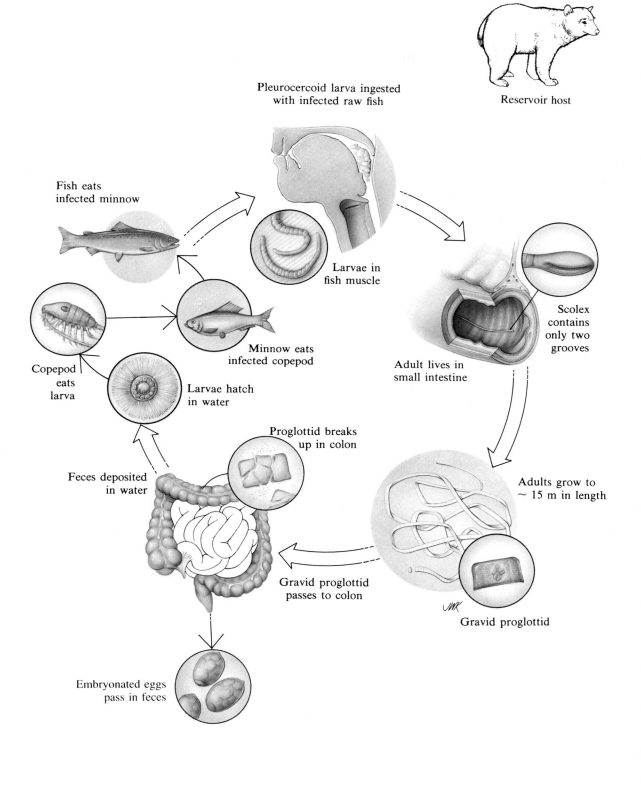

Reservoir host

Pleurocercoid larva ingested
with infected raw fish

Fish eats
infected minnow

Larvae in
fish muscle

Scolex
contains
only two
grooves

Adult lives in
small intestine

Minnow eats
infected copepod

Copepod
eats
larva

Larvae hatch
in water

Adults grow to
~ 15 m in length

Proglottid breaks
up in colon

Feces deposited
in water

Gravid proglottid
passes to colon

Gravid proglottid

Embryonated eggs
pass in feces

A

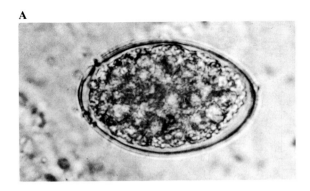

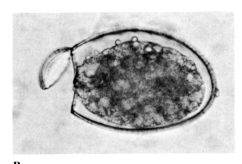

B

Figure 15.3. Eggs of *Diphyllobothrium latum*. **A.** An egg as seen in freshly passed stool. **B.** An egg that has begun to hatch. The embryo will emerge from the operculated end. **A, B,** ×625.

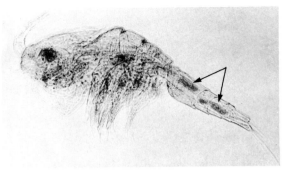

Figure 15.5. The procercoid larvae (*arrows*) of *Diphyllobothrium latum* lie within the body cavity of *Diaptemus* sp., their crustacean intermediate host. ×16.

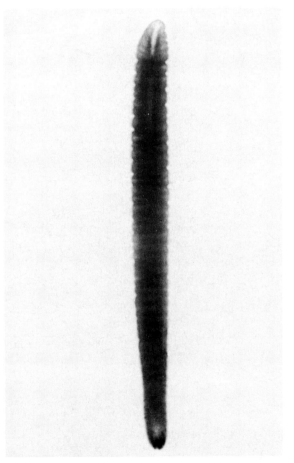

Figure 15.6. Pleurocercoid larva (i.e., infectious stage for man) of *Diphyllobothrium latum*. Note the grooved immature scolex, reminiscent of the adult. This larva lives between the muscle fibers of the second intermediate host, the fish. ×25.

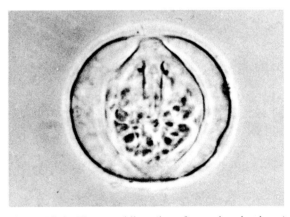

Figure 15.4. The coracidium (i.e., free-swimming larva) of *Diphyllobothrium latum* is ciliated. This stage is ingested by the first intermediate host, the copepod. ×1000.

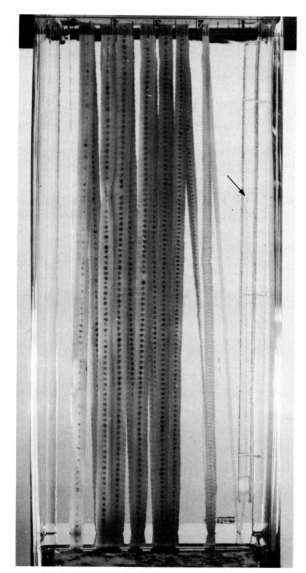

Figure 15.7. Whole adult *Diphyllobothrium latum* worm preserved in alcohol and displayed in a museum jar. This specimen measures over 9 m in length. *Arrow* points to the scolex.

factor than those who were free of anemia, but who also harbored the worm.[3]

Clinical Disease

The infected individuals usually become aware of the infection when they pass immature segments of the worm. Some patients have diarrhea.[4] Fewer than 2% of those infected with *D. latum* develop megaloblastic anemia, most common in the first 3 decades of life.

Diagnosis

Diagnosis is made by microscopic observation of the eggs (Fig. 15.3A) in the stool. There are no specific serological tests for infection with this parasite.

Treatment

The drug of choice is niclosamide.

Prevention and Control

The numerous reservoir hosts are potentially important in maintaining the life cycle in sylvatic settings. Interference with this aspect of the life cycle is difficult. However, proper disposal of human feces can have a major impact in reducing the prevalence of infection. On an individual basis, the best way to avoid infection with *D. latum* is to eat only well-cooked fish.

In Scandinavian countries, gravlox and a wide variety of other raw fish dishes are sources of infection with this tapeworm.

loblastic anemia among carriers of *D. latum* is not well understood. It may be related to the position of the worm in the intestine: those higher in the duodenum may absorb more of the vitamin. There may be some genetic predisposition on the part of the host as well. One study indicated that patients with megaloblastic anemia due to infection with *D. latum* had less intrinsic

References

1. Plater F: Praxeos seu de cognoscendis, praedicendis praecudensis curandiso affectibus homini incommodantibus tractatus tertius et ultimus. De vitiis, libris duobus agens: quorum primum corpis: secundus. Exretorum vitia continet. Chapter XIV, Basel, Typis Conradi Waldkirchii, 1609
2. Janicki C: Le cycle evolutif du *Dibothriocephalus latus L.* Societe Neuchateloise des Sciences naturelles Bulletin 42:19–53, 1916–1917

3. Salokannel J: Intrinsic factor in tapeworm anemia. Acta Med Scand (Suppl) 517:1–51, 1970

4. Saarni M, Nyberg W, Grasbeck R, et al.: Symptoms in carriers of *Diphyllobothrium latum* and in uninfected controls. Acta Med Scand 173:147–154, 1963

5. Nyberg W: Absorption and excretion of vitamin B$_{12}$ in subjects infected with *Diphyllobothrium latum* and in non-infected subjects following oral administration of radioactive B$_{12}$. Acta Haematol (Basel) 19:90–98, 1958

16. Larval Tapeworms

Many species of tapeworm of medical importance produce infections in animals other than man and use intermediate mammalian hosts. Infection in man resembles that of the intermediate host; i.e., man harbors only a larval stage of the worm. Included in the list of tapeworms that cause larval infections in human populations are *Taenia solium, Echinococcus granulosus, E. multilocularis, Multiceps multiceps, M. serialis, M. brauni*, and a group of related tapeworms of the genus Spirometra.

Only larval infections with *T. solium* (cysticercosis) and *E. granulosus* (hydatid disease) will be discussed fully.

Taenia solium (Linnaeus 1758)

Life Cycle

Disease produced by infection with larval *T. solium* is not uncommon in regions where *T. solium* adult infections exist. Therefore, it is found in the endemic areas listed in Chapter 14. The infection results from ingestion of eggs (Fig. 16.1) from a contaminated environment. It is also possible that eggs released from proglottids and regurgitated into the stomach reenter the small intestine and initiate the life cycle.

The larval tapeworm (i.e., oncosphere) penetrates the intestinal wall and enters the bloodstream. Eventually, it enters one of many tissues (e.g., striated muscles, heart, brain, eye, etc.) and encysts, developing into a cysticercus measuring approximately 5 mm × 10 mm (Fig. 16.2A and B).

Pathogenesis

Regardless of the tissue affected, pathological consequences are those of a space-occupying lesion. Cysticerci in brain tend to grow to a larger size than those in other tissues (Fig. 16.3). In addition, occasionally a cysticercus may develop within a ventricle of the brain, leading to hydrocephalus. There is no cellular response to living cysticerci. Ultimately, the cysticerci die and become calcified, usually within 2 years after the initial infection. The process of calcification may be accompanied by the release of antigens, thus inducing an acute local inflammatory reaction, which may be clinically significant in cerebral cysticercosis.[1]

Clinical Disease

The patient with cysticercosis is usually asymptomatic, but may notice painless subcutaneous nodules, or small, discrete swellings of particular muscles, in which cysticerci have lodged. If a cysticercus lodges in the eye, it invades the retina

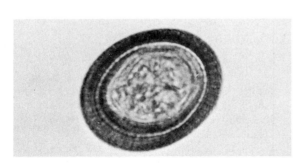

Figure 16.1. Egg of *Taenia solium*. This stage causes infections in the intermediate host (the pig) and larval in man. ×625.

Cysticercosis

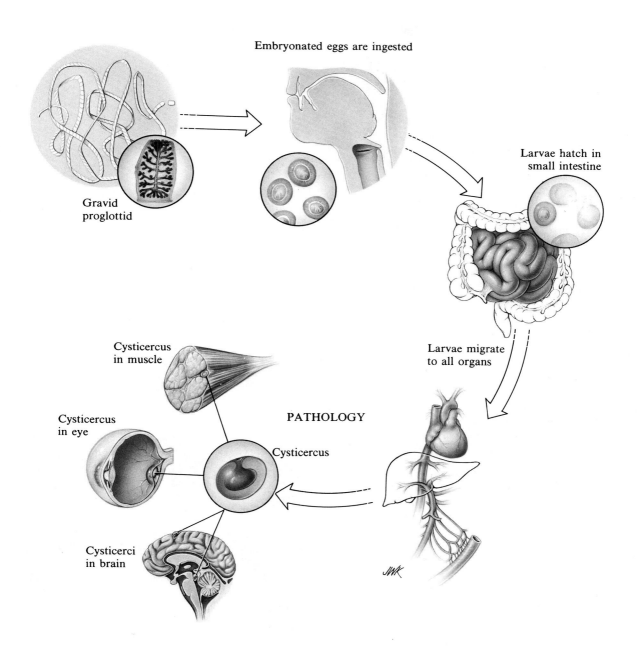

Embryonated eggs are ingested

Gravid
proglottid

Larvae hatch in
small intestine

Larvae migrate
to all organs

Cysticercus
in muscle

Cysticercus
in eye

PATHOLOGY

Cysticercus

Cysticerci
in brain

JWK

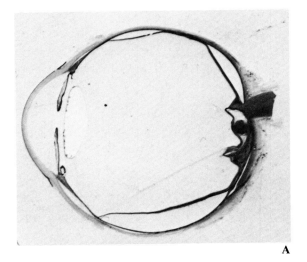

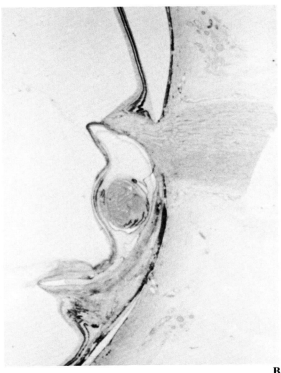

Figure 16.2. The cysticercus stage of *Taenia solium* can be found anywhere in the body. It causes serious clinical problems if it is located in the eye (**A** and **B**). Hooks are clearly visible in **B,** identifying this as a cyst of *T. solium*. **C.** Section of eye with a single cysticercus of *Taenia solium*. The presence of hooks (*arrow*) identifies the species of the larval tapeworm. **A,** ×4; **B,** ×16; **C,** ×52.

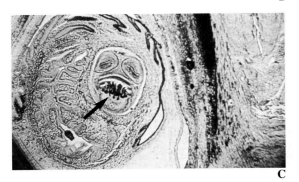

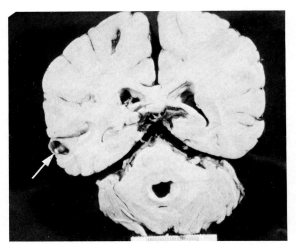

Figure 16.3. A single cysticercus of *Taenia solium* is seen in the left cerebral cortex (*arrow*). Five others were found in different parts of the brain. The patient died of a mesothelioma, an unrelated disease. The cysts were an incidental finding at autopsy.

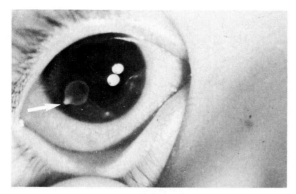

Figure 16.4. A free-floating cysticercus (*arrow*) in the anterior chamber of the eye. This patient also had lesions in the brain and throughout the musculoskeletal system.

(Fig. 16.2C). It may also invade the vitreous humour and the anterior chamber of the eye (Fig. 16.4), giving the patient impressions of shadows. Secondary reactions are expressed as conjunctivitis, retinitis, uveitis, and eventual atrophy of the choroid.

Cerebral cysticercosis can present as a space-occupying lesion and in every respect can mimic a tumor. Thus seizures, hydrocephalus, and focal neurological abnormalities can be the presenting signs.

Diagnosis

Specific diagnosis is difficult to establish, because cysticerci causing severe symptoms are not read-ily accessible to examination. If a patient suspected of cysticercosis also has an intestinal infection with *T. solium* (diagnosed by examination of a passed proglottid), the suspicion that the space-occupying lesion is a cysticercus is strengthened. Likewise, if in addition the patient presents with subcutaneous lesions, they can be biopsied and the diagnosis confirmed by locating the hooklets in section. Small punctate densities seen on a radiogram of the extremities can also help establish the diagnosis of cysticercosis. The lesions can usually be identified by computerized axial tomography or magnetic resonance imaging.[2] Immunodiagnosis is also available. It is based on the detection either of antibody[3], or of antigens[4] by a combination of test based on the ELISA technique.

Treatment

Cysticercosis, whether caused by *Taenia solium* or any other taeniid species, responds well to treatment with praziquantel.[5] The drug is given over a period of days and the death of the parasite is accompanied by a transient inflammatory response which may elicit neurological symptoms.

Prevention and Control

See Prevention and Control section in Chapter 13 (*Taenia saginata*).

Echinococcus granulosus (Batsch 1786)

Echinococcus granulosus, a parasite of dogs, is one of the smallest tapeworms, measuring only 5 mm in length and consisting of a scolex and only three segments. The adult lives in the small intestine of dogs and other canidae. Only the larval form of the infection is found in the human host and causes space-occupying lesions known as hydatid cysts. This infection is considered very serious and has resulted in fatalities.

The distribution of the adult and larval infections parallels sheep husbandry. Thus Greece, Rumania, Spain, Italy, Argentina, South Africa, U.S.S.R., Turkey, Lebanon, Syria, and Egypt are endemic foci of infection. In Lapland (i.e., northern Scandinavian countries), herding of reindeer is also associated with this infection. Small, endemic areas of infection exist in the United States, primarily in California, Utah, and Arizona, where Basques and American Indians are predominantly involved.[6]

Historical Information

As was true for other tapeworms, *E. granulosus* was recognized as a pathological entity (in this instance, the hydatid cysts) long before it was formally. described. In 1766 Pallas[7] described and sketched the hydatid cysts that he removed from the viscera of mice and compared them with those recovered by others from human infections. The larvae (i.e., protoscoleces) were depicted in detail in 1782 by Goeze[8] in his classic monograph. The adult worms in the dog were first reported by von Siebold[9] in 1853. Finally, Naunyn[10] in 1863 fed the contents of hydatid cysts derived from a human infection to dogs and recovered the adult tapeworms. Thus, these experiments provided the link between the animal and human infection cycles.

Life Cycle

The adult worm of *E. granulosus* (Fig. 16.5) lives in the small intestine of the dog, its definitive host. All domestic breeds of dog are susceptible to the infection. In addition, wild dogs, wolves, coyotes, and jackals can harbor the adult infection.

The gravid segment (one per adult tapeworm) breaks off and disintegrates in the large bowel, releasing hundreds of infective eggs that then pass out with the feces. The sheep, as well as other animals including man, acquire the larval stage by ingesting the egg (Fig. 13.4).

The oncosphere hatches in the small intestine and reaches the liver, the most commonly infected organ, by the hematogenous route. Once in the tissue, the larva secretes a hyaline membrane and become surrounded by it. This membrane eventually differentiates into an outer, acellular laminate structure and an inner, germinal layer. The inner surface of the germinal layer gives rise to protoscoleces (i.e., the units infectious for the definitive host) and more outer membrane material (Fig. 16.6A-C).

The hydatid cyst (Fig. 16.7) requires several months to mature. The fully grown cyst is filled with fluid and can contain hundreds of thousands of protoscoleces. The diameter of the mature outer cyst varies from 2 cm to 20 cm and sometimes is even larger. The fluid portion of the cyst contains both host and parasite components, and it is from this fluid that the antigen used in the serodiagnosis of this infection is derived.

For the life cycle to be completed, the hydatid cyst and its contents (i.e., the protoscoleces) must be ingested by a canine host. This commonly occurs when infected sheep are slaughtered and

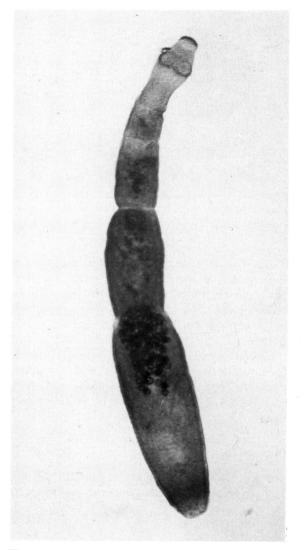

Figure 16.5. Adult *Echinococcus granulosus*. The entire worm consists of scolex and three proglottids. It lives in the small intestine of the dog. ×50.

organs containing hydatid cysts are fed to the sheepdogs.

The protoscolex released from the hydatid cyst attaches itself by its four suckers and a row of hooks to the wall of the small intestine. New, gravid proglottids are produced within about 2 months after ingestion of the protoscoleces.

The dogs do not seem to become ill from the effects of even heavy intestinal infections, which can exceed a million adult worms.

Echinococcus granulosus

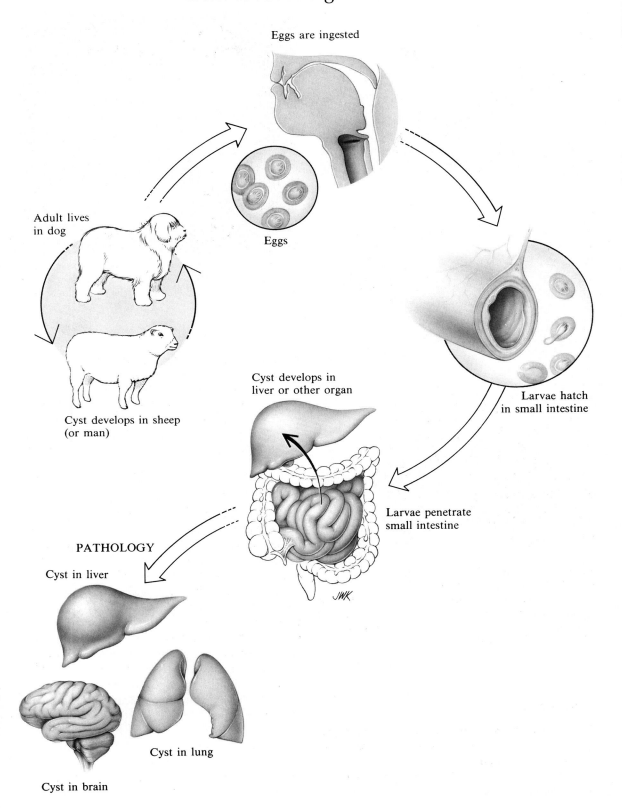

Eggs are ingested

Eggs

Adult lives
in dog

Cyst develops in sheep
(or man)

Cyst develops in
liver or other organ

Larvae hatch
in small intestine

Larvae penetrate
small intestine

JWK

PATHOLOGY

Cyst in liver

Cyst in lung

Cyst in brain

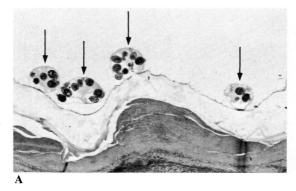

A

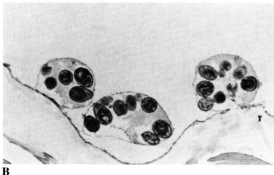

B

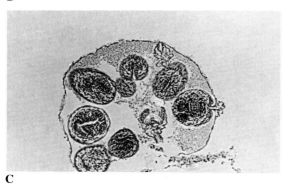

C

Figure 16.6. A, B, and C. The brood capsules (*arrows*) of the hydatid cyst of *Echinococcus granulosus* bud from the germinal membrane and are more clearly seen at higher magnifications (**B**). The protoscoleces are seen best in **C**; each can give rise to an adult tapeworm if it is eaten by a dog. **A,** ×22; **B,** ×48; **C,** ×105.

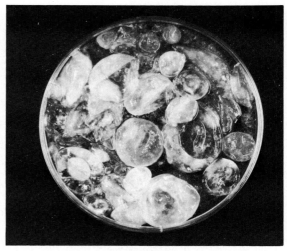

Figure 16.7. A dish with many daughter cysts of *Echinococcus granulosus* that were recovered from a single large hydatid cyst. ×0.33.

Pathogenesis

Hydatid disease develops as the result of rapid growth of the cyst, or of cysts, and subsequent expansion of the cyst wall.

When a cyst ruptures, the fluid content and the protoscoleces contained within it are released into the body. This can lead to an immediate anaphylactic reaction. Moreover, the cyst contents can seed the area and invade new tissues to produce second-generation hydatid cysts. Even a small piece of the germinal layer can reestablish an entire hydatid cyst. In this sense, *E. granulosus* is a metastatic parasite.

Clinical Disease

The symptoms are those of a large space-occupying lesion. If the liver is involved, it tends to become enlarged. The cyst presents as a palpable, soft, nontender, intrahepatic mass. The uninvolved bulk of the liver remains normal. Involvement of the lung is usually identified by a chance radiogram or the coughing up of bloody sputum in which protoscoleces or hooklets can be found. Rupture of a cyst, wherever it is lodged, may occur even after a relatively minor blunt trauma and often leads to an allergic reaction. It may be mild and limited to urticaria, or may take the form of anaphylactic shock, requiring immediate intervention.

Diagnosis

As in the case of any space-occupying lesion, diagnosis must be made by a variety of tests,

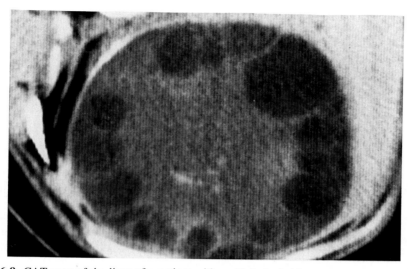

Figure 16.8. CAT scan of the liver of a patient with multiple hydatid cysts. (Courtesy of Dr. Ferrer)

most of them nonspecific. Scans, using radio-nuclides such as gallium or technetium, can identify such cysts; so can ultrasonography. Computerized axial tomography or magnetic resonance imaging (Fig. 16.8), not yet widely used in the diagnosis of hydatid cysts, will undoubtedly become prime diagnostic means for localization of the cysts. Plain radiograms can reveal only calcified cycts, which usually contain noninfective protoscoleces.

Immunoelectrophoresis is an important tool in the serodiagnosis of *E. granulosus,* and its use has improved laboratory testing in this disease. Hydatid cyst fluid is used as the antigen in electrophoresis, reacting with the patient's serum.[11] Arc 5 of the pattern is diagnostic for *E. granulosus* (Fig. 16.9). Almost all patients with active infections can be diagnosed by this method. Reliable complement fixation and indirect hemag-glutination tests are also available.[12] In old cases, in which the protoscoleces have died and the cyst itself has become calcified, finding hooklets is diagnostic for *E. granulosus* (Fig. 16.10). At this late stage of the disease, serological tests may be negative.

Most important to the diagnosis of hydatid disease is taking of an accurate case history. Ownership of dogs, life on a sheep farm, even in childhood, especially in endemic areas, and history of travel to endemic areas are all important factors suggesting the possibility that a suspected mass is indeed a hydatid cyst.

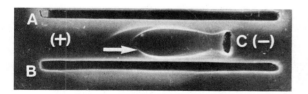

Figure 16.9. Immunoelectrophoretic pattern of serum from a patient with a viable hydatid cyst (*B*). The trough (*A*) contained a known positive serum. The antigen used was concentrated hydatid cyst fluid. Arc 5 (*arrow*) is diagnostic for infection with larval taeniid tapeworms. (Courtesy of Dr. P. Schantz)

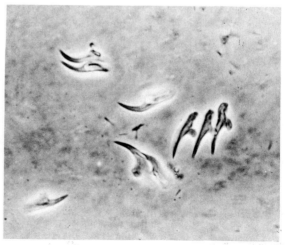

Figure 16.10. Hooklets of *Echinococcus granulosus* found in sputum of a patient who had hydatid disease. ×580.

Definitive diagnosis can be established only by microscopic identification of the hydatid tissue or its contents (Fig. 16.6).

Treatment

Cysts containing living protoscoleces should be removed surgically to prevent their inadvertent rupture. Obviously, the probability of a successful removal depends on the location of the cysts. If such a cyst is accessible, it must be handled gently to preclude rupture during surgery. A variety of means have been recommended for prevention of spillage and metastatic seeding of the cyst fluid. These include scolecidal solutions, such as hypertonic glucose or saline solution, 50% ethanol, or a 10% formaldehyde solution. After the cyst is exposed, a small amount of its content is aspirated and replaced with one of the scolecidal solutions. This procedure is repeated until the entire content of the cyst becomes filled with the solution. Alternatively, cryosurgery has been used.[13] When surgical removal is impossible, high doses of mebendazole (40 mg/kg/24 h) administered over a long period (1–6 months) have been tried with variable success.[14]

Prevention and Control

Infection of dogs with *E. granulosus* must be prevented. Control is best achieved through avoidance of feeding dogs any infected organs of the slaughtered sheep and other animals and by treatment of infected dogs with niclosamide.[15] A more effective method has been mass slaughter of infected dogs in isolated, well-defined ecosystems.[16] Public health education in endemic areas has led to decreased incidence.

Echinococcus multilocularis (Leuckart 1863)

The adult stage of *E. multilocularis* usually infects sylvatic canine mammals, such as fox, but may also infect wild and domesticated dogs. The intermediate hosts include a wide variety of rodents, such as voles, field mice, and ground squirrels. Infection in man is analogous to that in the intermediate host. Human infections have been reported in Alaska, North Dakota, and Minnesota, in the United States; in Manitoba, Saskatchewan, and Alberta, in Canada; in Siberia, in the U.S.S.R.; and in Europe.

Infection begins when the intermediate host has ingested the egg. The larva hatches in the small intestine and invades the liver by the hematogenous route. It develops in the liver into an alveolar type of cyst (Fig. 16.11). Ingestion of diseased liver by the definitive hosts leads to infections with the adult stage of the worm, which completes the life cycle.

In man, the incubation period of larval infection with *E. multilocularis* is probably quite long, because the initial exposure apparently occurs in childhood, whereas the disease has been recognized mainly in adults.[17] Lesions of the liver usually are only membranous, with no identifiable protoscoleces within.

No therapy has been fully effective, but mebendazole[18] or albendazole has been shown to be of some value when surgery cannot be performed. Rarely surgery can be effective[19].

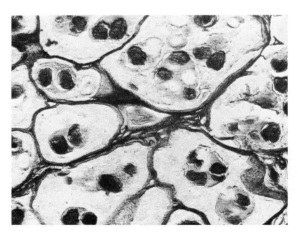

Figure 16.11. Section through the liver of a rodent (vole) infected with the alveolar cyst of *Echinococcus multilocularis*. In human alveolar infection, the germinal membrane and acellular laminate layer are present, but protoscoleces or hooklets are usually not recovered. ×63.

Multiceps spp.

Multiceps spp. are a group of tapeworms usually infecting dogs and other canidae, which are their definitive hosts. The intermediate hosts are domestic cattle, horses, and goats and some wild herbivorous game animals of Africa. Man acquires the larval infection, known as coenurus disease, which resembles cysts found in the intermediate hosts. Human infections have been largely confined to the African continent, but a few cases have been described from France, England, and North and South America.

The larva usually invades the brain. It must be distinguished from other space-occupying lesions due to parasites, such as cysticerci and hydatid cysts.

Diagnosis is based on clinical, epidemiological, and laboratory findings. No serological tests are currently available.

Treatment involves surgery if the lesion is accessible. No chemotherapy is available. Prevention is not possible, because reservoir hosts include a large number of species of wild animals.

Spirometra spp.

Sparganosis represents an infection with the larval stages of tapeworms, all of which belong to the genus Spirometra. The definitive hosts for many of the species of spirometra have not been identified. Cats and dogs have been shown to harbor adult *S. mansonoides*. Moreover, cats can be experimentally infected with *S. ranorum*. Cases of sparganosis have been reported from Southeast Asia, Japan, China, and Africa. The intermediate hosts represent a broad spectrum of vertebrates, viz. amphibia, reptiles, birds, or mammals.

Human infection results from ingestion of raw or undercooked flesh of any of the numerous intermediate hosts and from application of such flesh as poultices. The larval worms usually migrate into the subcutaneous tissues and grow into irregular nodules. The surrounding tissues become edematous and painful.

Treatment is surgical; there is no effective chemotherapy. Prevention is difficult, because of the entrenched dietary habits and other customs.

References

1. Sparks AK, Neafie RC, Connor DH: Cysticercosis. In Binford CH, Connor DH (eds): Pathology of Tropical and Extraordinary Diseases. Washington, DC, Armed Forces Institute for Pathology, 1976, pp 539–543

2. Carbajal JR, Palacios E, Azar-Kia B, et al.: Radiology of cysticercosis of the central nervous system, including computed tomography. J Radiol 125:127–131, 1977

3. Coker-Vann M, Brown P, Gajdusek C: Serodiagnosis of human cysticercosis using a chromatofocused antigenic preparation of *Taenia solium* cysticerci in an enzyme-linked immunosorbent assay (ELISA). Trans Roy Soc Trop Med Hyg 78:491–496, 1984

4. Estrada JJ, Kuhn RE: Immunochemical detection of antigens of larval *Taenia solium* and antilarval antibodies in the cerebrospinal fluid of patients with neurocysticercosis. J Neurol Sci 71:39–48, 1985

5. Webbe G: Cestodal infections of Man. In: Chemotherapy of Parasitic Diseases. (Campbell WC, Rew RS, eds). Plenum Press, New York and London, 1986, pp 457–478

6. Schantz PM: Echinococcosis in American Indians living in Arizona and New Mexico. A review of recent studies. Am J. Epi. 106:370–379, 1977

7. Pallas PS: Miscellanea Zoologica: Quibus Novae Imprimis Atque Obscure Animalium Species Describuntur Et Observationibus Iconibusque Illustrantur. Hagae Comitum Petrum van Cleff, 1766

8. Goeze JAE: Versuch einer Naturgeschichte der Eingeweidewurme Thierischer Körper. Blankenburg, P. A. Pape, 1782

9. von Siebold CT: Über die Verwandlung der Echinococcus-brut in Taenien. Ztschr Wissensch Zool 4:409–424, 1853

10. Naunyn B: Über die zu *Echinococcus hominis* gehörige Taenie. Arch Anat Physiol Wissensch Med 412–416, 1863

11. Pozzuoli R, Musiani P, Arru E, et al: *Echinococcus granulosus:* Isolation and characterization of sheep hydatid fluid antigens. Exp Parasitol 32:45–55, 1972

12. Schantz PM, Gottstein B: Echinococcosis (Hydatidosis). In: Immunodiagnosis of Parasitic Diseases (Walls KW, Schantz PM, eds.). Academic Press, Orlando and New York, 1986, pp 69–108

13. Saio F, Nazarian I: Surgical treatment of hydatid cysts by freezing of cyst's wall and instillation of 0.5% of silver nitrate solution. N Engl J Med 284:1346, 1971

14. Pawlowski ZS: Chemotherapy of human echinococcosis. Proceedings of the XIII Congresco International de Hydatidologia, pp 346–347. Madrid, Spain.

15. Schwabe CW: Epidemiological aspects of the planning and evaluation of hydatid disease control. Austral Vet J 55:109–117, 1979

16. Beard TC: The elimination of echinococcosis from Iceland. Bull WHO 48:653–660, 1973

17. Lukaschenko NP: Problems of epidemiology and prophylaxis of alveococcosis (multilocular echinococcosis): A general review—with particular reference to the U.S.S.R. Int J Parasitol 1:125–134, 1971

18. Wilson JF, Davidson M, Rausch RL: A clinical trial of mebendazole in the treatment of alveolar hydatid disease. Ann Rev Resp Dis 118:747–757, 1978

19. Gamble WG, Segal M, Schantz PM, et al.: Alveolar hydatid disease in Minnesota. First human case acquired in the contiguous United States. JAMA 241:904–907, 1979

17. Tapeworms of Minor Medical Importance

Hymenolepis nana (Siebold 1852)

Historical Information

This cyclophyllidean tapeworm was identified as a pathogen by Bilharz[1] in 1852 during an autopsy of a child. It is now known to be a cosmopolitan parasite. *Hymenolepis nana* is small, measuring 35–45 mm in length. The adult consists of 150–200 proglottids and lives loosely attached to the wall of the small intestine.

the segments break off from the strobila and disintegrate in the small intestine, the eggs are freed and either pass out with feces or hatch in the small intestine, and reinfect the villous tissue. In some cases, hundreds of adult *H. nana* can be found in individuals in whom this process of autoinfection takes place. Eggs deposited in the

Life Cycle

Infection with *H. nana* is acquired by the ingestion of embryonated eggs (Fig. 17.1). When the eggs hatch in the small intestine, the larva, known as an oncosphere, penetrates the lamina propria of a villus and undergoes development into the pre-adult cysticercoid (Fig. 17.2). The cysticercoid then enters the intestinal lumen and attaches to the surface of the villous tissue, where it finally develops, after approximately 3 weeks, into a mature adult (Fig. 17.3). The adult worm remains attached to the villus with the aid of four suckers and hooklets on its scolex (Fig. 17.4).

Self-mating between adjacent proglottids results in production of hundreds of fertilized eggs. As

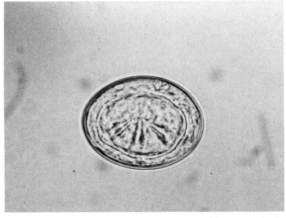

Figure 17.1. Embryonated infectious egg of *Hymenolepis nana*. × 1000.

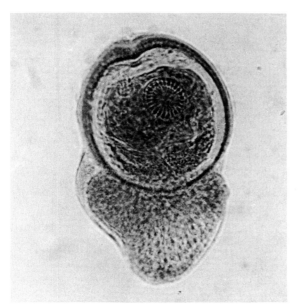

Figure 17.2. Cysticercoid of *Hymenolepis nana*. This stage develops in the villous tissue of the small intestine. ×200.

feces continue the cycle if they are ingested by man or a small rodent.

Pathogenesis

In light infections, there is no tissue damage. When the infection is heavy, as in cases of autoinfection, there may be sufficient damage to the mucosal surface to cause diarrhea.

Infection in adult patients, but not in young children, is usually self-limited, probably reflecting the ability of the host to develop protective immunity. In experimental infections of rodent hosts, antibodies protect against reinfection.[2]

Clinical Disease

Diarrhea is the most prominent symptom of heavy infection. Although headaches and convulsions have been attributed to this infection, there is no evidence of a causal relationship.

Diagnosis

Discovery of embryonated eggs (Fig. 17.1) in the stool provides definitive diagnosis. When whole pieces of strobila are passed, they can be identi-

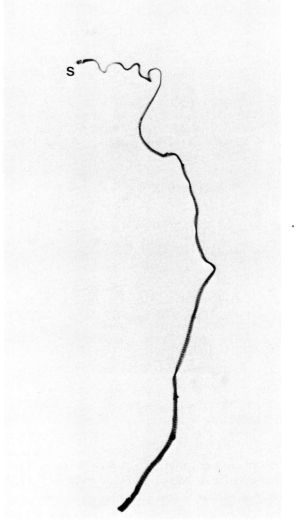

Figure 17.3. Entire adult of *Hymenolepis nana*. **S,** scolex. ×11.

fied directly, or the eggs can be expressed from the gravid proglottids and then identified.

Treatment

Niclosamide is the drug of choice, but it is less effective than in therapy of *T. saginata* (Chapter 13) because of autoinfection. Therefore, reexamination of the patient's stool following therapy is important because an additional course of therapy may be necessary. It may be prudent to accept failure of therapy in patients who are asymptomatic.

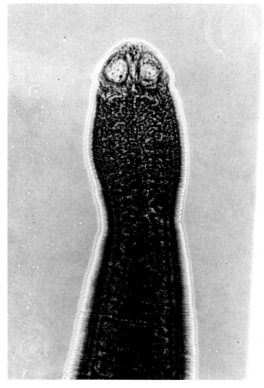

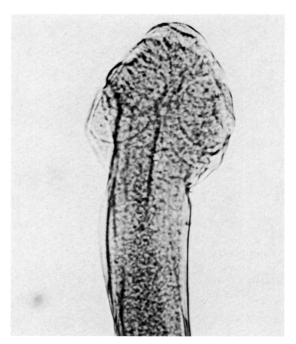

Figure 17.5. Scolex of *Hymenolepis diminuta*. ×210.

Figure 17.4. Scolex of *Hymenolepis nana*. ×150.

Prevention and Control

Control is best effected by prevention of contamination with human feces of food and water supplies. Owing to the mechanism of autoinfection, it is difficult sometimes to eradicate the worms from individual patients. Rodent reservoir hosts contaminate the environment and cannot be controlled readily.

Hymenolepis diminuta (Rudolphi 1819)

Historical Information

Hymenolepis diminuta was formally described by Rudolphi[3] in 1819, but credit is given to Weinland[4] for first describing the infection in man in 1858.

Life Cycle

The adult worm measures about 50 cm in length. The scolex (Fig. 17.5) has four suckers, but no hooklets and the strobila contains about 1000 proglottids (Fig. 17.6A-C).

   H. diminuta is acquired by ingestion of the cysticercoid stage. The cysticercoid lives within the body cavity of a wide variety of insects including immature fleas and flour beetles, which are the intermediate hosts.

   Once ingested by man, the cysticercoid is freed from invertebrate tissues by the digestive processes of the host. It then everts its scolex and grows into an adult, which matures within 25 days.

   After fertilization each gravid proglottid breaks off from the strobila and disintegrates in the small intestine. The eggs are passed with the

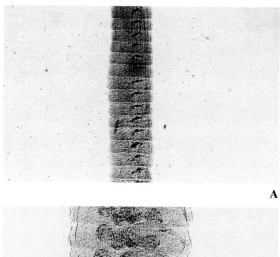

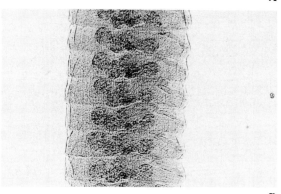

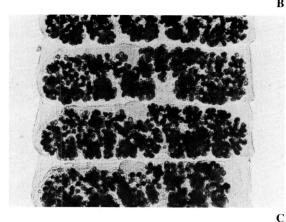

Figure 17.6. Proglottids of *Hymenolepis diminuta*. **A.** Immature proglottids; **B.** mature proglottids; **C.** gravid proglottids. **A, B,** and **C,** ×22.

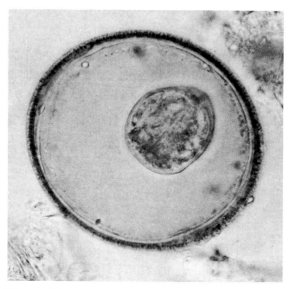

Figure 17.7. Embryonated infectious egg of *Hymenolepis diminuta*. ×1000.

are inadvertently eaten by man. Other vertebrates (e.g., rats, mice, and dogs) also serve as definitive hosts.

Pathogenesis

H. diminuta induces no tissue damage.

Clinical Disease

There are no clinical symptoms attributable to this infection.

Diagnosis

Identification of eggs (Fig. 17.7) in the stool is the definitive method of diagnosis. Occasionally, whole segments of adult worms, which can be identified directly, are also passed in the feces. It is possible to extract eggs from such gravid segments and identify them.

Treatment

Niclosamide is the drug of choice.

Prevention and Control

H. diminuta, like *H. nana*, must be controlled both in the infected individual and in the reservoir host, but the latter is highly unlikely.

feces and are ingested by the invertebrate intermediate host (usually an insect) to continue the life cycle. The eggs hatch within the lumen of the invertebrate gut tract, and the freed oncosphere penetrates its body cavity and develops into the cysticercoid, the stage infective for man. The life cycle is completed when infected insects

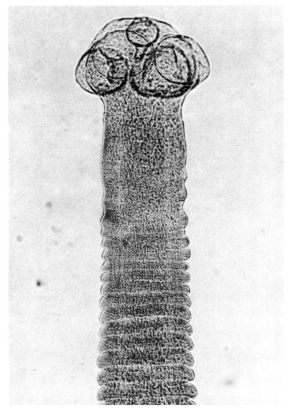

Figure 17.8. Scolex of adult *Dipylidium caninum*. ×156.

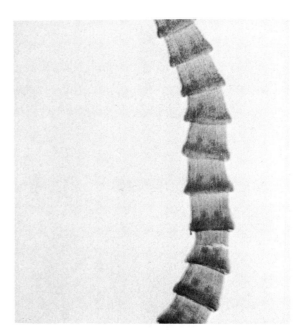

Figure 17.9. Immature proglottids of *Dipylidium caninum*. ×30.

Treatment of infected pets, particularly dogs, and rodents with niclosamide will aid in prevention of this infection.

Community efforts to curtail contamination of food, especially whole grains and processed flour, by insects containing the intermediate stage of the worm is an effective control measure.

Dipylidium caninum (Linnaeus 1758)

Dipylidium caninum lives as an adult in the lumen of the small intestine of the dog, cat, fox, hyena, and occasionally, man. It requires a flea as its intermediate host. The name of the genus is of Greek origin, and means double pore or opening.

Life Cycle

The infection is acquired by ingestion of an infected adult flea, usually *Ctenocephalides canis* or *C. felis* (see Chapter 38). The cysticercoid larva is released from the flea by the action of diges- tive enzymes of the host, attaches to the villous surface of the small intestine, and grows to an adult worm (Figs. 17.8–17.10), which can reach 50 cm in length within 25 days, when it begins to shed gravid proglottids (Fig. 17.10). The gravid proglottids disintegrate and release the eggs (Fig. 17.11), which accumulate in the feces and are passed to the external environment, where they are eaten by the larval flea. As in the case of *H. diminuta*, the oncosphere penetrates the body cavity of the immature flea and develops into the cysticercoid larva, the infective stage for man. Small children are frequently infected when they

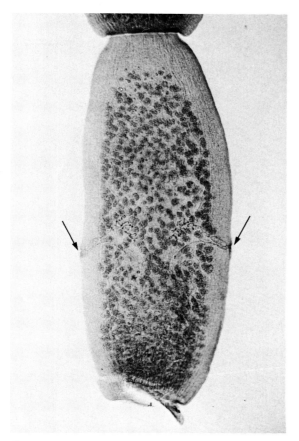

Figure 17.10. Gravid proglottid of *Dipylidium caninum*. Note the two lateral pores (*arrows*). ×26.

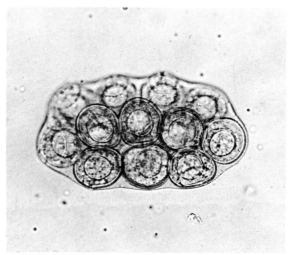

Figure 17.11. Eggs of *Dipylidium caninum*. Many eggs are contained within each packet in the gravid proglottid. They are infectious for the intermediate host, the flea. ×280.

are in close contact with dogs or cats and inadvertently swallow an infected adult flea.

Pathogenesis

There are no known pathogenic effects of this infection in man.

Diagnosis

Diagnosis is made by microscopic examination of the stool. The characteristic morphology of the clusters of eggs (Fig. 17.11) in the stool facilitates identification. If whole proglottids are found, they are also readily identifiable (Fig. 17.10).

Treatment

The drug of choice is niclosamide.

Prevention and Control

Eradication of fleas in pets and treatment of infected animals with niclosamide will reduce the chances of human infection.

References

1. Bilharz T: Ein Beitrag zur Helminographia humana. Ztschr Wissensch Zool 4:53–76, 1852
2. Weinmann CJ: Cestodes and acanthocephala. In Jackson GJ, Herman R, Singer I (eds): Immunity to Parasitic Animals, Vol 2. New York, Appleton-Century-Crofts, 1970, pp 1021–1059
3. Rudolphi CA: Entozoorum Synopsis cui Accedunt Mantissa Duplex et Indeces Locupletissimi. Berolini, 1819
4. Weinland DF: An essay on the tapeworms of man. Cambridge, Massachusetts, 1858

III
The Trematodes

Introduction

Phylum Platyhelminthes

The class Trematoda is divided into two orders, Monogenea and Digenea, both of which consist of obligate parasites. All of the trematodes of medical importance are classified within the order Digenea, and include the blood flukes, the intestinal flukes, and the tissue flukes. They are mainly found throughout the tropics and subtropics and only rarely are encountered in the temperate zones.

Anatomy and Physiology

Flukes of the order Digenea possess one of two reproductive styles. They are either monoecious, in which case the sexes are combined in single individuals, or dioecious, in which case the sexes are separate.

The outer surface of the adult worm consists of tegument, which serves as an absorbing surface for nutrients. It is covered by microvilli, underneath which there are mitochondria, pinocytes, and other structures promoting absorption. Pinocytosis and active transport of low-molecular weight nutrients enable the worm to be nourished by the digested foodstuffs in the small intestine of the host. In addition, the flukes have a functional gut tract, into which they ingest tissues of the host.

The tegument covers several layers of muscles. The muscle layers are innervated by a pair of dorsal ganglia, which give rise to lateral peripheral nerves running the length of the body. Commissures from the lateral nerves innervate various organs including the musculature, gut tract, and reproductive organs.

The gut tract originates at the oral cavity, which is enveloped by the anterior sucker. The ingested matter is pumped down into a bifurcated, intestinal tract, which ends blindly. Digestion, aided by enzymes, which include a variety of proteases, lipases, aminopeptidases, and esterases, takes place within this structure.

The flukes have no body cavity; the organs are embedded in the parenchyma.

Trematodes excrete solid wastes by reverse peristalsis in the gut tract, and liquids by a network of tubules that connect collecting organelles, known as flame cells, with the excretory pore of the parasite.

Monoecious trematodes reproduce by self-fertilization or by cross-fertilization. The eggs, supplied with yolk from the vitelline glands, are fertilized within the uterus and surrounded by a shell in the Mehlis' gland. They must be shed into a suitable environment to continue the life cycle.

Dioecious trematodes, which include the blood flukes, live *in copula* as separate sexes. They produce eggs and fertilize them continuously.

18. The Schistosomes: *Schistosoma mansoni* (Sambon 1907), *Schistosoma japonicum* (Katsurada 1904), and *Schistosoma haematobium* (Bilharz 1852)

Schistosomiasis is an infection caused by three species belonging to the genus Schistosoma: *S. mansoni*, *S. japonicum*, and *S. haematobium*. In addition, *S. intercalatum* has been identified as a pathogen in certain regions of West Africa. The World Health Organization estimates that at present 200–300 million people are infected with one or more of these species. The geographic distribution of these parasites reflects that of their specific snail vectors.

Infections with *S. mansoni* prevail throughout tropical and subtropical Africa, South America, and the Caribbean. The parasite is transmitted from man to man through snails belonging to the genus Biomphalaria. There are only a few known reservoir hosts, such as baboons and monkeys in Africa, and they usually do not transmit the infection to man.

S. japonicum is found only in the Orient, primarily in China, Malaysia, the Philippines, and, to a small extent, in Japan. Its snail intermediate hosts belong to the genus Onchomelania. Dogs, monkeys, rats, pigs, and cattle serve as its important reservoir hosts. It is uncertain whether *S. mekongi*, found in northeastern Thailand, Laos, and Cambodia, is a separate species or a variant of *S. japonicum*.

S. haematobium is prevalent in Africa, the Middle East, and southwestern India. The intermediate hosts are members of the genus Bulinus. It has no important reservoir hosts, although during an epidemic of the infection in the Omo River Valley of Ethiopia the origin of *S. haematobium* was traced to monkeys.[1]

Historical Information

Bilharz, in a succession of letters written between 1851 and 1853 to his friend and mentor, von Siebold, accurately described many helminths infecting man, including *S. haematobium*. In 1902, Manson described a case of schistosomiasis in an Englishman who traveled extensively throughout the Caribbean and who had many eggs with lateral spines in his feces but not in his urine.[2] Sambon[3], in 1907, recognized that there were two blood flukes on the basis of morphology and origin of the eggs in stool and urine. In tribute to Manson, Sambon named this new organism after him. Shortly thereafter, in 1908, *S. mansoni* was also discovered in South America by Piraja da Silva.[4] In 1915, Leiper[5] conducted extensive investigations on schistosomiasis and reported the life cycle of *S. mansoni*. He accurately described its snail intermediate host and morphology of the adult worms.

In 1904, Katsurada[6] described and named the adult worms of *S. japonicum*, which he found in a naturally infected cat. Coincidentally, Catto, a Scotsman working in Singapore, described an identical adult worm in a patient who died of cholera.[7] He proposed for it the name *S. cattoi*, but his publication was delayed. Earlier, in 1888, Majima[8] observed eggs of *S. japonicum* in the liver he examined at autopsy. He was unaware of the adult worms, but correctly deduced that the eggs had, in some way, caused the cirrhosis. The connection between the clinical disease, Katayama fever, and the presence of *S. japonicum* infection was made by Kawanishi,[9] in 1904, when he found eggs of this blood fluke in the stools of patients suffering from the acute phase of the infection. The details of the life cycle were worked out by Fujinami and Nakamura[10] in 1909 and by Miyagawa[11] in 1912. *Onchomelania* sp. snails were identified as vectors by Miyairi and Suzuki[12] in 1914.

Ancient Egyptians believed that the advent of manhood was signaled by the appearance of blood in the urine, analogously to the advent of womanhood, signaled by menstruation. The hematuria, in fact, represented a late manifestation of *S. haematobium* infection. Autopsies of mummies conducted in modern times indicate that this infection was present at least as long ago as 1200 b.c. Clinical disease and its pathology were described in detail by Griesinger[13] in 1854. He noted the relationship of the infection to the involvement of the bladder and ureters. Leiper[5] in 1915 described the life cycle of *S. haematobium*, its intermediate host, and its morphology. He also investigated susceptibility of various indigenous

Schistosoma mansoni

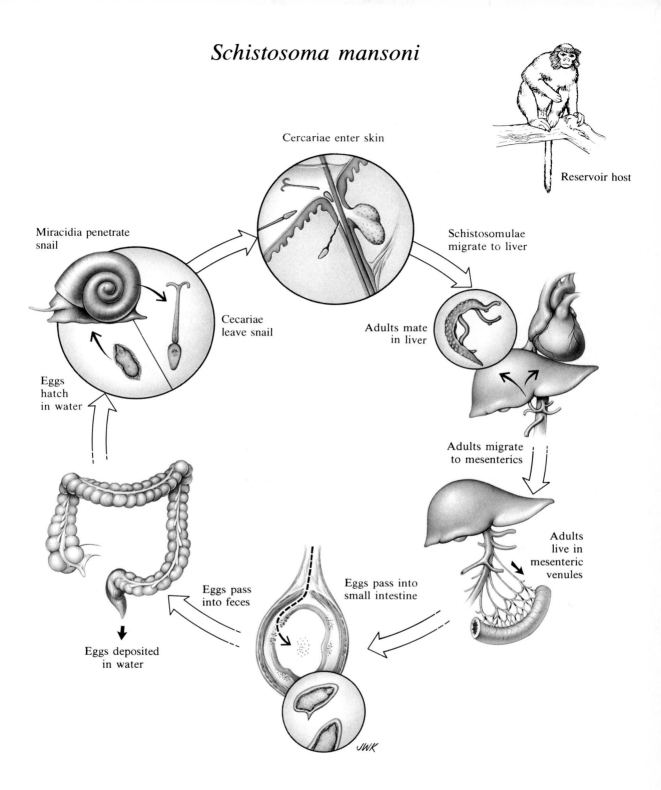

Cercariae enter skin

Reservoir host

Miracidia penetrate snail

Schistosomulae migrate to liver

Cecariae leave snail

Adults mate in liver

Eggs hatch in water

Adults migrate to mesenterics

Eggs pass into feces

Eggs pass into small intestine

Adults live in mesenteric venules

Eggs deposited in water

JWK

animals of northern Egypt to infection with *S. haematobium* and found that rats and mice were susceptible.

Life Cycle

Unlike other trematodes, schistosomes have separate sexes. The females are larger than the males, measuring 15 mm in length; the males measure 10 mm. The adult schistosome species are most easily distinguished by the morphology of the males. The outer tegumental surface of the male *S. mansoni* (Fig. 18.1A) is covered with papillae; the male *S. japonicum* is smooth; the male *S. haematobium* has widely spaced tubercles, which are shorter than the papillae of *S. mansoni*.

The schistosomes remain *in copula* (Fig. 18.1B) during their life span. The habitat of *S. mansoni* is the inferior mesenteric veins (Fig. 18.2). *S. japonicum* lives in the superior mesenteric veins, but some worms find their way to the choroid plexus, venules around the spinal column, and other ectopic locations. *S. haematobium* is

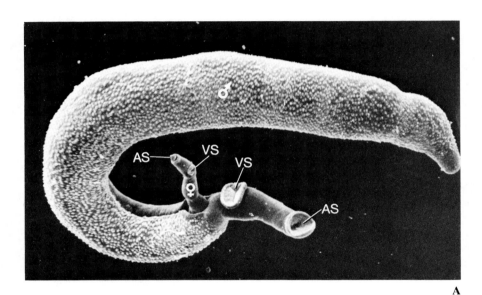

A

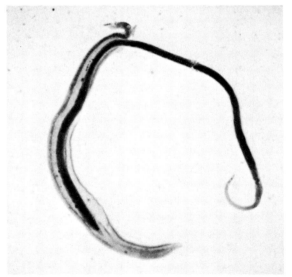

B

Figure 18.1. A. Scanning electron micrograph of adult (♂♀) *Schistosoma mansoni*. Note ventral suckers (*VS*) and anterior suckers (*AS*) on each adult worm. **B.** A pair of adult worms as they appear under the light microscope. **A,** ×42; **B,** ×7.5. (**A:** From Kessel RG, Shih CY: Scanning Electron Microscopy in Biology. New York, Springer-Verlag, 1976. Reproduced with permission.)

Schistosoma japonicum

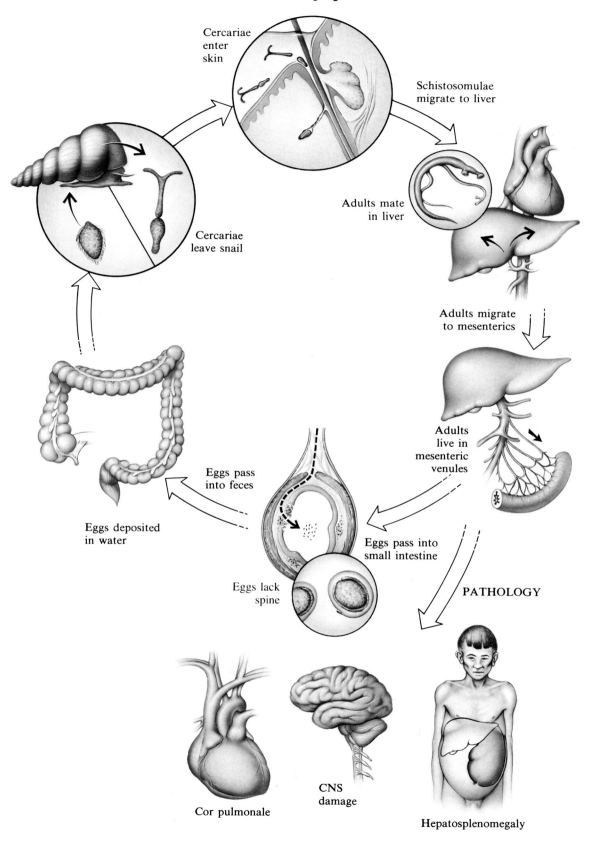

Cercariae enter skin

Schistosomulae migrate to liver

Cercariae leave snail

Adults mate in liver

Adults migrate to mesenterics

Adults live in mesenteric venules

Eggs pass into feces

Eggs pass into small intestine

Eggs deposited in water

Eggs lack spine

PATHOLOGY

Cor pulmonale

CNS damage

Hepatosplenomegaly

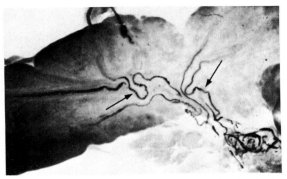

Figure 18.2. Adult *Schistosoma mansoni* in situ in the mesenteric venules of an infected mouse. Only the darkened, egg-laden uteri of the females are visible (*arrows*). ×5.2.

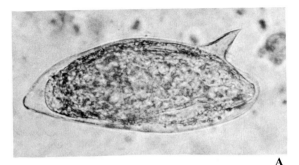

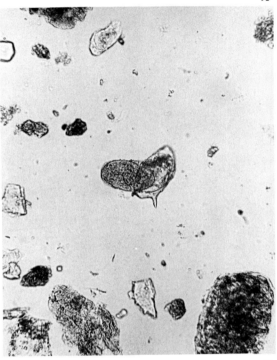

Figure 18.3. A. Embryonated egg of *Schistosoma mansoni*. Note the characteristic lateral spine. **B.** The egg hatches upon contact with fresh water. **A** ×300. **B.** ×50

found in the venus plexus surrounding the urinary bladder, but the route by which it arrives at this site is unknown.

The nutritional requirements of the three species are served by hemoglobin.[14] They split apart the hemoglobin molecule enzymatically,[15] digest the globin portion, and regurgitate the heme moiety into the bloodstream. They also absorb low-molecular weight nutrients such as free amino acids and sugars by active transport through the tegumental surface and store glycogen as a reserve source of energy. Their energy metabolism is facilitated largely through glycolysis. The worms live, on the average, 5–8 years; some live as long as 37 years.[16]

The worms mate continuously as the male surrounds the female with his gynocophoric canal. The females lay eggs throughout their lives. The eggs of *S. mansoni* (Fig. 18.3A and B) are oval and possess a lateral spine; those of *S. japonicum* (Fig. 18.4) are globular and lack a spine; those of *S. haematobium* (Fig. 18.5) are oval, with a terminal spine. The female *S. mansoni* produces approximately 300 eggs every day; *S. japonicum*, 1500–3000; the egg production of *S. haematobium* has not been determined. The eggs pass through the birth pore located above the posterior sucker. When the worm applies the sucker to the endothelial surface of the vein, the fully embryonated eggs penetrate the endothelium and enter the surrounding connective tissue. The secretions of the miracidium (i.e., the larval stage) (Fig. 18.6), within the egg, contain proteolytic enzymes that lyse tissue and facilitate this pro-

cess. The eggs tend to collect in the submucosa (Fig. 18.7) before breaking out into the lumen.

When the adult worms move to another location within the vein, they raise the posterior sucker from the endothelial surface, thus allowing eggs to be swept with the flow of blood to the liver. In *S. mansoni* infections 50% of all eggs produced reach the liver. Eggs that reach the lumen of the small intestine are included in the fecal mass. Eggs reaching the bladder are swept out with the urine. For the life cycle to continue, the feces or the urine must be deposited in fresh

Schistosoma haematobium

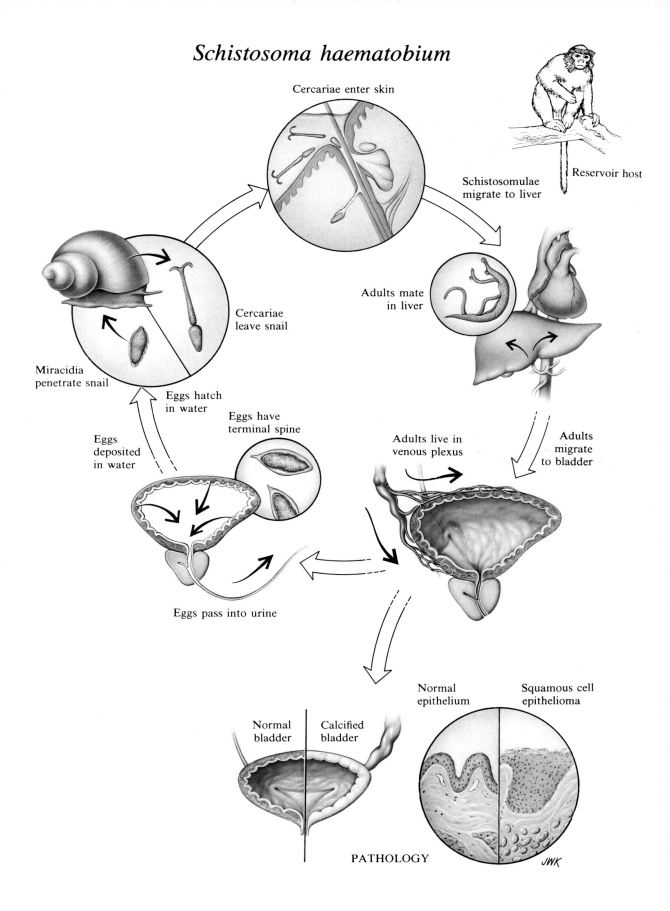

Cercariae enter skin

Reservoir host

Schistosomulae migrate to liver

Adults mate in liver

Cercariae leave snail

Miracidia penetrate snail

Eggs hatch in water

Eggs deposited in water

Eggs have terminal spine

Adults live in venous plexus

Adults migrate to bladder

Eggs pass into urine

Normal bladder

Calcified bladder

Normal epithelium

Squamous cell epithelioma

PATHOLOGY

JWK

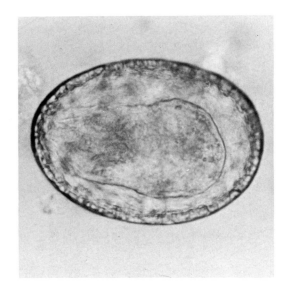

Figure 18.4. Embryonated egg of *Schistosoma japonicum*. × 700.

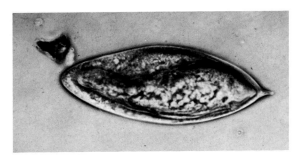

Figure 18.5. Embryonated egg of *Schistosoma haematobium*. Note the characteristic terminal spine. × 340.

water so that the miracidia can hatch and reach the appropriate snail (Figs. 18.8 and 18.9).

The miracidium seeks out its snail host by chemotaxis and enters the soft, fleshy parts of the snail, facilitating the passage by the use of proteolytic enzymes. Within the snail, the miracidium invades first lymph spaces and later the hepatopancreas. Infection proceeds by sequential stages of development beginning with the sporocyst, followed by the daughter sporocyst, and fi-

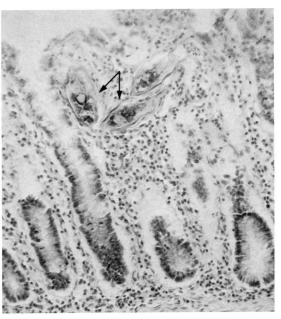

Figure 18.7. Eggs (*arrows*) of *Schistosoma mansoni* in the villi of the small intestine. × 118.

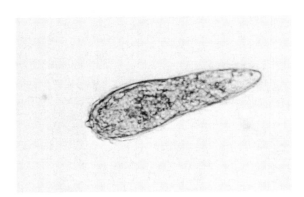

Figure 18.6. Ciliated miracidium of *Schistosoma mansoni*. × 300.

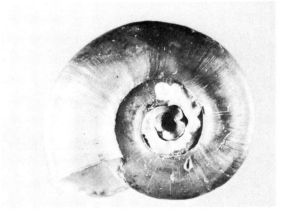

Figure 18.8. The most common intermediate host for *Schistosoma mansoni, Biomphalaria glabrata.* × 2.5.

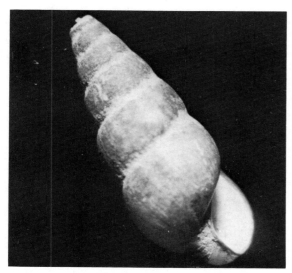

Figure 18.9. The intermediate host of *Schistosoma japonicum, Onchomelania* sp. ×8.

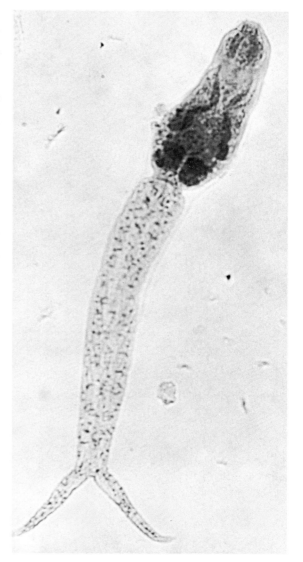

Figure 18.10. Cercaria of *Schistosoma mansoni.* ×250.

nally the cercaria (Fig. 18.10). During each stage of the development, there is an increase in the number of individuals and, ultimately, in *S. mansoni*, some 4000 cercariae are produced from a single miracidium. Each miracidium gives rise to either male or female cercariae. The cercariae exit from the snail, aided by the proteolytic enzymes. An infected snail can produce up to 40,000 cercariae before it becomes overwhelmed and dies.

The cercariae of *S. mansoni* are positively phototropic and negatively geotropic, and therefore accumulate at the surface of water. The tropisms of the other two species are not so well understood, but their cercariae also are found at the surface. The cercariae actively swim until they come in contact with the definitive host, whom they must reach within 8 h; otherwise they exhaust their reserve glycogen and die.

Infection is initiated when the cercariae penetrate human skin through a hair follicle; this step requires about one-half hour. They shed their tails on penetration and are rapidly transformed within the dermal layer of skin into the schistosomula stage. After approximately 2 days, the schistosomulae migrate through the bloodstream to the capillaries of the lung, then into the heart and the liver parenchyma, and mature to adult worms (Fig. 18.11).

The proportion of cercariae that eventually become adult schistosomes is small. For *S. mansoni* it has been estimated to be in the range of 20%.[17]

Other mammalian species, including baboons, rhesus monkeys, chimpanzees, mice, and rats, can be experimentally infected with the cercariae of *S. mansoni*. In the rat few viable eggs are produced.

Pathogenesis

Penetration of the skin by cercariae causes no major reaction, but repeated exposure leads to

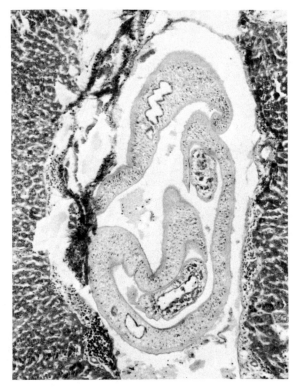

Figure 18.11. Adult *Schistosoma mansoni* in the liver. × 100.

actually loses immunogenicity of its surface components during long-term infections.

It is the egg of the schistosome that is primarily responsible for host reactions associated with the infection. The damage caused by the eggs is related to the host response to the secretions of the egg, or soluble egg antigens (SEA).[20] In the intestine, erosion of the submucosa and villous tissue by secreted proteolytic enzymes results in inflammation of the submucosa and sloughing of cells. Gastrointestinal hemorrhage can result from the damage to the submucosa.

Eggs swept back into the liver block the presinusoidal capillaries and, at the same time, the SEA elicit T-cell-dependent granulomas (Fig. 18.12) that accumulate around each egg.[21] These granulomas eventually kill the egg, become fibrosed, and obstruct the capillary. Fibrosis of the portal areas incorporating the blood vessels leads to pipe stem cirrhosis and, ultimately, to portal hypertension. Development of collateral circulation, which includes formation of esophageal varices, follows. Parenchymal liver cells are unaffected by the granulomas and liver function re-

sensitization and the development of a maculopapular rash.

Many schistosomes parasitic for animals can infect man, but fail to complete their life cycle. They also cause a hypersensitivity skin reaction, known as "clam digger's itch" or "swimmer's itch." There are no major reactions to the developing worms in the liver or to the adult worms in the mesenteries.

The development of protective immunity may be directly related to immunological reactions against the schistosomulae in the dermis, and probably involves both eosinophils and antibodies.[18] The schistosomula is the stage against which the protective immune responses of the host are primarily directed. One theory suggests that immunological reactions against the adult schistosome do not result in expulsion of the worms because the worms incorporate certain proteins of the host into the outer tegumental surface, thus camouflaging themselves.[19] This may not be the only mechanism of protection. Experimental evidence suggests that the worm

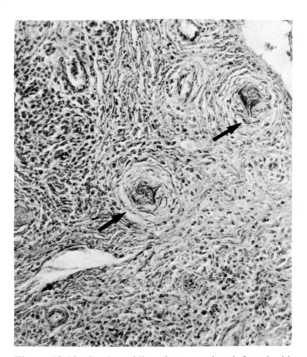

Figure 18.12. Section of liver from a patient infected with *Schistosoma mansoni*. The eggs (*arrows*) have become surrounded by granulomas that have become fibrosed. × 100.

mains normal. The eggs are also carried to the spleen, which becomes hyperplastic and contributes to the increased pressure in portal circulation.

Collateral circulation washes eggs into the capillary bed of the lungs, which leads to pulmonary fibrosis and consequent cor pulmonale.

Although hepatosplenic schistosomiasis is caused by the immunological reactions against the eggs, Spencer and Gibson[22] claim that dead adult worms that wash back into the liver disintegrate and cause additional damage.

Accumulation of eggs of *S. haematobium* around the bladder (Fig. 18.13) and ureters leads to formation of granulomas and ultimately fibrosis. In addition, calcification of old eggs that remain in the wall results in rigidity of the bladder wall and subsequent increase of pressure in the ureters and kidneys. The bladder epithelium develops pseudopolyps, which can transform into squamous cell carcinoma in untreated patients.

Clinical Disease

Clinical schistosomiasis occurs only in relatively heavily infected individuals. Thus, the disease is rare in an occasional traveler through the endemic

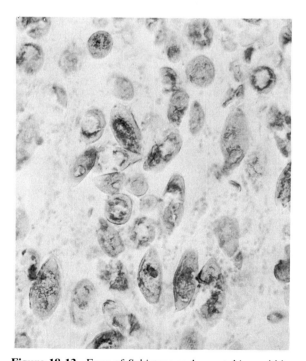

Figure 18.13. Eggs of *Schistosoma haematobium* within the wall of the bladder. ×110.

areas. Clinical manifestations are correlated with the life cycle. Within 24 h of penetration of the skin by the cercariae, the patient develops cercarial dermatitis and experiences itching, which may last for 2 or 3 days.

During the migratory phase in the sensitized individuals, systemic reactions develop, which include eosinophilia, approaching 30%; chills and fever, associated with sweating; diarrhea, and cough. During the acute phase the patient has fever, generalized lymphadenopathy, hepatomegaly, and splenomegaly. This stage, known as Katayama fever, in patients infected with *S. japonicum* begins suddenly 2–3 weeks after the initial infection and may last for 1 or 2 months. It may resemble typhoid fever. Although spontaneous recovery is the usual fate of such a patient, in cases of heavy infections with *S. japonicum,* Katayama fever can lead to death.

Neither the initial swimmer's itch nor the subsequent Katayama fever constitutes a major problem in schistosomiasis. The fundamental clinical disease is the chronic stage, directly related to the intensity of infection. It is caused by the granulomatous inflammation as host reaction to the deposited eggs. Hepatomegaly represents the clinical manifestation of portal fibrosis. Splenomegaly follows and, in advanced cases, the spleen may fill much of the left side of the abdomen. The patient may also develop symptoms of hypersplenism.

Portal obstructive disease due to schistosomiasis is no different from that of portal hypertension due to other causes in that it leads to hematemesis from ruptured esophageal varices.

As the result of portal hypertension and the consequent development of collateral circulation, schistosome eggs are washed into the lungs, where they induce granulomatous inflammation and lead to obstructive disease and eventually cor pulmonale. *S. haematobium* is much less likely to induce pulmonary schistosomiasis than the other two schistosomes, because only small numbers of eggs are washed into the lungs from the venus plexus through the inferior vena cava.

Rarely, all three schistosomes may induce focal inflammatory reactions within the central nervous system, caused by deposition of eggs in the spinal cord and in the brain.[23] *S. mansoni* and *S. haematobium* are more likely to do so in the spinal cord and *S. japonicum* in the brain. The inflammatory reaction in response to deposition of the eggs may cause focal transverse myelitis and encephalopathy.

S. haematobium, unlike the other two schistosomes, causes involvement of the urinary tract, characterized by an inflammation of the bladder, that can result years later in malignant squamous cell epithelioma. Obstruction of the ureter due to inflammatory changes and fibrosis is also seen and leads to hydronephrosis. Symptoms of dysuria are common. Eggs deposited in the walls of the bladder and the ureter die, become calcified, and thus appear as radiopaque patches on radiograms of the urinary tract. Cystoscopic examination reveals characteristic granules, described as sand. This obstructive disease of the urinary tract often leads to secondary bacterial infections. Infections with *S. mansoni*[24] and *S. japonicum*[25] have been associated with nephrotic syndrome, caused by the deposition of immune complexes on the glomerular membrane.

Diagnosis

The definitive diagnosis is made by identification, with the aid of a microscope, of schistosome eggs (Fig. 18.3–18.5) in the stool. If a casual examination is negative, concentration of the specimen is required, because the number of eggs in the stool is relatively small. It is important to determine viability of eggs to decide whether the patient continues to harbor live worms. If eggs cannot be found in the stool specimen, a rectal biopsy (Fig. 18.14) must be carried out. In this case it is mandatory to examine the biopsied epithelium, before it is fixed in formalin. This is accomplished by squashing the tissue between two microscope slides and examining it under the low-power lens of a microscope. It is helpful to refer to the specimen as a "rectal snip" rather than a biopsy to preclude its fixation and subsequent sectioning, which would make identificaiton of the eggs difficult and determination of their viability impossible.

In the case of *S. haematobium,* urine is examined for the presence of eggs. It can be concentrated by sedimentation. *S. haematobium* eggs may also be seen in stool and rectal snip specimens, but their numbers will be small.

Immunological tests are available, but they do not distinguish active—and extensive—disease from simple light infection of no consequence.

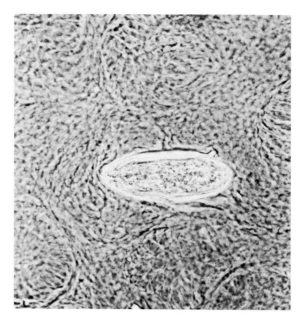

Figure 18.14. Rectal snip from a patient infected with *Schistosoma mansoni.* The snip is positive for eggs. The lateral spine is diagnostic for this species. × 250.

Indirect immunofluorescence, ELISA, and circumoval precipitin tests are available. The reactions are positive in nearly all infected individuals. The ELISA test is particularly useful in conducting epidemiological surveys.

The extent of the disease, particularly presence of portal hypertension and esophageal varices, must be assessed by the usual diagnostic modalities.

Radiological studies can lead to the suspicion of *S. haematobium,* particularly in old cases in which the adult worms have died and are therefore no longer producing eggs. The bladder shows a crescent of calcification, and the ureters may be distended and calcified as well.

Treatment

The decision to treat must be made only after a thorough assessment of the patient and usually on the advice of a consultant familiar with this disease. It is rarely necessary to treat immediately and therefore there usually is an opportunity to seek an appropriate consultation; if a consultant is not available nearby, the advice can be obtained by telephone or mail. Only in the case of focal encephalopathy or transverse myelitis must therapy be started quickly, because it may arrest, or even reverse, these very serious manifestations.

Treatment should be undertaken only in individuals who still harbor live worms. Praziquantel is effective against all four species of schistosomes infecting man. The drug is well tolerated, with few, minor side effects.[26] These include nausea, epigastric pain, dizziness, and general malaise. All of these symptoms disappear within 48 hours after treatment. Because the drug is effective in a single dose it has been used in control programs.[27] There is evidence that part of its effectiveness is due to synergism with the host's humoral immune response.[28] Oxamniquine is considered a second drug of choice for treatment of infections with *S. mansoni*.

Surgical treatment of *S. mansoni* infections, which involves an intravenous injection of tartar emetic, followed by extracorporeal filtration of the bloodstream, can reduce the number of worms, but is technically complicated and therefore cannot be recommended as standard therapy. Portacaval or splenorenal shunts should be avoided in untreated schistosomiasis, because they increase the probability of deposition of eggs in the lungs. If such a shunt is mandated by the intensity of portal hypertension, it should be preceded by chemotherapy of schistosomiasis.

Prevention and Control

Schistosoma spp. have complex biologies and therefore appear to present numerous weak points against which control programs can be directed. However, the fact that the number of these serious infections is increasing, rather than the reverse, suggests that effective eradication of either the snail vectors or the schistosomes themselves has not yet been achieved. Control of schistosomiasis at the community level has been directed at: (1) eradication of snail vectors with molluscicides[29] and biological agents[30]; (2) public health education; (3) sanitation,[31] or other engineering interventions, concerning freshwater supplies; and with the advent of praziquantel and oxamniquine, (4) chemotherapy.

Internationally funded research programs, aimed at vaccine development and serodiagnosis, offer promise of control or even prevention of this important worldwide health problem. However, it is clear from these studies that intervention strategies dependent on vaccination, however promising,[32,33] are years away from practical application.

Prevention of schistosomiasis on an individual level requires that the person never come in contact with infested freshwater, or that all individuals defecate and urinate in sanitary facilities. These suggestions are impossible to carry out in much of the world, because of many complex economic, cultural, and behavioral patterns. In addition, it is necessary for many people to be in contact with freshwater for agricultural or other food-gathering purposes. Temporary visitors to endemic areas, however, can heed the advice to avoid potential sources of infection. Control of *S. japonicum* is complicated by the fact that water buffalo and cattle serve as reservoir hosts in many regions of the Orient, particularly in China.

References

1. Fuller GK, Lemma A, Trinidad H: Schistosomiasis in Omo National Park of Southwest Ethiopia. Am J Trop Med Hyg 28:467–471, 1979
2. Manson P: Report of the case of bilharzia from the West Indies. Br Med J 2:1894–1895, 1902
3. Sambon LW: New or little known African entozoa. J Trop Med Hyg 10:117, 1907
4. Piraja da Silva MA: Contribucao para o estudo da schistosomiase na Bahia. Brazil-Medico 2:281–283, 1908
5. Leiper RT: Researches on Egyptian Bilharziosis. London, John Bale Sons and Danielsson, 1918
6. Katsurada F: The etiology of a parasitic disease. Iji Shimbun 669:1325–1332, 1904
7. Catto J: *Schistosoma cattoi*, a new blood fluke of man. Br Med J 1:11–13, 1905
8. Majima T: A strange case of liver cirrhosis caused by parasitic ova. Tokyo Ig Za 2:898–901, 1888
9. Kawanishi K: A report on a study of the "Katayama Disease" in Higo-No-Kuni. Tokyo Ig Za 18:31–48, 1904
10. Fujinami K, Nakamura H: Katayama disease in Hiroshima prefecture. Route of infection, development of the worm in the host and animals in Katayama disease in Hiroshima prefecture (Japanese blood sucking worm disease—schistosomiasis japonica). Kyoto Ig Za 6:224–252, 1909
11. Miyagawa Y: Über den Wanderungsweg des *Schistosomum japonicum* von der Haut bis zum Pfortadersystem und über die Körperkonstitution der jungsten Würmer zur Zeit der Hautinvasion. Zentralbl Bakteriol Parasitenkun Infektionskrankh 66:406–417, 1912

12. Miyairi K, Suzuki M: Der Zwischenwirt der *Schistosomum japonicum* Katsurada. Mitteilungen der Medizinischen Fakultät Kaiserlichen Universität Kyushu 1:187–197, 1914

13. Griesinger W: Klinische und anatomische Beobachtungen über die Krankheiten von Aegypten. Arch Physiol Heilk 13:528–575, 1854

14. Lawrence JD: The ingestion of red blood cells by *Schistosoma mansoni*. J Parsitol 59:60–63, 1973

15. Senft AW, Maddison SE: Hypersensitivity to parasite proteolytic enzymes in schistosomiasis. Am J Trop Med Hyg 24:83–89, 1975

16. Vermund SH, Bradley DJ, Ruiz-Triben E: Survival of *Schistosoma mansoni* in the human host: estimates from a community-based prospective study in Puerto Rico. Am J. Trop Med Hyg 32:1040–1048, 1983

17. Marcial-Rojas RA: Schistosomiasis mansoni. In Marcial-Rojas RA (ed): Pathology of Protozoal and Helminthic Diseases with Clinical Correlation. Baltimore, Williams & Wilkins, 1971, pp 373–413

18. von Lichtenberg F, Scher A, Gibbons N et al.: Eosinophil-enriched inflammatory response to schistosomula in the skin of mice immune to *Schistosoma mansoni*. Am J Pathol 84:479–500, 1976

19. Smithers SR, Terry RJ: The immunology of schistosomiasis. Adv Parasitol 7:41–93, 1969

20. Warren KS: The pathology of schistosome infections. Helminth Abstr Series A 42:591–633, 1973

21. Davis BH, Mahmoud AAF, Warren KS: Granulomatous hypersensitivity to *Schistosoma mansoni* eggs in thymectomized and bursectomized chickens. J Immunol 113:1064–1067, 1974

22. Spencer H, Gibson JB: Schistosomiasis. In Spencer H, Dyan AD, Gibson JB (eds): Tropical Pathology. New York, Heidelberg, Springer-Verlag, 1973, pp 561–595

23. Scrimgeour EM, Gajdusek CD: Involvement of the central nervous system in *Schistosoma mansoni* and *S. haematobium* infection. Brain 108:1023–1038, 1985

24. Andrade ZA, Rocha H. Schistosomal glomerulopathy. Kidney Internat. 16:23–29, 1979

25. Watt G, Long GW, Caluboquib C, et al.: Prevalence of renal involvement in *Schistosoma japonicum* infection. Trans Roy Soc Trop Med Hyg 82:339–342, 1987

26. Polderman AM, Gryseek B, Gerold JL et al.: Side effects of praziquantel in the treatment of *Schistosoma mansoni* in Maniema, Zaire. Trans Roy Soc Trop Med Hyg 98:752–754, 1984

27. Yogore MG Jr, Lewert RM, Blas BL.: Seroepidemiology of Schistosomiasis *japonica* by ELISA in the Philippines. Am J Trop Med Hyg 33:882–890, 1984

28. Brindly PJ, Sher A.: The chemotherapeutic effect of praziquantel against *Schistosoma mansoni* is dependent on host antibody response. J Immunol 139:215–220, 1987

29. Jordan P: Schistosomiasis—research to control. Am J Trop Med Hyg 26:877–885, 1977

30. Jobin WR, Brown RA, Velez SP, et al.: Biological control of *Biomphalaria glabrata* in major reservoirs of Puerto Rico. J Trop Med Hyg 26:1018–1024, 1977

31. Unrau GO: Individual household water supplies in rural St. Lucia as a control measure against *Schistosoma mansoni*. Bull WHO 52:1–8, 1975

32. Smithers SR: Parasitology. Improving prospects for a schistosomiasis vaccine (News). Nature 323:205–206, 1987

33. Capron A, Dessaint TP, Capron M, et al.: Immunity to schistosomes: Progress towards a vaccine. Science 238:1065–1072, 1987

19. *Clonorchis sinensis* (Loos 1907)

Clonorchis sinensis infections are endemic in Japan, Korea, Vietnam, and China. In addition to infecting man, clonorchis can also infect dogs and cats. *Opisthorchis felineus,* a closely related species of trematode, which infects various carnivores, including man, occurs throughout the Philippines, India, Japan, Vietnam, and eastern Europe, particularly Poland and Western U.S.S.R. *O. viverrini* is found in northern Thailand[1] and Laos. The biology, pathogenesis, and clinical disease caused by these three parasites are so similar that no separate description will be given for *O. felineus* and *O. viverrini*.

Historical Information

The adult *C. sinensis* was first described by McConnell[2], in 1875, but Loos is given credit for naming it. Many of the details of its life history were determined by Japanese parasitologists.

Clonorchis sinensis

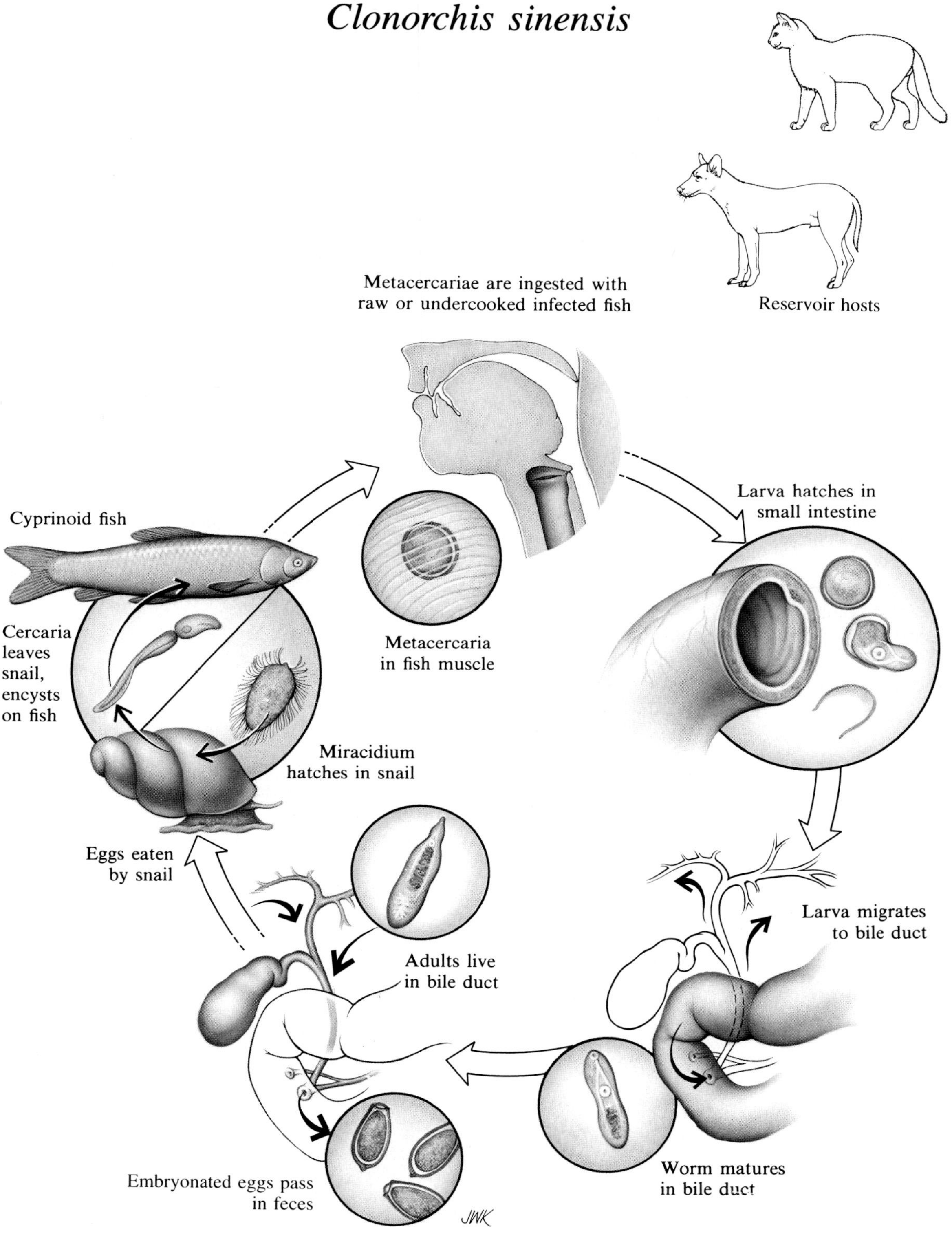

Metacercariae are ingested with
raw or undercooked infected fish

Reservoir hosts

Larva hatches in
small intestine

Cyprinoid fish

Metacercaria
in fish muscle

Cercaria
leaves
snail,
encysts
on fish

Miracidium
hatches in snail

Larva migrates
to bile duct

Eggs eaten
by snail

Adults live
in bile duct

Embryonated eggs pass
in feces

Worm matures
in bile duct

JWK

Ijima[3], in 1887, discovered that *C. sinensis* could infect animals other than man and thus established the concept of reservoir hosts for this parasite. Kobayashi, in 1914, found that freshwater fish was the intermediate vertebrate host, and 4 years later Muto[4] extended these findings by identifying certain genera of snails (e.g., Bulimus) as the first intermediate hosts. The genus of snails that are the first intermediate host varies with geographic locale.

Life Cycle

The adult fluke (Fig. 19.1) measures approximately 19 mm by 3.5 mm and lives within the bile ducts, where it feeds on epithelium.

Embryonated eggs (Fig. 19.2) pass from the common bile duct into the small intestine and are excreted with the feces. They must reach freshwater to continue the life cycle. Experimental infections of dogs, cats, rabbits, and guinea pigs showed that an adult worm produces between 1,000 and 4,000 eggs per day; there is no corresponding information for human infections.

The eggs are eaten by the snail intermediate host in which they hatch, stimulating release of the miracidium. The miracidium penetrates the hepatopancreas where it undergoes development through the sporocyst and redia stages. The cercariae emerge from the snail and encyst under the scales of freshwater fish of the family Cyprinidae and under the exoskeleton of various freshwater crustaceae. The encysted metacercariae (Fig. 19.3), ingested by man during consumption of raw or undercooked fish or crustaceae, excyst in the small intestine. The immature flukes crawl into the common bile duct and eventually attach to its epithelial surface. After growing to maturity, the adult flukes fertilize their own eggs, thus reinitiating the cycle.

Pathogenesis

Any damage to the infected host (Fig. 19.4) occurs as a result of inflammatory changes induced by the attachment and feeding behavior of the adult worms. These changes are clinically significant only in heavy infections. They include proliferation and desquamation of the biliary epithelium, formation of crypts, and metaplasia.[5]

Clonorchis infection has been claimed responsible, by association, for a variety of disease

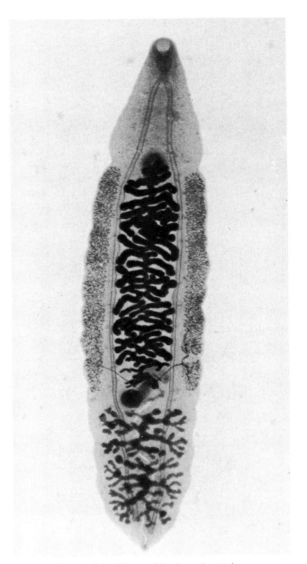

Figure 19.1. Adult *Clonorchis sinensis*. ×4.

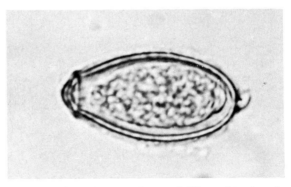

Figure 19.2. Embryonated egg of *Clonorchis sinensis*. ×1400.

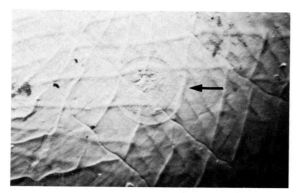

Figure 19.3. Metacercaria (*arrow*) of *Clonorchis sinensis* as seen under the scales of one of its intermediate hosts, a cyprinoid fish. × 110.

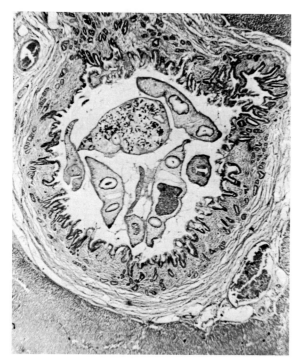

Figure 19.4. Sections of adult *Clonorchis sinensis* in the common bile duct. × 23.

states, among them cholangiocarcinoma and hepatocarcinoma. There is no evidence that the latter bears any relationship to the infection with this fluke.[6] On the other hand, cholangiocarcinoma may be related, although the evidence is based only on correlations, supported by animal experiments.[7] An etiological relationship between clonorchis infection and pancreatitis has been suggested,[8] but a group of patients who harbored these worms for more than 40 years remained free of any disease attributable to clonorchis.[9]

Clinical Disease

There is no unequivocal evidence that clonorchis infection is symptomatic. Light infections certainly do not cause any disease. Heavy, chronic infection can cause recurrent pyogenic cholangitis and pancreatitis.[5]

Treatment

Praziquantel is an excellent, widely used drug against *C. sinensis*.[10,11]

Diagnosis

Stool examination will reveal the characteristic eggs of Clonorchis (Fig 19.2).

Prevention and Control

Ingestion of infected raw, undercooked, pickled, salted, frozen, or dried freshwater fish and crustacea is the cause of clonorchiasis.

Aquaculture of the cyprinoid fishes in areas where human feces are used as fertilizers and the presence in the same environment of the animal reservoir hosts make any control measures difficult.

Molluscicides have not been fully effective, but their use, coupled with regular draining of fish ponds, has been moderately successful in the reduction of the prevalence of metacercariae on the fish. Ammonium sulfate added to feces kills *C. sinensis* eggs. It is therefore recommended for pretreatment of human excrement used as fertilizer.

In individual cases, prevention can be achieved by thorough cooking of freshwater fish.

References

1. Kurathong S, Lerdverasirikul P, Wongpaitoon V, et al.: *Opisthorchis viverrini* infection in rural and urban communities in Northeast Thailand. Trans Roy Soc Trop Med Hyg 81:411–414, 1987
2. McConnell JFP: Anatomy and pathological relations of a new species of liver fluke. Lancet 2:271–274, 1875
3. Ijima I: Notes on *Distoma endemicum*. Baelz J Coll Sci Imperial University, Japan 1:47–59, 1887

4. Muto S: On the primary intermediate host of *Clonorchis sinensis*. Chuo Igakkai Zasshi 25:49–52, 1918

5. Sun T: Pathology and immunology of *Clonorchis sinensis* infection in the liver. Am Clin Lab Sci 14:208–215, 1984

6. Gibson JB: Parasites, liver disease and liver cancer. In: Liver Cancer, I. A. R. C. Scientific Publ. No. 1. Lyon, WHO and International Agency for Research on Cancer, 1971

7. Hou PC: Hepatic clonorchiasis and carcinoma of the bile duct in a dog. J Pathol Bacteriol 89:365, 1965

8. McFadzean AJS, Yeung RTT: Acute pancreatitis due to *Clonorchis sinensis*. Trans Roy Soc Trop Med Hyg 60:466, 1966

9. Strauss WG: Clinical manifestations of clonorchiasis. A controlled study of 105 cases. Am J Trop Med Hyg 11:625–630, 1962

10. Hsu CCS, Kron MA: Clonorchiasis and praziquantel. Arch Int. Med 145:1002–1003, 1985

11. Campbell WC, Garcia EG: Trematode infections of man in: Chemotherapy of Parasitic diseases. (Campbell WC, Rew RS, eds). Plenum Press, New York and London, 1986, pp 385–400

20. *Fasciola hepatica* (Linnaeus 1758)

Fasciola hepatica, the sheep liver fluke, is found throughout Latin America, the southeastern United States, South America, Africa, Europe, and China. The sheep serves as the common definitive host for *F. hepatica*, but other mammals, including man, can also be infected. Its monoecious life style insures that each infection results in the production of fertilized eggs.

F. gigantica, a closely related species inhabiting the lumen of the small intestine, is found throughout Asia and Africa in cattle, and rarely in man.

Historical Information

Fasciola was well known to shepherds in France as early as 1379. Writings of de Brie indicate not only an awareness of the infection, but also that its source was consumption of contaminated watercress.[1]

Much later, in 1684, Redi[2] accurately described an adult *F. hepatica*, which he found in a rabbit. Linnaeus gave this fluke its current name in 1758, and Leuckart[3] and Thomas[4] in 1881 provided partial descriptions of the life cycle. It was Lutz[5] who showed that the adult of *F. hepatica* was acquired by swallowing the infective stage, a fact that could probably have been deduced from the early description by de Brie.

Life Cycle

The adult worm (Fig. 20.1) measures approximately 35 mm by 15 mm. It lives in the parenchyma of the liver and feeds on the hepatocytes and blood. The worm burrows through the liver and creates tunnels behind itself, into which it deposits its excretions and the fertilized eggs (Fig. 20.2).

The eggs leave the liver through the common duct, enter the small intestine, and become included in the fecal mass. The embryonated eggs must be deposited in freshwater for the cycle to continue. After an incubation period of 9–15 days, the miracidium (Fig. 20.3) emerges from the operculated egg, swims around until it finds its snail host, penetrates its body wall, and enters the hepatopancreas. The most common species of snail host for *F. hepatica* is *Lymnea truncatula*, but many other species of Lymnea can also serve this purpose.

Following development first into the sporocysts and then into rediae, the cercariae (Fig. 20.4) emerge from the snail and attach themselves to the surfaces of littoral vegetation, where they become encysted. Within the cyst they transform into the infective stage, the metacercariae (Fig. 20.5).

The ingested metacercariae excyst in the small intestine, penetrate the intestinal wall, and migrate in the peritoneal cavity to the surface of the liver. There they penetrate the liver and begin a process of maturation into reproductive adults, which takes up to 5 months.

Pathogenesis

The adult fasciola consumes large quantities of liver tissue, which creates tunnels (Fig. 20.6) and abscesses filled with debris of necrotic tissue,

Fasciola hepatica

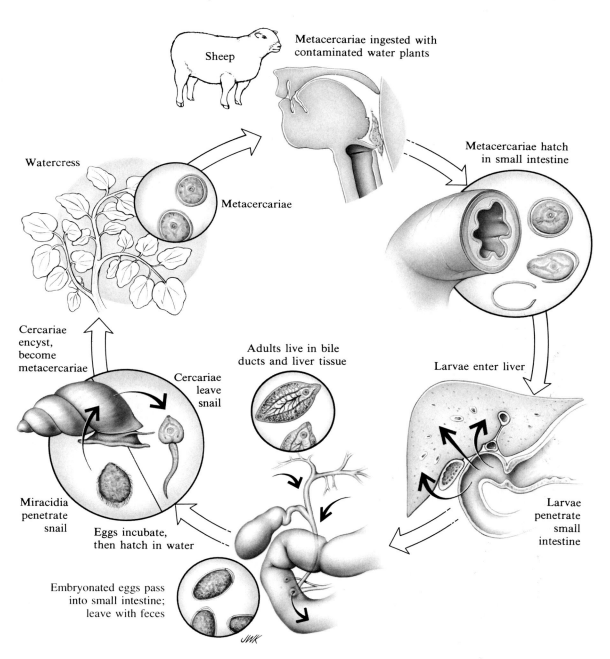
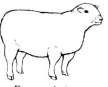

Reservoir host

Sheep

Metacercariae ingested with contaminated water plants

Metacercariae hatch in small intestine

Watercress

Metacercariae

Larvae enter liver

Cercariae encyst, become metacercariae

Cercariae leave snail

Adults live in bile ducts and liver tissue

Larvae penetrate small intestine

Miracidia penetrate snail

Eggs incubate, then hatch in water

Embryonated eggs pass into small intestine; leave with feces

worm excreta, and fertilized eggs. In addition to
the liver, other sites in the body, such as the
brain and the lung, can also become infected.[6] A
variant of fascioliasis, limited to the Middle East,
is halzoun, or pharyngitis and laryngeal edema,
caused by an adult fasciola adhering to the posterior pharyngeal wall. The condition is caused
by consumption of raw, infected sheep liver.[7]

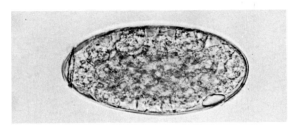

Figure 20.2. Fertilized egg of *Fasciola hepatica*. ×315.

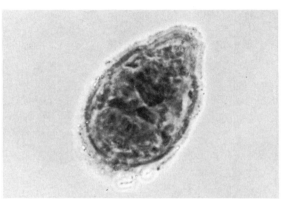

Figure 20.3. Miracidium of *Fasciola hepatica*. Note cilia
that cover the outer surface. ×880.

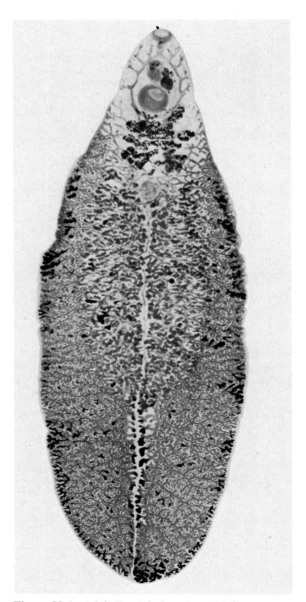

Figure 20.1. Adult *Fasciola hepatica*. ×4.8.

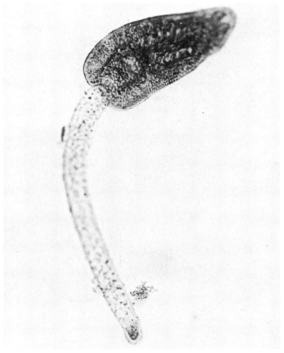

Figure 20.4. Cercaria of *Fasciola hepatica*. ×195.

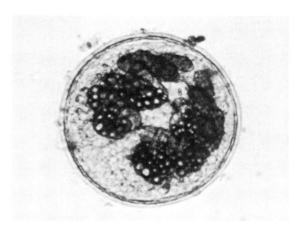

Figure 20.5. Metacercaria of *Fasciola hepatica*. × 165.

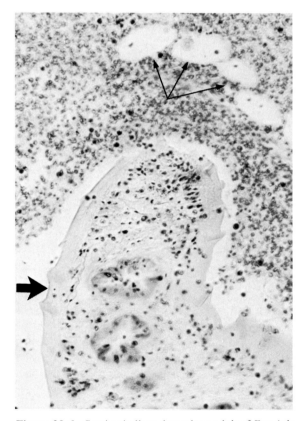

Figure 20.6. Section in liver through an adult of *Fasciola hepatica*. The worm has lysed a tunnel through the liver tissue. Eggs originally present (*arrow*) in this section were inadvertently removed in the process of fixation. × 100.

Clinical Disease

Approximately 1 month after ingestion of an infested vegetable, man may develop symptoms related to the migration of the worms. Although many infected people are asymptomatic during this phase of the infection, others experience fever, pain in the right upper quandrant of the abdomen, and general malaise of varying degree, including myalgia and urticaria. In those heavily infected, the liver is enlarged and tender. These symptoms subside within a month or so. About 3 months later, the clinical disease, now related to the presence of mature worms in the bile ducts, is proportional to the number of worms. There may be symptoms referable to obstruction of bile ducts, but these are quite rare. Fasciola in sites other than liver may cause no symptoms, or it may be present as a small tumor mass; if the parasite invades the brain, it can induce focal neurological abnormalities. Halzoun causes intense pain in the back of the throat. Extensive edema may lead to laryngeal obstruction.

Diagnosis

Microscopic identification of eggs in the stool provides the most accurate diagnosis. However, worms present in ectopic locations may not pass eggs into the feces and the diagnosis may be missed. CT scan and other methods of imaging are helpful in the differential diagnosis of fascioliasis.

If no eggs have been found in the stool, one can resort to immunodiagnosis. Counterimmunoelectrophoresis and ELISA tests are both rapid and tend to be positive during the actue phase of the infection, i.e. between the fifth and the 20th weeks.[8] There are nevertheless crossreactions with antibodies to group specific antigens of trematodes, which can confuse the diagnosis.

Treatment

Bithionol is the only drug effective against fascioliasis[9]. Praziquantel—excellent in treatment of infections with other flukes—is ineffective against fasciola.[10]

Prevention and Control

Fasciola can be controlled by draining of ponds, protection of water supplies from sheep livestock, and regular surveys of herds and herders for presence of the parasites followed by appropriate treatment. However, use of molluscicides and drug treatment of livestock is the most effective measure against this parasite. Education of farm personnel regarding the mode of acquisition of the infection, in association with the other methods, is essential.

References

1. de Brie J: Le bon berger ou le vray regime et gouvenement de bergers et bergeres: Compose par le rustique Jehan de Brie le bon berger (1379). Paris, Isidor Liseux, 1879
2. Redi F: Osservazioni di Franceso Redi: Intorno agli animali viventi che si trovano negli animali viventi. Florence, Piero Matini, 1684
3. Leuckart FR: Zur Entwicklungsgeschichte des Leberegels. Zool Anzeiger 4:641–646, 1881
4. Thomas APW: Report of experiments on the development of the liver fluke, *Fasciola hepatica*. J R Agric Soc Engl 17:1–28, 1881
5. Lutz A: Zur Lebensgeschichte des *Distoma hepaticum*. Zentralbl Bakteriol Parasitenkunde 11:783–796, 1892
6. Catchpole BN, Snow D: Human ectopic fascioliasis. Lancet 2:711–712, 1952
7. Schacher JF, Saab S, Germanos R, et al.: Experimental lymphaedema in dogs infected with *Brugia* spp. Trans Roy Soc Trop Med Hyg 63:854–858, 1969
8. Hillyer GV: Fascioliasis, Paragonomiasis, Clonorchiasis, and Opisthorchiasis. In: Immunodiagnosis of Parasitic Diseases (Walls KW, Schantz PM, eds). Academic Press, Orlando and New York, 1987, pp 39–69
9. Campbell WC, Garcia EG: Tremotode infections of man in: Chemotherapy of Parasitic diseases. (Campbell WC, Rew RS, eds). Plenum Press, New York and London, 1986, pp 385–400
10. Farid A, Trabolsi B, Boctor F, and Hafez, A: Unsucessful use of praziquantel to treat acute Fascioliasis in children J Inf Dis 154:920–922, 1986

21. *Paragonimus westermani* (Kerbert 1878)

The human lung fluke, *Paragonimus westermani*, is widely distributed throughout the Orient and the Indian subcontinent. It is found in Japan, China, Micronesia, New Guinea, Korea, Vietnam, Thailand, Cambodia, India, and the Philippines. In addition, a related species of paragonimus parasitic for man is found in the Cameroons, Nigeria, and Zaire. *P. westermani* can also infect other wild and domestic mammals, such as foxes, civets, tigers, leopards, panthers, mongooses, wolves, pigs, dogs, and cats.

Historical Information

Kerbert,[1] in 1878, provided the morphological description of the adult worm, which he recovered at an autopsy of a Bengal tiger. However, according to Leuckart, Nakahama had previously described an identical trematode, which he had found at an autopsy of a man.

The life cycle of *P. westermani* was largely worked out by Japanese parasitologists. Nakagawa,[2] in 1916, implicated the crab as the intermediate host in the transmission of *P. westermani*, and Yokogawa,[3] in 1915, determined the correct route of migration of the immature adult fluke in the mammalian host. Most of the early descriptions of the clinical disease were provided in 1880 by von Baelz[4] and Manson,[5] who also identified eggs of *P. westermani* in the sputum of patients with hemoptysis.

Life Cycle

The adult *P. westermani* (Fig. 21.1) measures 10–12 mm in length and 5–7 mm in width. It lives within a fibrotic capsule of tissue at the periphery of the lung (Fig. 21.2). Usually, two adult worms are found within the same capsule. The worms pass fertilized eggs (Fig. 21.3) into the surrounding tissue. Eventually, these eggs reach the bronchioles and are included in the sputum, which also contains blood and debris from the necrotic lesions created by the adults. The number of eggs produced by each worm is unknown. Because the patients swallow some of

Paragonimus westermani

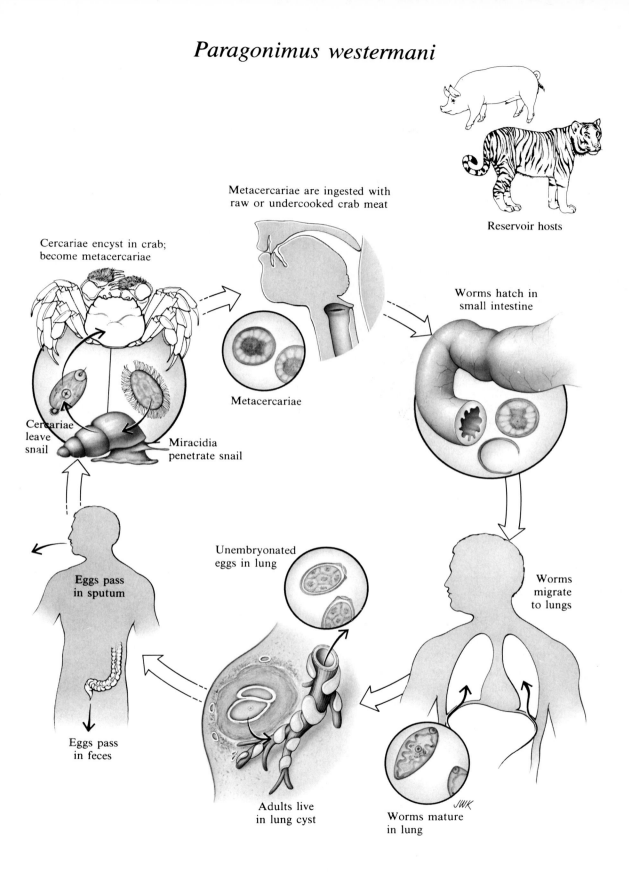

Reservoir hosts

Metacercariae are ingested with
raw or undercooked crab meat

Cercariae encyst in crab;
become metacercariae

Metacercariae

Worms hatch in
small intestine

Cercariae
leave
snail

Miracidia
penetrate snail

Unembryonated
eggs in lung

Worms
migrate
to lungs

Eggs pass
in sputum

Eggs pass
in feces

Adults live
in lung cyst

Worms mature
in lung

JWK

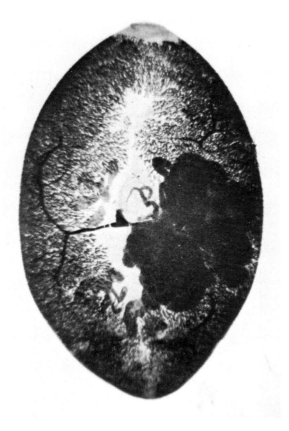

Figure 21.1. Adult *Paragonimus westermani.* ×7.8.

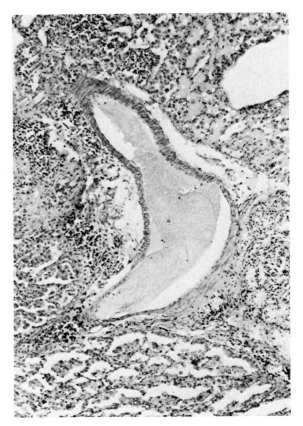

Figure 21.2. Section of an adult *Paragonimus westermani* in lung. ×100.

the sputum, the eggs become incorporated into the feces. The eggs must reach freshwater to embryonate. They hatch within 3 weeks, yielding miracidia, which penetrate appropriate snail hosts, e.g., *Melania sp., Semisulcospira* sp. and *Thiara* sp. (Fig. 21.4). They develop into cercariae through the sporocyst and redia stages, culminating in the production of cercariae within several weeks after initial infection. The cercariae exit from the snail and encyst upon and within the crustacean intermediate host, the freshwater crab. All organs of the crab can harbor the encysted metacercariae (Fig. 21.5). The crab, eaten raw or undercooked, then passes the infection to the definitive mammalian host. The metacercariae excyst in the small intestine, and the immature adult flukes penetrate the abdominal cavity, where they undergo further development. After several days, the worms actively penetrate the diaphragm and the lung, forming burrows in the lung tissue.

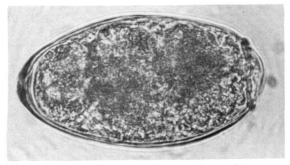

Figure 21.3. Fertilized, unembryonated egg of *Paragonimus westermani.* ×580.

Adult worms have also been reported at aberrant sites in the body including the brain, liver, intestines, muscles, skin, and testes. Egg production begins about 30 days after ingestion of the metacercariae.

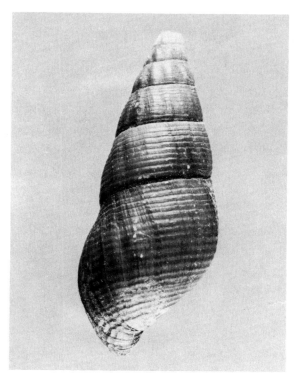

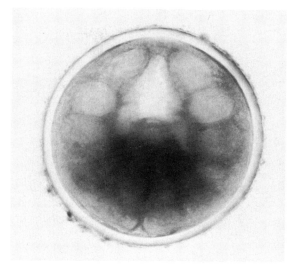

Figure 21.5. Metacercaria of *Paragonimus westermani*. This stage encysts on or inside various large crustaceans. ×170.

Figure 21.4. A snail intermediate host of *Paragonimus westermani*, *Melania* sp. ×3.1.

Pathogenesis

Little damage is done by the migration of immature adult worms, either on their way from the small intestine to the abdominal cavity or during their final journey to the lung tissue. Worms migrating to ectopic sites, such as the brain, do cause damage. In the lung, fibrotic lesions elicited by metabolic products of the worms and their eggs develop around each adult or pair of adults (Fig. 21.2). Communication between the capsules and the bronchioles leads to secondary bacterial infections. The inflammatory response is characterized by a variety of cells, but eosinophils usually predominate. Therefore, Charcot-Leyden crystals (see Fig. 25.8A) can frequently be found in the sputum of patients with paragonimiasis. In old infections (i.e., older than 1 year), the adult worms within the capsules may die and the lesions calcify.

Clinical Disease

The disease is insidious, beginning with nonspecific cough that becomes chronic and is produc-

tive of blood-tinged sputum, known as "endemic hemoptysis." The patient experiences pleural pain and dyspnea. These primary manifestations can be complicated by recurrent bacterial pneumonitis and lung abscess. Depending on the severity of the infection and the frequency of bacterial superinfections, there may be pneumothorax and pleural effusion, with consequent pleural adhesions. Chronically infected patients often have clubbing of fingers and toes.

Lesions in the brain can lead to seizures.

Diagnosis

Clinical diagnosis depends on suspicion of paragonimiasis in any patient from the endemic area who has the characteristic pulmonary disease. Pulmonary paragonimiasis must be distinguished from chronic bronchiectasis, lung abscess due to other causes, and tuberculosis. Cerebral paragonimiasis must be distinguished from the more likely brain tumors and lesions caused by other helminths, i.e., larval tapeworms and fasciola.

Diagnosis can be best confirmed by microscopical observation of the eggs (Fig. 21.3) in the sputum. In heavily infected patients the eggs that were swallowed can also be seen in the stools.

The complement fixation test can be useful in

evaluating severity of disease because elevated titers correlate well with heavy worm burden.[6]

Treatment

The drug of choice against *Paragonimus westermani* is praziquantel.[7]

Prevention and Control

Because of numerous reservoir hosts, control of *P. westermani* is nearly impossible.

The metacercariae can be killed by boiling the crabs for several minutes until the meat has congealed and turned opaque.

References

1. Kerbert C: Zur Trematoden-kenntnis. Zool Anzeiger 1:271–273, 1878

2. Nakagawa K: The mode of infection in pulmonary distomiasis. Certain freshwater crabs as intermediate hosts of *Paragonimus westermanii*. J Infect Dis 18:131–142, 1916

3. Yokogawa S: On the route of migration of *Paragonimus westermani* in the definitive host. Taiwan Igakkai Zasshi, 152:685–700, 1915

4. von Baelz EOE: Über Parasitare Haemoptoe (gregarinosis pulmonum). Zentralbl Med Wissensch 18:721–722, 1880

5. Manson P: *Distoma ringeri:* Medical Report for the half year ended 30 September 1880. Published by the order of the Inspector General Shanghai; Imperial Maritime Customs (China). Special Series No. 2. 20th Issue, pp 10–12, 1880

6. Johnson RJ, Johnson JR: Paragonimiasis in Indochinese refugees. Roentgenographic findings in clinical correlations. Am Rev Resp Dis 128:534–538, 1983

7. Johnson RJ, Jong EC: Paragonimiasis: diagnosis and the use of praziquantel in treatment. Rev Infect Dis 7:200–206, 1985

22. Trematodes of Minor Medical Importance

Fasciolopsis buski (Lankaster 1857)

The adult worm lives attached to the columnar epithelium of the small intestine. *Fasciolopsis buski* is a pathogen restricted to the Orient and the Indian subcontinent. It is found in China, India, Vietnam, and Thailand. Reservoir hosts include dogs and rabbits.

Life Cycle

The adult (Fig. 22.1) resembles *F. hepatica* (see Chapter 20). It is somewhat larger, measuring 20–30 mm by 10 mm. Its eggs are laid unembryonated and pass out with the fecal mass. If they reach warm (i.e., 25°–30°C) freshwater, the eggs (Fig. 22.2) undergo embryogenesis and hatch within 5–8 weeks. The miracidium that emerges (Fig. 22.3) penetrates snails (e.g., Segmentina and Heppentis) and develops sequentially into sporocysts, rediae, and cercariae (Fig. 22.4).

After leaving the snail, the cercariae come to rest on littoral vegetation such as water chestnuts and bamboos. The metacercariae are found are on the husks of the seeds of these plants. Once eaten, the metacercariae excyst in the small intestine and attach themselves to the lumenal surface. They mature to egg-laying adults within 2–4 months.

Pathogenesis and Clinical Disease

The worm feeds on columnar epithelial cells and thus injures the tissue. In massive infections with thousands of worms, obstruction of the ampula of Vater, common bile duct, and small intestine can occur. The patients may experience abdominal pain simulating that due to peptic ulcer. Hypoproteinemia and edema have been described in children with this infection, but multiple causes of these have not been ruled out. Eosinophilia is a common feature. Fatalities attributed to this infection have never been confirmed.

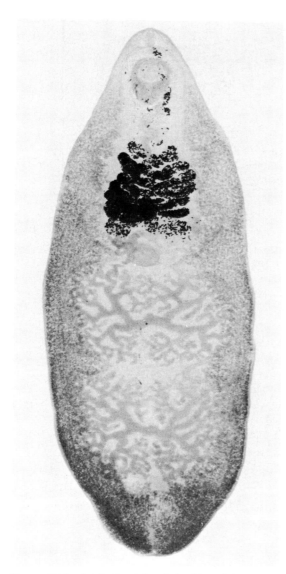

Figure 22.1. Adult *Fasciolopsis buski*. ×4.4.

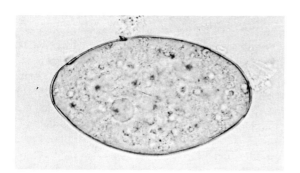

Figure 22.2. Fertilized, nonembryonated egg of *Fasciolopsis buski*. ×378.

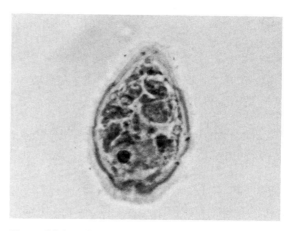

Figure 22.3. Miracidium of *Fasciolopsis buski*. Note cilia that completely cover the outside of the organism. ×464.

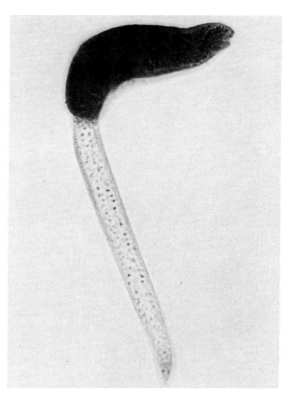

Figure 22.4. Side view of the cercaria of *Fasciolopsis buski*. ×210.

Diagnosis

Diagnosis depends on microscopic examination of the stool and identification of the characteristic eggs (Fig. 22.2).

Treatment

Treatment consists of administration of praziquantel.

Prevention and Control

Prevention of contamination of water supplies with fecal matter is the primary method of control. Thus, dumping of raw sewage or defecation into water used for cultivating water plants should

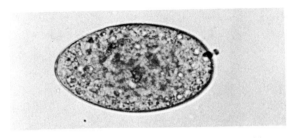

Figure 22.5. Egg of *Echinostoma ilocanum*. This egg closely resembles that of *F. buski* (see Fig. 22.2). ×540. (Courtesy of Dr. L. Ash)

be proscribed. Reservoir hosts apparently play only a minor role in the maintenance of this parasite in the environment.

Echinostoma ilocanum (Garrison 1908)

Echinostoma ilocanum is found mainly in the Philippines and Indonesia. Its life cycle is similar to that of fasciolopsis, except that the metacercariae encyst in various species of freshwater molluscs.

Adult worms live in the small intestine and the symptoms they cause are dependent on the number of these flukes present. Diarrhea seems to be the only adverse effect of infection, although the full pathogenic extent of echinostomiasis has not been sufficiently investigated.

Diagnosis is made by identification of the eggs (Fig. 22.5) in the stool. The eggs are often confused with those of *F. buski* (Fig. 22.2).

Treatment with praziquantel is effective.

Heterophyes heterophyes (Siebold 1852) and *Metagonimus yokogawai* (Katsurada 1912)

Life Cycles

These two small flukes live in the small intestine of man. They cause little damage. *Heterophyes heterophyes* is found throughout the Orient, the Middle East, and Africa. *Metagonimus yokogawai* is also common in the Orient, but foci of infections have been reported in Spain and the U.S.S.R.

Their life cycles are similar. The adult worms (Figs. 22.6 and 22.7) are attached by their two suckers to the columnar epithelium of the small intestine. The embryonated eggs pass out with the fecal mass into fresh or brackish water. *H. heterophyes* primarily infects snails of the genus Cerithidia; *M. yokogawai* infects those of the genera Semisulcospira and Thiara.

The embryonated eggs (Figs. 22.8 and 22.9) are ingested by their respective snail hosts and hatch to release miracidia. The miracidia begin sequential development in the snail into sporocysts, rediae, and cercariae. The cercariae break out of the snail and, like those of *Clonorchis sinensis*, encyst under the scales of various fish. The species of fish intermediate hosts for both of these parasitess varies with the geographic locale. In the Orient, the intermediate hosts are the cyprinoid and salmonid fish; in the Middle East, the mullet and tilapia.

After raw or undercooked infected fish is ingested by the host, the metacercariae excyst in the small intestine and develop into adult worms,

which begin laying eggs. The length of time between ingestion of the infected fish and oviposition is 7–12 days.

Pathogenesis and Clinical Disease

Only heavily infected individuals are symptomatic, developing nonspecific diarrhea, often associated with cramping abdominal pain. Young children tend to have more severe symptoms,
because they are more likely to experience dehydration and electrolyte imbalance. Occasionally,
eggs are swept into the circulation and reach vital

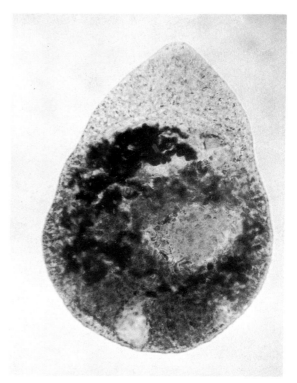

Figure 22.7. Adult *Metagonimus yokogawai.* × 110.

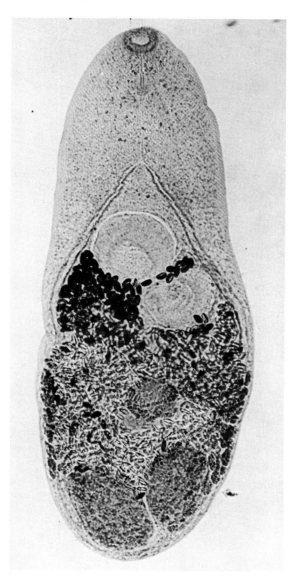

Figure 22.6. Adult *Heterophyes heterophyes.* × 100.

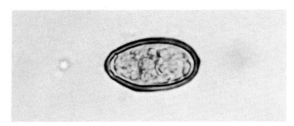

Figure 22.8. Egg of *Heterophyes heterophyes.* × 830.
(Courtesy of Dr. L. Ash)

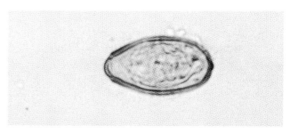

Figure 22.9. Egg of *Metagonimus yokogawai.* × 1070.
(Courtesy of Dr. L. Ash)

organs, such as the heart or the brain, where they cause focal granulomas, with variable clinical consequences.

Diagnosis

The eggs of *H. heterophyes* (Fig. 22.8) and *M. yokogawai* (Fig. 22.9) resemble those of *C. si-* *nensis* (Fig. 19.2). They must be carefully differentiated by the absence of a terminal knob and a collar at the operculum.

Treatment

The drug of choice is praziquantel.

IV
The Protozoa

Introduction

Protozoans are an extremely diverse group of unicellular animals. As free-living organisms they are found in virtually every ecological niche, such as bottoms of the deepest marine trenches, salt lakes, edges of ice flows, and even certain thermal springs. As parasites, they infect all species of vertebrates and many invertebrates, in which they have adapted to life in nearly all available sites within the body of the host.

There are about 66,000 documented species, of which about half are represented in fossils. Of the living species, about 10,000 are parasitic. Unlike most of the helminths, these organisms replicate within the host to produce hundreds of thousands of their kind within a few days of the infection.

Parasitic protozoans have a major influence on human existence. For example, the trypanosomes that infect cattle in Africa interfere with animal husbandry throughout most of the central savanna regions and thus limit the economic growth of these vast areas. Malaria is responsible for more human deaths in the world than any other cause.

Anatomy and Physiology

All protozoa are enveloped by a unit membrane, across which nutrients can be actively transported, phagocytized, or moved by pinocytosis. Many of these organisms also possess various surface coats consisting of materials derived from the host or secreted by the parasite. The protozoa are eukaryotic; a few are multinucleate. Their cytoplasm contains a wide variety of subcellular organelles, such as the Golgi apparatus, lysosomes, mitochondria, rough and smooth endoplasmic reticulum, and secretory granules of specialized function (e.g., the hydrogenosome of *Trichomonas vaginalis*). All of these cytoplasmic inclusions enable the organism to respire, digest foods, generate energy, reproduce, and grow. The protozoa that lack mitochondria are usually anaerobic.

Protozoans digest particulate material by lysozymal enzymes within the phagolysosome. *Entamoeba histolytica*, however, appears to secrete digestive enzymes directly into the phagosome without the participation of the lysosomes. Protozoans excrete wastes either by diffusion or by reversal of phagocytosis, exocytosis.

These organisms are motile and can be grouped according to their mechanisms of locomotion, such as cilia, flagella, and pseudopods.

Protozoans use two mechanisms of reproduction, the asexual and the sexual. Asexual reproduction usually involves binary fission, but in some organisms is complex and includes multiple karyokinesis followed by cytokinesis. Sexual reproduction always takes place within the definitive host, and results in the formation of a zygote.

23. *Trichomonas vaginalis* (Donne 1836)

Trichomonas vaginalis is a sexually transmitted flagellate. Members of both sexes are equally susceptible to this infection, but women tend to remain infected for longer periods of time (years) unless they are treated. Trichomoniasis in men has not been well studied, but subclinical infections are thought to be self-limited.[1]

Historical Information

Donne[2], in 1837, presented the first formal description of *T. vaginalis* infection and cited Dujardin's unpublished morphological description of this organism. Dujardin considered it as a composite combining the characteristics of both monas and tricodes groups, hence the original name *Tricomonas vaginale,* which was later changed by Ehrenberg[3] to the current one. Although presence of the organism is usually associated with changes in the vaginal mucosa, proof that *T. vaginalis* is indeed a pathogen came much later, in 1940, when healthy volunteers were inoculated with *T. vaginalis* and developed all the signs and symptoms of the disease previously noted in patients who harbored this organism.[4] This study also provided an accurate description of the pathological findings in this disease.

Life Cycle

The amorphous trophozoite of *T. vaginalis* (Figs. 23.1 and 23.2) measures 10–25 μm by 7–8 μm. It has no cyst stage, a feature common to all members of the genus Trichomonas. *T. vaginalis* possesses four flagella, an undulating membrane, and a rigid axostyle. A prominent nucleus occupies the anterior third of the cytoplasm. *T. vaginalis* is anaerobic; therefore its cytoplasm contains no mitochondria. Instead, specialized granules, the hydrogenosomes,[5] are distributed throughout the region of cytoplasm adjacent to the axostyle (Fig. 23.3). They are responsible for the secretion of molecular hydrogen. In accord with its anaerobic state, trichomonas derives its carbon from reduction of glycogen and glucose to succinate, acetate, malate, and hydrogen. In addition, it produces some CO_2, but not through the Krebs cycle pathway.[6]

The trophozoite lives in a close association with, and at times even attached to, the epithelium of the urogenital tract, whence it derives most of its nutrition. It reproduces by binary fission. The infection is usually transmitted by sexual intercourse. Continual reinfection of one sexual partner by the other—the so-called "ping-pong" infection—can be an obstacle to therapy. Newborn girls can acquire the infection from their infected mothers during passage through the birth canal.[7] In such cases the infection tends to remain asymptomatic until puberty.

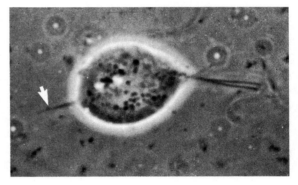

Figure 23.1. Trophozoite of *Trichomonas vaginalis*. Note flagella and axostyle (*arrow*). Phase contrast, × 2000.

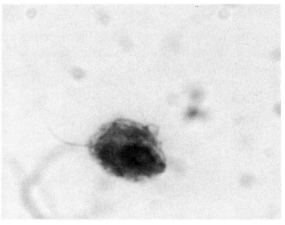

Figure 23.2. Trophozoite of *Trichomonas vaginalis* (Giema stain). Only a few structures can be seen in this preparation. × 1500.

Trichomonas vaginalis

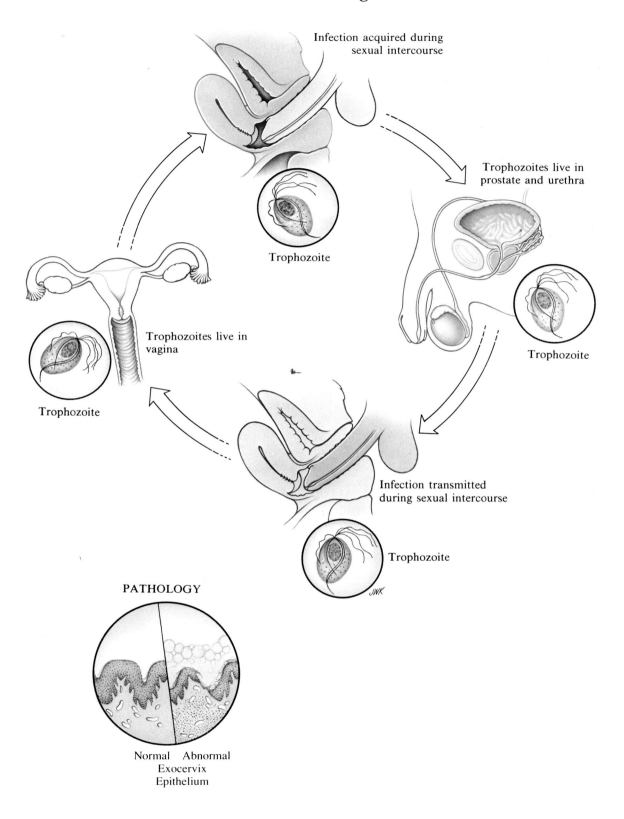

Infection acquired during
sexual intercourse

Trophozoites live in
prostate and urethra

Trophozoite

Trophozoites live in
vagina

Trophozoite

Trophozoite

Infection transmitted
during sexual intercourse

Trophozoite

PATHOLOGY

Normal   Abnormal
Exocervix
Epithelium

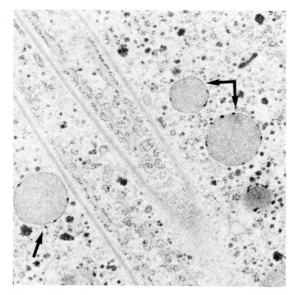

Figure 23.3. Transmission electron micrograph of a portion of the trophozoite of *Trichomonas vaginalis*. The *arrows* point to the hydrogenosomes. ×9000. (Courtesy of Dr. M. Müller)

Pathogenesis

Pathogenicity of *T. vaginalis* apparently varies with the strain of the organism and results from a contact-dependent cytotoxicity, the mechanism of which is still unknown.[8,9] Only some of the numerous serotypes that have been described throughout the world cause serious clinical disease.[10] Two-thirds of the infected women show some pathological findings.[1] These include edema, and inflammation of squamous epithelium, and, less frequently, basal hyperactivity and even metaplasia (although there is no evidence of any causal association of cervical carcinoma or other malignancies with trichomonas infections). The cells themselves are affected, exhibiting enlargement, cytolysis, and hyalinization; there is also enlargement of the nuclei, with bi- and trinucleation and fragmentation.

In addition, the infection can be compounded by changes in bacterial flora, with proliferation of streptococci and diphtheroids, which change the pH of the vagina to a more alkaline one than normal. Thus, it is possible that pathogenesis of clinical disease depends on these interactions, as well as on the strain of the trichomonas.

Lastly, certain host factors, such as secretion of hormones and synthesis of secretory immunoglobulin, affect the host-pathogen interaction.

Clinical Disease

Some 20% of the infected women are asymptomatic; the others experience a wide range of symptoms from mild vaginal discomfort and dyspareunia to an incapacitating illness. The most common presentation is vaginal itching or burning associated with thick, yellow, blood-tinged discharge. There may also be some burning on urination and urethral discharge. All of these symptoms are exacerbated during menstruation. In men, the infection is usually asymptomatic; when the prostate is invaded by the organism, pain in the groin and on urination may be the presenting symptom.

Diagnosis

Direct microscopic examination of the discharge, diluted by a drop of warm saline solution mixed with methylene blue, can usually reveal motile organisms. For confirmation, the secretion can be dried on a microscope slide and then stained with one of the standard solutions containing methylene blue, such as the trichrome, Giemsa, or Wright's stain. It is also possible to culture trichomonas, and thus the diagnosis can be made after several days in those patients with characteristic symptoms whose direct examination is negative. Trichomonas is often discovered on the routine Papanicolaou smears. There are no routine serodiagnostic tests, but they are likely to be developed in the future. In men, the diagnosis can be made by examining expressed urethral fluid after massaging the prostate.

Treatment

Symptomatic women should be treated with metronidazole. The potential side effects are discussed in Chapter 24. Symptomatic men should also be treated; asymptomatic men can transmit the infection, and therefore should be considered candidates for treatment for that reason. Strains of *T. vaginalis* resistant to metronidazole have been reported.[11]

Prevention and Control

Use of a condom during sexual intercourse for as long as either partner is infected is the most reliable method of prevention. Recently, attempts at treating sexual partners by a single administration of 1 g of metronidazole to both simultaneously has been suggested. The effectiveness of such a treatment remains to be assessed. As in other sexually transmitted diseases, identification and treatment of all the partners is necessary.

References

1. Honigberg BM: Trichomonads of importance in human medicine. In Kreier JP (ed): Parasitic Protozoa, Vol 2. New York, Academic Press, 1978, pp 275–454
2. Donne A: Animalcules observes dans la matieres purulentes et le produit des secretions des organes genitaux de l'homme et de la femme. C R Hebdomad Seanc Acad Sci 3:385–386, 1837
3. Ehrenberg CG: Die Infusionsthierchen als vollkommenen Organismen. Leipzig, Voss, 1838
4. Kessel JF, Gafford JA: Observations on the pathology of trichomonas vaginitis and on vaginal implants with *Trichomonas vaginalis* and *Trichomonas intestinalis*. Am J Obstet Gynecol 39:1005–1014, 1940
5. Müller M: The hydrogenosome. In Gooday GW, Lloyd D, Trinc APJ (eds): The Eukaryotic Microbial Cell. Symposium 30. Cambridge, Cambridge University Press, 1980, pp 127–142
6. Mack SR, Müller M: End products of carbohydrate metabolism in *Trichomonas vaginalis.* Comp Biochem Physiol 67B:213–216, 1980
7. Littlewood JM, Kohler HG: Urinary tract infection by *Trichomonas vaginalis* in a newborn baby. Arch Dis Child 41:693–695, 1966
8. Alderete JF, Garza GE: Specific nature of *Trichomonas vaginalis* parasitism of host cell surfaces. Infect Immun 50:701–708, 1985
9. Krieger NJ, Ravdin JI, Rein MF: Contact-dependent cytopathogenic mechanisms of *Trichomonas vaginalis.* Infect Immun 50:778–786, 1985
10. Krieger JN, Holmes KK, Spence MR, et al.: Geographic variation among isolates of *Trichomonas vaginalis:* demonstration of antigenic heterogenicity by using monoclonal antibodies and the indirect fluorescence test. J Infect Dis 152:979–984, 1985
11. Müller M, Meingassner JG, Miller WA, et al.: Three metronidazole-resistant strains of *Trichomonas vaginalis* from the United States. Am J Obstet Gynecol 138:808–812, 1980

24. *Giardia lamblia* (Stiles 1915)

Giardia lamblia is a ubiquitously distributed flagellated protozoan that inhabits the small intestine of its host, where it is attached to the surface of columnar epithelial cells. The infection with giardia, transmitted through fecal contamination of food[1] and drinking water,[2] is endemic in many regions of the world, but it also occurs in sporadic epidemic bursts. Giardiasis is one of several diseases with increased prevalence among male homosexuals.[3] It is also prevalent in children attending day care centers.[4,5] In addition to man, the domestic dog and certain wild animals, such as beavers and muskrats, serve as hosts for *G. lamblia.*[6]

Using restriction endonuclease digestion of giardia DNA and an analysis of the digests, it has been possible to distinguish a number of different patterns among the various isolates. Most of the isolates, regardless of their human or animal source and their geographic origin, were quite similar. A few, however, differed so greatly that they might even be considered a separate species.[7] This method is useful in tracing the sources of this infection in an epidemic.

Historical Information

Van Leeuwenhoek, in a letter written to Hooke at the Royal Society in 1681, accurately described the motile trophozoite of *G. lamblia,* which he observed in a sample of his own stool, as "animalcules a-moving very prettily . . . Their bodies

were somewhat longer than broad, and their bel-
ly, which was flatlike, furnisht with sundry little
paws . . . and albeit they made a quick motion
with their paws, yet for all that they made but
slow progress."[8]

The descriptive information of this historic letter was not widely distributed. The fact that van
Leeuwenhoek did not submit drawings of the
creatures he observed further detracted from the
impact of his report.

Thus, it is Lambl who is credited with the full
description of the trophozoite, which he identified
in 1859 in the stools of various pediatric patients
in Prague.[9] His published observations were accompanied by drawings of three views of these
organisms based on his many observations
through the microscope. The current name of the
parasite was given it by Stiles in 1915 and the
details of its morphology were elaborated by Simon in 1921.[10]

Life Cycle

G. lamblia exists in two forms, the trophozoite
(Fig. 24.1) and the cyst (Fig. 24.2). The former
is pear-shaped and motile, 10–20 μm long and
7–10 μm in diameter. The trophozoite possesses
eight flagellae and is bi-nucleate. In addition, it
contains two rigid structures called blepharoplasts

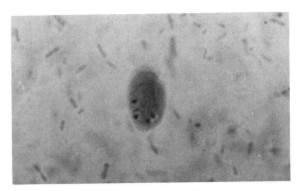

Figure 24.2. Cyst of *Giardia lamblia*. Two nuclei are
shown (*arrow*); the other two are not seen because they
are out of the focal plane. × 2,000.

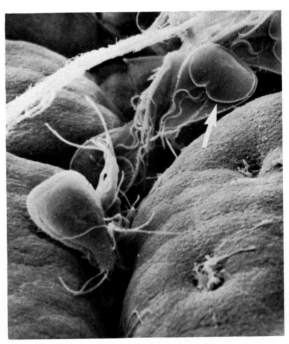

Figure 24.3. Scanning electron micrograph of the trophozoite of *Giardia lamblia* showing the ventral sucker
disc (*arrow*). × 1,600. (Courtesy of Drs. R Owen and L
Brandborg)

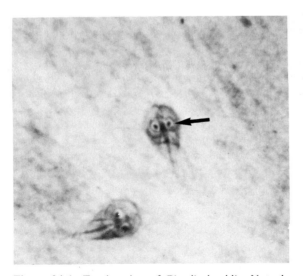

Figure 24.1. Trophozoites of *Giardia lamblia*. Note the
two nuclei (*arrow*). × 800. (Courtesy of Dr. D Lindmark)

which occupy the entire length of the organism.
Its anterior region has a disk-like depression (Fig.
24.3) that the trophozoite uses for attachment to
the surface of epithelial cells. Like *Entamoeba
histolytica* and the trichomonads, *G. lamblia* derives all of its energy from anaerobic metabolism.

Giardia lamblia

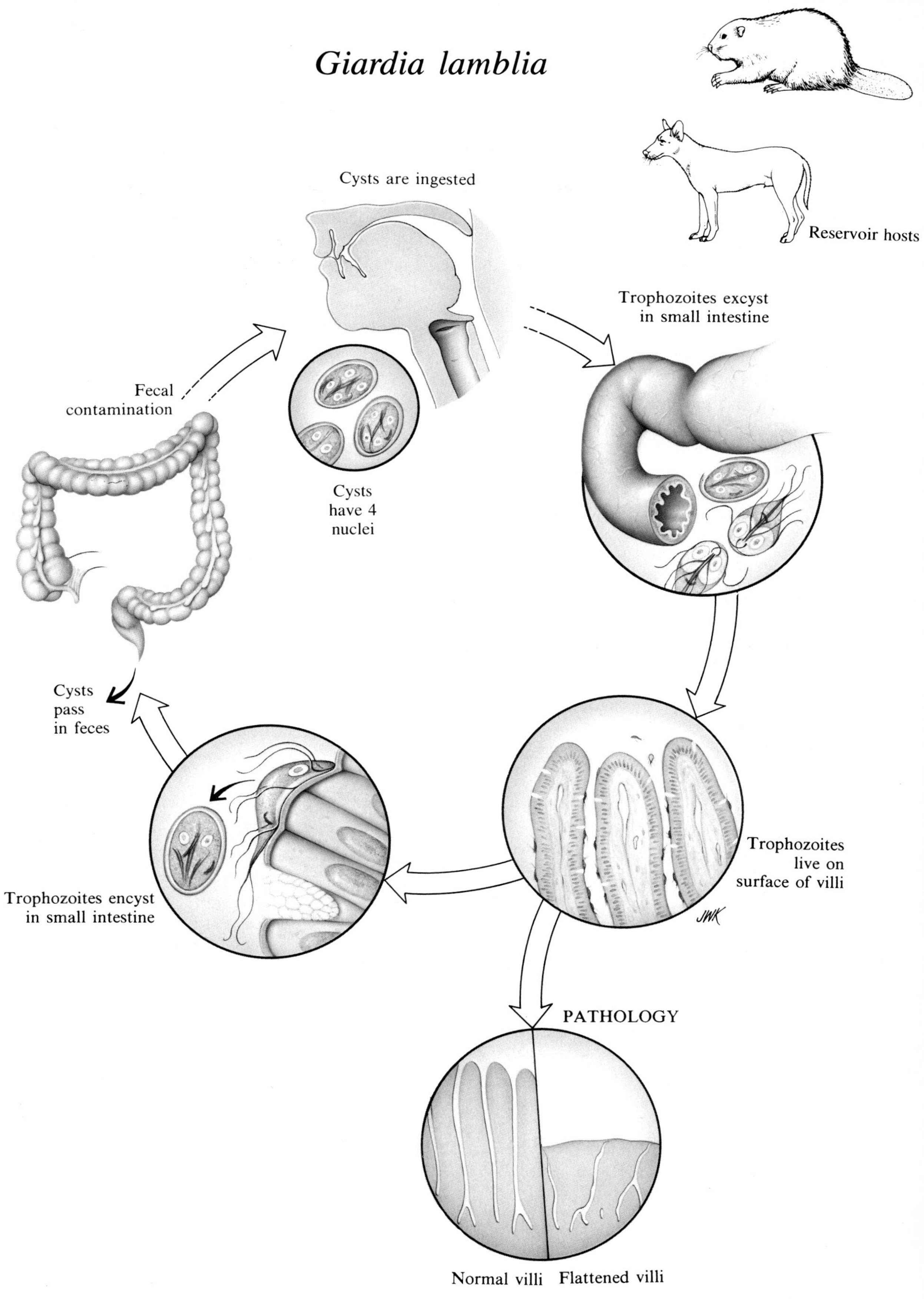

Cysts are ingested

Reservoir hosts

Trophozoites excyst
in small intestine

Fecal
contamination

Cysts
have 4
nuclei

Cysts
pass
in feces

Trophozoites encyst
in small intestine

Trophozoites
live on
surface of villi

PATHOLOGY

Normal villi   Flattened villi

In vitro, *G. lamblia* takes up glucose and absorbs certain lipids.[11] Its nutritional requirements in vivo are unknown.

The cyst is oval and has four nuclei, attenuated flagella, and blepharoplasts. In spite of its anaerobic nature, *G. lamblia* has no hydrogenosomes or related subcellular organelles.

The cyst represents the resting stage of the organism. Its rigid outer wall protects the organism against changes in environmental temperatures, dehydration, and such disinfectants as chlorine, all of which would destroy the trophozoite. The cyst is also the infective stage, transmitted from individual to individual by water and food contaminated by feces. After the cyst is ingested, its cytoplasm differentiates into two motile, fully formed trophozoites, which then come out of the cyst wall and attach themselves to the epithelial surface of the small intestine (Fig. 24.4). Subsequently they multiply by binary fission. The mechanisms governing in vivo excystation are not known, but in vitro studies strongly suggest that hatching proceeds only after the cyst has encountered an acidic environment,[12] such as the stomach. Within days after the infection, many millions of trophozoites develop, often covering completely a part of the small intestinal epithelial surface. *G. lamblia* is not considered a tissue parasite, but its ability to adhere closely to the columnar cells at the level of the microvilli results in antigenic stimulation of the host.

Cysts form in the lumen of the small intestine, but the stimulus for this process is not known. The trophozoites of *G. lamblia* can be grown in vitro axenically[13] (Fig. 24.5).

Pathogenesis

Malabsorption syndrome is characteristic of giardiasis.[14] Atrophy of the villi (Fig. 24.6A and B), a major pathological consequence of heavy infection with *G. lamblia,* is frequent, though not invariable.[15] The two are not necessarily causally related, because many patients with malabsorption

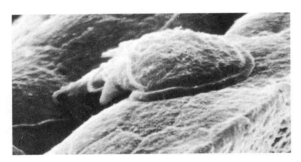

Figure 24.4. Scanning electron micrograph of a biopsy specimen of the duodenum with a trophozoite of *Giardia lamblia* attached to the surface of the columnar epithelium. ×2,500. (Courtesy of Dr. R Owen)

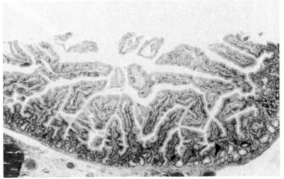

A

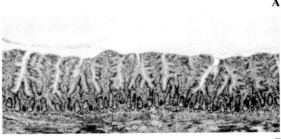

B

Figure 24.6. **A.** Normal villi from the small intestine. **B.** Flattened villi from the small intestine of a patient with malabsorption syndrome due to *Giardia lamblia.* ×80. (Courtesy of Dr. M Wolff)

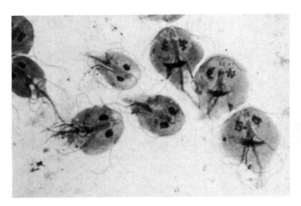

Figure 24.5. Trophozoites of *Giardia lamblia* in culture. ×1000. (Courtesy of Dr. D Lindmark)

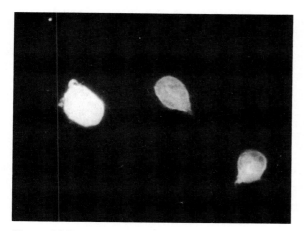

Figure 24.7. Fluorescent antibody test for *Giardia lamblia*. The patient's serum was placed on top of a layer of cultured trophozoites that were fixed on coverslips. Antihuman goat antibodies labeled with fluorescene isothiacyante detect human antibodies attached to this organism. ×600. (Courtesy of Dr. G Huldt)

due to giardia have normal mucosa.[12] The mechanisms by which *G. lamblia* induces malabsorption are unknown. It is possible that the trophozoites closely adhering to the epithelial surface interfere mechanically with absorption. However, the fact that antibodies are formed against surface components of the trophozoite (Fig. 24.7) suggests that there may be more complex interactions between the parasite and the intestinal surface than mere physical contact.

The immune status of the host appears to play a major role in pathogenesis of giardiasis. Individuals who are deficient in secretory IgA develop heavier and longer lasting infections than those who are not.[16] This clinical observation is supported by experimental studies. Host defense against giardiasis in mice is mediated by T-cell-dependent antibodies and may involve antibody-mediated cytotoxicity.[17] Mother's milk is protective, as well, because it contains antibodies of the IgA class.[18] Moreover, products of lipid hydrolysis of the milk in the normal digestive tract are toxic to giardia.[19,20,21]

Clinical Disease

The most prominent symptom of giardia infection is protracted diarrhea. It can be mild and produce semisolid stools, or it can be intensive and debilitating when the stools become watery and voluminous. Untreated, this type of diarrhea may last for weeks or months, although it may vary in intensity, with exacerbations and remissions. Chronic infections are characterized by steatorrhea, accompanied by a classic malabsorption syndrome with substantial weight loss, general debility, and consequent fatigue. Hypoproteinemia[22] and vitamin A deficiency[23] in such patients has been reported. In addition, some people at any stage of intensity of this infection may have epigastric discomfort, anorexia, and even pain. Cholecystitis has been attributed to giardiasis in rare instances, when giardia organisms were found in the gall bladder. Nevertheless, a causal relationship has not been established. There are many asymptomatic carriers of *G. lamblia*. One recent study of children in day care centers in Israel suggested that asymptomatic carriers of giardia had better growth rates and fewer respiratory infections than those who were apparently free of giardia[4]. Confirmation of the validity and the determination of the potential significance of this observation await further studies.

Diagnosis

In any case of protracted diarrhea, infection with giardia must be considered a possible cause. Casual examination of the stools may reveal either trophozoites (Fig. 24.1) or cysts (Fig. 24.8) of giardia. This finding, especially in the absence of

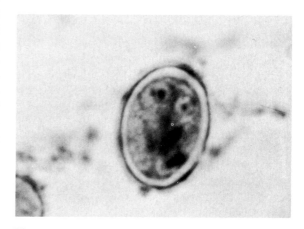

Figure 24.8. Cyst of *Giardia lamblia* recovered from the stool of an infected patient. Two of the four nuclei are visible in this view. ×2600.

any other explanation for the diarrhea, should prompt treatment, and, if the latter is successful, one may reasonably assume a causal relationship between the organism and the previous disease. Failure to find giardia in a casual stool examination does not rule out this diagnosis. It is often necessary to examine many specimens and, indeed, even obtain a duodenal aspirate or a biopsy of the small intestinal mucosa to make the diagnosis. In one relevant study, among patients in whom the organism was identified on small intestinal biopsy, the parasite was noted in the duodenal aspirate of only 75%, and in the stool examination of only 50%.[24] Obviously, probability of identifying giardia in any of the specimens depends on the care with which it is examined in the laboratory, and the percentages cited here may not represent a universal situation. Nevertheless, the above results strongly suggest that giardiasis may not be ''ruled out'' by stool examination, or even duodenal aspiration. The string test,[25] a technique for sampling duodenal mucosal surface, has reduced the requirement for small intestinal biopsies. Immunological tests are all based on the detection of giardia antigen in stools by the capture ELISA technique. There are commercially available kits for this purpose.[26,27] The usefulness of this method of diagnosis has not been evaluated vis-a-vis the direct detection by microscopic examination of the stool, or the duodenal contents.

Treatment

All symptomatic patients infected with giardia should be treated. The drug of choice is quinacrine HCl. Side effects include dizziness, headache, nausea and vomiting, and yellow staining of the skin. Although these side effects are not uncommon, they rarely prevent satisfactory completion of therapy. Persons with exfoliative dermatitis can develop severe exacerbation of their skin disease and therefore should not receive this drug. Inadvertent overdosage can lead to insomnia, bizarre dreams, and even frank psychosis; in very rare instances such symptoms can also occur with the conventional dose. Because quinacrine accumulates in the liver and has a long half-life, these untoward symptoms may last for several days after discontinuation of the drug.

Metronidazole is an alternative drug of choice. It should not be used by pregnant women, particularly during the first trimester. Side effects include nausea, dryness of the mouth, perception of metallic taste and consequent anorexia, and an intolerance for alcohol, of the type experienced with disulfiram. Either drug controls clinical symptoms of giardiasis in 80% of the recipients; in case of failure, repetition of therapy after 1 or 2 weeks will usually be effective. Obviously, because of the relative difficulty of diagnosing giardiasis, eradication of this organism cannot be absolutely confirmed. A reasonable rule in clinical management of patients with this infection is that disappearance of symptoms after therapy and failure to detect giardia organisms in the stools may be accepted as a satisfactory result. Recurrence of symptoms should be treated in the same manner as the original infection.

Furazolidone is a newer drug, found to be effective and well tolerated in clinical studies. At the present time it is the only drug against giardia that is available as a suspension in the United States, which makes it useful in administration to young children. Side effects are relatively frequent and include nausea, vomiting, diarrhea, and fever. Moreover, there have been rare hypersensitivity reactions, such as urticaria, hypotension, and serum sickness. In individuals deficient in glucose-6-phosphate dehydrogenase, it causes mild hemolysis. It causes malignant tumors in rats. Although it is approved in the United States for treatment of giardiasis, warnings of its potential oncogenicity are included in the inserts. On balance, in view of its potential danger and the availability of quinacrine for the majority of patients, this drug cannot be recommended for treatment of giardiasis.

Prevention and Control

Prevention of individual disease involves measures described in the chapter on amebiasis (Chapter 25). Control in the community is more difficult to achieve, because of the presence of reservoir hosts, as previously mentioned. Proper maintenance of community water supplies, purification systems, and delivery systems is essential to prevention of outbreaks of giardiasis.

References

1. Osterholm MT, Forfang JC, Ristinen TL, et al.: An outbreak of food-borne giardiasis. N Engl J Med 304:24–28, 1981

2. Shaw PK, Brodsky RE, Lyman DO, et al.: A communitywide outbreak of giardiasis with evidence of transmission by a municipal water supply. Ann Intern Med 87:421–426, 1977

3. Schmerin MJ, Jones TC, Klein H: Giardiasis: Association with homosexuality. Ann Intern Med 88:801–803, 1978

4. Sagi EF, Shapiro M, Deckelbaum, R: *Giardia lamblia:* Prevalence, influence on growth, and symptomatology in healthy nursery children. Israel J Med Sci 19:815–817, 1983

5. Pickering LK, Woodward WE, Dupont HL, et al.: Occurrence of *Giardia lamblia* in children in day care centers. J Pediatr 104:522–526, 1984

6. Davies RB, Hibler CP: Animal reservoirs and cross-species transmission of Giardia. In Jakubowski W, Hoff JC (eds): Waterborne Transmission of Giardiasis. EPA 600/9–79–001, 1979, pp 104–126

7. Nash TE, McCutchan T, Keister D et al.: Restriction–endonuclease analysis of DNA from 15 giardia isolates obtained from humans and animals. J Infect Dis 152:64–73, 1985

8. van Leeuwenhoek A: cited by Dobell C. In: Antony van Leeuwenhoek and His "Little Animals." New York, Dover Publications, 1960, p 224

9. Lambl VDF: Mikroskopische Untersuchungen der Darm-Excrete. Beitrag zur Pathologie des Darms und zur Diagnostik am Krankenbette. Vierteljahrschrift für die Praktische Heilkunde. Med Fac Prague 1:1–58, 1859

10. Simon CE: *Giardia enterica,* a parasitic intestinal flagellate of man. Am J Hyg 1:440–491, 1921

11. Lindmark DJ: Energy metabolism of the anaerobic protozoan *Giardia lamblia*. Mol Biochem Parasitol 1:1–12, 1980

12. Bingham AK, Jarroll EL Jr, Meyer EA, et al.: *Giardia* sp.: Physical factors of excystation in vitro, and excystation vs. eosin exclusion as determinants of viability. Exp Parasitol 47:284–291, 1979

13. Meyer EA: *Giardia lamblia:* Isolation and axenic cultivation. Exp Parasitol 39:101–105, 1976

14. Brasitus TA: Parasites and malabsorption. Amer J Med 67:1058–1065, 1979

15. Levinson JD, Nastro LJ: Giardiasis with total villous atrophy. Gastroenterology 74:271–275, 1978

16. Ament ME, Rubin CE: Relation of giardiasis to abnormal intestinal structure and function in gastrointestinal immuno-deficiency syndrome. Gastroenterology 62:216–226, 1972

17. Smith PD: Pathophysiology and immunology of giardiasis. Annu Rev Med 36:295–307, 1985

18. Nayak N, Ganguly NK, Walia BNS, et al.: Specific secretory IgA in the milk of *Giardia lamblia*-infected and uninfected women. J Infect Dis 155:724–727, 1987

19. Gillin FD, Reiner DS, Gault, MJ: Cholate–dependent killing of *Giardia lamblia* by human milk. Infect Imm 47:619–622, 1985

20. Hernell O, Ward H, Blackberg L et al.: Killing of *Giardia lamblia* by human milk lipases: an effect mediated by lipolysis of milk lipids. J Inf Dis 153:715–720, 1986

21. Reiner DS, Wang CS, Gillin FS: Human milk kills *Giarda lamblia* by generating toxic lipolytic products. J Infect Dis 154:825–832, 1986

22. Okeahialom TC: Giardiasis in protein energy malnutrition. E Afr Med J 59:765–770, 1982

23. Mahalanabis D, Simpson TW, Chakrabosty ML, et al.: Malabsorption of water miscible vitamin A in children with giardiasis and ascariasis. Am J Clin Nutr 32:313–318, 1979

24. Kumath KR, Murugasu R: A comparative study of four methods for detecting *Giardia lamblia* in children with diarrheal disease and malabsorption. Gastroenterology 66:16–21, 1974

25. Bezjak B: Evaluation of a new technique for sampling duodenal contents in parasitologic diagnosis. Am J Digest Dis 17:848–850, 1972

26. Ungar BL, Yolken RH, Nash TE et al.: Enzyme-linked immunosorbent assay for the detection of *Giardia lamblia* in fecal specimens. J Infect Dis 149:90–97, 1984

27. Green EL, Miles MA, Warhurst DC: Immunodiagnostic detection of giardia antigen in faeces by a rapid visual enzyme-linked immunosorbent assay. Lancet 28:691–693, 1985

25. *Entamoeba histolytica* (Schaudinn 1903)

Infection with *Entamoeba histolytica* has worldwide distribution. It is estimated that the world prevalence exceeds 500 million infections.[1] It is the causative agent of amebic dysentery and inhabits the lumen and mucosa of the large intestine, predominantly the transverse colon and cecum. Less frequently, it also causes extraintestinal infections, being capable of invading virtually any tissue and organ. Members of all age groups and both sexes are infected, but there is a higher prevalence of amebiasis among adult men, who have an increased risk of exposure in the agricultural occupations. An increased prevalence of this infection is also found in male homosexuals,[2] however this protozoan may be less pathogenic in this population.[3,4] Animals other than man, such as dogs and monkeys, harbor an ameba that is indistinguishable from *E. histolytica*. Nevertheless, they do not constitute an important reservoir for human infections.

Historical Information

Losch is given credit both for having described in 1875 the clinical manifestations of infection with *E. histolytica* and for reproducing the disease in dogs by infecting them with amebae derived from human cases.[5] Quincke and Roos, in 1893, distinguished this pathogenic ameba from that of *E. coli*,[6] a harmless commensal often found in the stool of healthy individuals. A later paper by Schaudinn,[7] in 1903, also accurately depicted trophozoites and cysts of *E. histolytica*. Schaudinn died at the age of 35 of overwhelming amebiasis, as a result of self-experimentation with this pathogen. Councilman and Lafleur, in 1891, described pathogenesis of *E. histolytica* infection,[8] and Walker and Sellards described the clinical disease in 1913.[9] In vitro cultivation of *E. histolytica* was first achieved by Boeck, in 1925,[10] and its life cycle was elucidated by Dobell in 1928.[11]

Life Cycle

The anaerobic trophozoite is motile, measures 20-30 μm in diameter, and possesses a single nucleus with a centrally located karyosome (nucleolus) (Fig. 25.1A and B; see also Fig. 25.8B). The cytoplasm of the trophozoite may also con-

tain partially digested or whole erythrocytes (Fig. 25.2; see also Fig. 25.8B). The ameba is nourished by these erythrocytes and by other cells, but it also feeds on bacteria, which can sometimes be seen in the cytoplasm. *E. histolytica* is an anaerobe, and therefore lacks mitochondria. Although it possesses the ability to lyse tissues, no lysosomes have been seen under an electron microscope. Strains of *E. histolytica* vary in their pathogenicity; the location of the amebae in the large intestine varies from strain to strain. Trophozoites of the pathogenic strains live within

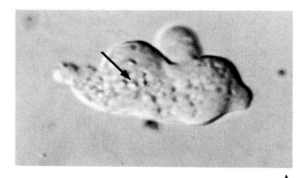

A

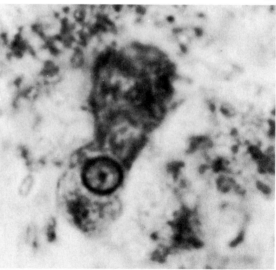

B

Figure 25.1. A. Trophozoite of *Entamoeba histolytica* as it appears in culture. **B.** Trophozoite of *Entamoeba histolytica*. Note the characteristic central karyosome and peripheral chromatin of the nucleus distributed in clumps of equal density. **A,** phase contrast, × 1,000; **B,** trichrome stain, × 1,000.

Entamoeba histolytica

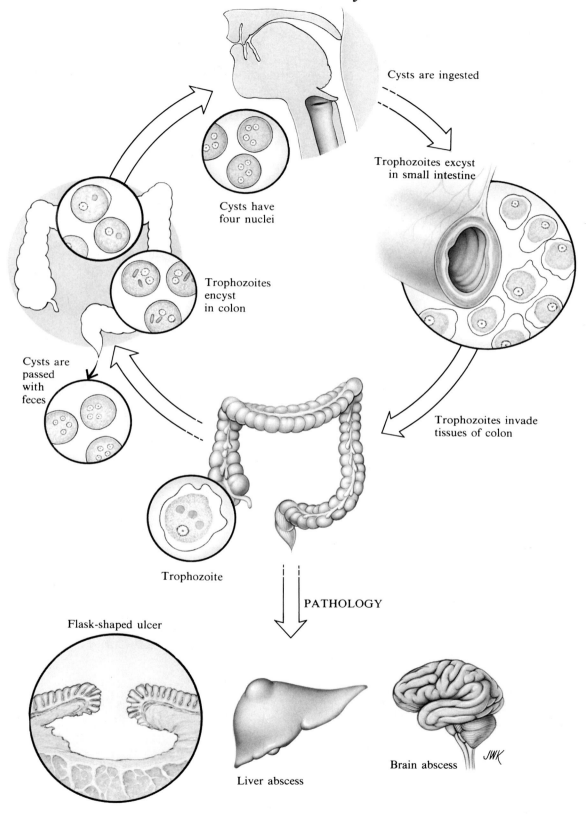

Cysts are ingested

Trophozoites excyst
in small intestine

Cysts have
four nuclei

Trophozoites
encyst
in colon

Trophozoites invade
tissues of colon

Cysts are
passed
with
feces

Trophozoite

PATHOLOGY

Flask-shaped ulcer

Liver abscess

Brain abscess

JWK

flask-shaped ulcers (Fig. 25.3) in the mucosa, which result from disruption of its surface by lysis induced by the ameba. The trophozoites are found at the margin of the ulcer next to the healthy tissue. Nonpathogenic strains of *E. histolytica* are often found in the lumen of the large intestine or at the mucosal surface. The trophozoites divide by binary fission.

E. histolytica forms cysts (Fig. 25.4 A–C) measuring 10–15 μm in diameter. The process of formation of the cyst begins when the trophozoite first rounds up into a precyst and secretes an

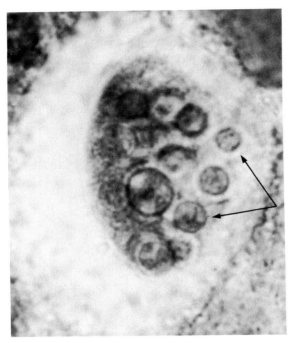

Figure 25.2. Trophozoite of *Entamoeba histolytica*. The cytoplasm is filled with ingested red blood cells (*arrows*). The nucleus is in the lower right portion of the trophozoite. ×1,285.

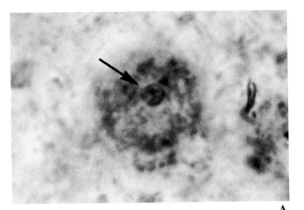

A

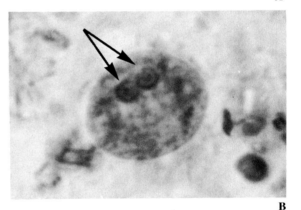

B

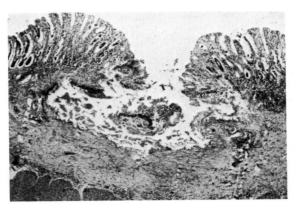

Figure 25.3. Section of large intestine showing a flask-shaped ulcer resulting from infection with *Entamoeba histolytica*. The organisms, not visible at this magnification, can be found at the margin of the ulcer, between the heatlhy tissue and the necrotic debris. ×66.

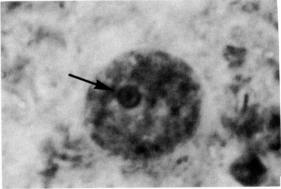

C

Figure 25.4. Cyst stage of *Entamoeba histolytica*. Four nuclei are present (*arrows*), as seen in this series of light photomicrographs taken at different focal planes. **A, B,** and **C,** trichrome stain, ×1,000.

impermeable outer cyst wall. Within the cyst the nucleus undergoes two division cycles, giving rise to four small nuclei. At the same time the ribosomes accumulate into aggregates called chromatoidal bodies (Fig. 25.5). When nuclear division is finished, encystment is completed. Cysts are sturdy and resist adverse environmental condi-

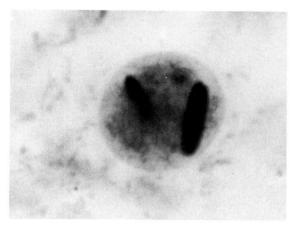

Figure 25.5. Precyst stage of *Entamoeba histolytica.* Chromatoidal bodies (collections of ribosomes) and a single nucleus are characteristic of this stage of cyst formation. ×1,000.

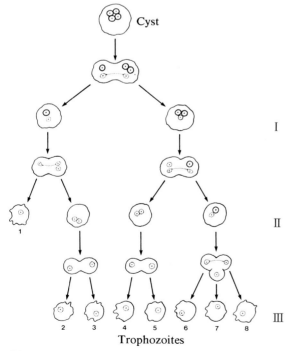

Figure 25.6. Division cycle of *Entamoeba histolytica* after excystation. Eight trophozoites are produced from a single quadrinucleate cyst.

tions. After the cyst is ingested by a susceptible host, its wall is disrupted by the formation of a small opening through which a quadrinucleate ameba emerges. The ameba then divides serially through three cycles, giving rise to a total of eight uninucleate trophozoites from one cyst (Fig. 25.6). Some of these trophozoites then invade the tissues of the large intestine and may erode them so extensively that they gain entrance into the bloodstream. Thus, amebae can reach all parts of the body, but most commonly establish extraintestinal infection in the right lobe of the liver, which they reach by portal vessels.

In extraintestinal amebiasis, no cysts are produced. Rather, the trophozoites continue to divide by binary fission.

Pathogenesis

Not all strains of *E. histolytica* are pathogenic. Studies of isoenzymes by electrophoresis have revealed differences in their mobility, which could be correlated with clinical expression of the infection with this protozoan.[12,13] There is no evidence, however, that these distinguishing isoenzymes are directly responsible for pathogenicity; they are only markers.

The pathogenic effects result from a cytolytic process that disrupts membranes of the cells when they come in contact with the parasite.[14] The cells thus disrupted are digested by the host's lysosomal enzymes. The intial cytopathic effect is probably mediated by a phospholipase A, associated with the plasma membrane and dependent on the calcium ion. Attachment of *E. histolytica* to host cells is mediated by a molecule containing N-acetyl-glucosamine.[15]

E. histolytica also produces cytotoxins that destroy white cells.[16] Although an exception is the ameboma, a large, tumor-like lesion, usually in the submucosa of the large intestine. Amebomas arise as the result of long-term "smoldering" infections in the intestine and represent an area of lysis that has resolved into a large, usually necrotic, lesion filled with neutrophils, eosinophils, and lymphocytes. These large masses may be mistaken for malignant tumors of the large bowel.

In any lesion induced by *E. histolytica,* the amebae inhabit only the perimeter of the necrotic tissue (i.e., the transition zone between healthy and dead tissue), because they feed only on living cells.

Clinical Disease

The majority of infected individuals are free of symptoms. Those who are symptomatic experience a wide range of manifestations. The most common and least problematic is nonspecific diarrhea, but one lasting more than the usual few days. Ulcerative colitis represents the next stage of severity. It can be quite localized and cause few or no symptoms, but it can also be quite extensive, involving most of the colon. This is usually associated with colicky pain, flatulation, and alteration in the pattern of bowel movements, bloody stools, and—eventually—dysentery.

On physical examination, one may detect generalized abdominal tenderness, with particular accentuation in the iliac fossae. If the disease has lasted for months, or years, in a subacute or asymptomatic state, and there is an ameboma, it may be palpable.

If the disease progresses unchecked, either for lack of therapy or because host response has been insufficient to render it chronic, the colon may become atonic and may perforate in one or several points of ulceration (Fig. 25.7). If this happens, symptoms and signs of peritonitis develop.

As an associated phenomenon, the perforated, inflamed bowel may adhere to the abdominal wall and the perforation may extend to the skin, causing cutaneous amebiasis, which can extend rapidly. This may also occur in the perianal area, as the result of invasion of the skin by the amebic trophozoites emerging from the rectum.

Extraintestinal amebiasis can affect any organ or tissue. The one most frequently involved is the liver. Invasion of this organ by amebae may occur in the wake of frank colonic amebiasis, but also in cases where the colonic infection was asymptomatic. Nearly half of all patients with amebic liver abscess do not give a history suggestive of amebic colitis.

Hepatic amebiasis is a slowly progressive, insidious disease, which may begin as a nonspecific febrile illness with pain and tenderness in the right upper portion of the abdomen. Examination at that time may reveal only a slightly enlarged liver, which is tender, but may also show a mass. If the amebic abscess perforates through the diaphragm, this is associated with characteristic right pleuritic pain and pain referred to the shoulder. Although the majority of patients with hepatic amebiasis have an involvement of the right lobe of this

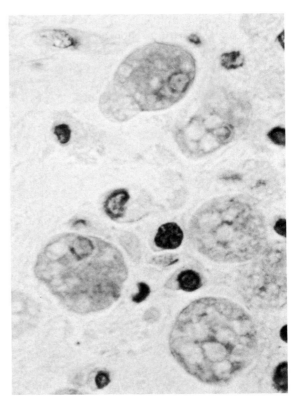

Figure 25.7. Section of an ulcer in the colon of a patient infected with *Entamoeba histolytica*. The organisms are clearly visible at this high magnification. × 500.

organ, some have the abscess only in the left lobe and therefore the enlargement and tenderness can be central, or even left-sided.

Laboratory results may reveal an increase in the erythrocyte sedimentation rate and a low degree of polymorphonuclear leukocytosis. A radiogram of the abdomen may show an enlargment of the liver but, more important, a fixed, raised diaphragm. In cases of perforation of the diaphragm, there may be evidence of consolidation of the left lower lobe of the lung, or its lower segment, and a pleural effusion. A radionuclide scan, a sonogram, or a computerized axial tomogram will show an abscess and help to define its extent; it may also reveal additional abscesses, which are rare. The direct extension to the right pleural space and the lung is the most common form of intrathoracic amebiasis, but hematogenous spread may cause metastatic amebiasis in other portions of the lung and the pleura, as well as in other organs, notably the brain. Amebic pericarditis can also occur in the same manner. Both of these latter conditions are extremely dangerous; they must be recognized quickly and treated. There are no reports of survival of patients with an amebic brain abscess, but a quick aspiration of the expanding pericardial effusion, combined with antiamebic therapy, has saved lives of patients with amebic pericarditis.

Diagnosis

Intestinal amebiasis must always be considered in any patient with protracted diarrhea and in all patients with dysentery. This diagnosis must also be considered in patients presenting with intraluminal colonic masses, because amebomas may resemble carcinoma of the colon. With respect to extraintestinal amebiasis, identification of the lesion by the various modalities suggested above, in the presence of a history compatible with amebiasis and in parallel with identification of amebae in the colon, points to the diagnosis. Amebic liver abscess should not be aspirated for diagnostic purposes alone.

Examination of fresh stool for the presence of cysts and trophozoites is mandatory and should be carried out immediately as the diagnosis is suspected. Presence of amebae—either trophozoites or cysts—together with a compatible clinical disease provides an excellent presumptive diagnostic indication of amebiasis. If amebae are not discovered on a casual stool examination, a purged stool specimen should be obtained and examined immediately. Because the amebae tend to be more concentrated in the cecum in light infections, it is the second and third expulsions of the stool, after administration of a purgative, that are most likely to yield amebae. If only casual stools can be obtained, then six consecutive daily stool examinations will reveal the infection in more than 90% of all patients harboring the ameba.[18]

Microscopic examination of stool for amebae is a difficult procedure requiring considerable technical expertise. False positive results, in which polymorphonuclear leukocytes, macrophages, or *E. coli* are mistaken for *E. histolytica* are as common as false negative results in which amebae fail o be recognized. If no expert laboratory is available in the immediate vicinity, it is possible to preserve the fresh stool specimens in formalin (for subsequent examination for cysts) and polyvinyl alcohol (for subsequent examination for trophozoites and cysts). Such preserved specimens may then be dispatched to the nearest regional laboratory (see Appendix III).

Charcot-Leyden crystals (Fig. 25.8A and B), which are products of degenerated eosinophils, are usually present in colonic infection with *E. histolytica*. They provide an indirect evidence of infection. However, they are also found in trichuriasis, paragonimiasis, certain allergic diatheses, and many other conditions.

Serological tests can be quite helpful, and include the indirect hemagglutination, complement fixation, and counterimmunoelectrophoresis tests.[19] In cases of noninvasive colonic amebiasis, about 40% or fewer patients will have a positive test. In invasive amebiasis, more than 95% of the patients have positive serological tests. Positive serology persists for many years. Therefore, it would be interpreted correctly only in the

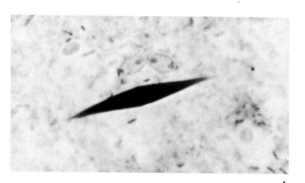

A

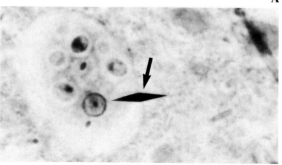

B

Figure 25.8. A. Charcot-Leyden crystal from the stool of a patient with amebiasis. **B.** Trophozoite of *Entamoeba histolytica* showing characteristic nucleus, red cells in cytoplasm, and Charcot-Leyden crystal overlying its plasma membrane. **A,** Giemsa stain, ×1,600; **B,** ×600.

context of the patient's past history. In more than 50% of all patients with extraintestinal amebiasis, no amebae can be found in the large intestine.

Treatment

An ideal treatment is yet to be devised; therefore there is some controversy over a correct approach to management of clinical amebiasis. In endemic areas, only patients with symptomatic amebiasis should be treated, because of the frequency of reinfection. In nonendemic areas, *every* patient with amebiasis should be treated.

Asymptomatic individuals and those with non-dysenteric amebic colitis should receive iodoquinol. In cases of invasive amebiasis, which include severe colitis with ulcerations and dysentery, hepatic abscess, and involvement of other extraintestinal sites, the patient should receive metronidazole. In addition, these patients must receive simultaneously, or sequentially, iodoquinol. Patients who are too ill to take oral metronidazole must be treated with emetine. Dehydroemetine, which is somewhat less toxic but not currently available in the United States, may be substituted.

The reason for the recommendation of iodoquinol in conjunction with metronidazole is that there have been cases reported of a successful completion of therapy of the extraintestinal amebiasis, which was then followed by a recurrence of the extraintestinal infection or by colonic amebiasis, in situations where reexposure to amebae was unlikely. This has suggested the possibility that metronidazole, although very effective in the treatment of the primary disease, may be unable to eradicate amebae from the colon. Iodoquinol is a relatively nontoxic drug, but occasionally causes rash, an exacerbation of exfoliative dermatitis, and in very rare instances may cause upper gastrointestinal disturbances, such as nausea and vomiting. In doses much higher than those prescribed for amebiasis and in cases where the drug was continued for several months or longer, iodoquinol—like its more famous congener clioquinol—has caused subacute myeloptic neuritis (SMON). There has been no case of SMON reported as a consequence of correctly administered antiamebic therapy.

Metronidazole also has a number of side effects (see Treatment section, Chapter 24). This drug should be reserved for cases of extraintestinal amebiasis and severe intestinal disease.

Emetine and dehydroemetine cause cardiac arrhythmias and even asystole. They also cause precordial pain, muscle weakness, and an intense inflammation at the site of the injection. Because of this high toxicity, these drugs must be reserved for patients in imminent danger of death due to amebiasis.

Although aspiration of the liver abscess is not recommended for diagnostic purposes, it may rarely be necessary for therapy. This is indicated when the abscess is extremely tense and so tender and painful that the patient may not tolerate awaiting resolution of it by chemotherapy. In most of such cases a percutaneous aspiration will suffice. The danger that one can spread the amebic infection must be considered, but because the number of amebae within the aspirate is exceedingly small—the trophozoites tend to be localized at the perimeter of the abscess—aspiration is quite safe. Nevertheless, it should be done by the most experienced person, usually a surgeon or a physician who has treated many patients with this disease.

Prevention and Control

In situations where amebiasis is transmitted by contaminated water, purification of the water or elimination of the source of fecal contamination is required to control spread of the infection.

A thorough screening of food handlers by stool examinations can identify some carriers whose occupations would place the general public at risk. Recurrent outbreaks of amebiasis in mental institutions can be prevented by routine stool examinations of the patients, followed by the appropriate treatment.

Prevention of the spread of amebiasis among male homosexuals presents a new set of problems for public health epidemiologists.

References

1. Guerrant FL: The global problem of amoebiasis: current status, research needs, and opportunities for progress. Rev Infect Dis 8:218–227, 1986
2. Pomerantz BM, Marr JS, Goldman WD: Amebiasis in New York City 1958–1978: Identification of the

male homosexual high risk population. Bull NY Acad Med 56:232–244, 1980

3. Goldmeier D, Sargeaunt PG, Price AB, et al.: Is *Entamoeba histolytica* in homosexual men a pathogen? Lancet 1:641–644, 1986

4. Allison-Jones E, Mindel A, Sargeaunt P et al.: *Entamoeba histolytica* as a commensal intestinal parasite in homosexual men. N Eng J Med 315:353–356, 1986

5. Losch FA: Massenhafte Entwicklung von Amöben in Dickdarm. Arch Pathol Anat Phys Klin Med Virchow 65:196–211, 1875

6. Quincke HI, Roos E: Über Amöben-enteritis. Berl Klin Wochenschr 30:1089–1094, 1893

7. Schaudinn F: Untersuchungen über Fortpflanzung einiger Rhizopoden (vorläufige Mitteilung). Arbeiten aus dem Kaiserlichen Gesundheitsamte 19:547–576, 1903

8. Councilman WT, Lafleur HA: Amebic dysentery. Johns Hopkins Hosp Rep 2:395–548, 1891

9. Walker EL, Sellards AW: Experimental entamoebic dysentery. Philip J Sci Trop Med 8:230–253, 1913

10. Boeck WC: Cultivation of *Entamoeba histolytica*. Am J Hyg 5:371–407, 1925

11. Dobell C: Researches on the intestinal protozoa of monkeys and man. Parasitology 20:357–412, 1928

12. Sargeaunt PG, Williams JE, Grene JD: The differentiation of invasive and non-invasive *Entamoeba histolytica* by isoenzyme electrophoresis. Trans Roy Soc Trop Med Hyg 72:519–521, 1978

13. Farri TA, Sargeaunt PG, Warhurst DC et al.: Electrophoretic studies of the hexokinase of *Entamoeba histolytica* groups I and IV. Trans Roy Soc Trop Med Hyg 78:672–673, 1980

14. Ravdin JI: Pathogenesis of disease caused by *Entamoeba histolytica*: studies of adherence, secreted toxins and contact-dependent cytolysis. Rev Infect Dis 8:247–260, 1986

15. Ravdin JI, Murphy CF, Salata RA, et al.: *N*-acetyl-D-galactosamine-inhibiting adherence lectin of *Entamoeba histolytica*. I. Partial purification and relation of ameoebic virulence in vitro. J Infect Dis 151:804–815, 1985

16. Ravdin JI, Guerrant RL: Studies on the cytopathogenicity of *Entamoeba histolytica*. Arch Invest Med (Mexico) (Suppl. 1) 11:123–128, 1980

17. Salata R, Ravdin JR: Reviews of the human immune mechanisms directed against *Entamoeba histolytica*. Rev Infect Dis 8:261–272, 1986

18. Sawitz WG, Faust EC: The probability of detecting intestinal protozoa by successive stool examinations. Am J Trop Med 22:131–136, 1942

19. Kagan IG: Serodiagnosis of parasitic diseases. In Rose NR, Friedman H (eds): Manual of Clinical Immunology, 2nd edition. Washington, DC, American Society for Microbiology, 1980, pp 573–604

26. *Balantidium coli* (Malmsten 1857)

Balantidium coli is widely distributed throughout the world, but the prevalence of human infection is not known. Endemic foci have been reported from New Guinea, Micronesia, Seychelles Islands, and Central and South America.[1] Sporadic epidemics have occurred in institutionalized populations. Infected individuals harbor the parasite in the colon, the infection being self-limited and only rarely associated with any symptoms. The parasite is capable of infecting a wide range of domesticated and wild mammals, including guinea pigs, horses, cattle, pigs, and rats.

Historical Information

The discovery of *B. coli* in association with human disease is attributed to Malmsten,[2] who in 1857 described two patients in Sweden with this infection. One recovered and the other died. In both, Malmsten found ciliates, which he carefully described and depicted in drawings.

Life Cycle

B. coli has two forms, the trophozoite (Fig. 26.1) and the cyst (Fig. 26.2). The cyst measures 55 μm in diameter and the trophozoite, ovoid in shape, is 70 μm in length and 45 μm in width. The cyst is the infective stage and is usually ingested in contaminated food or water. Excystation takes place in the small intestine and the released trophozoite takes up residence in the large intestine, invading the walls of the transverse and descending colon. In this regard it is similar to

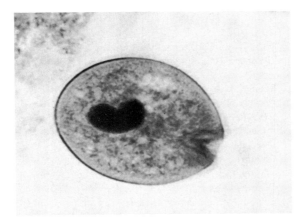

Figure 26.1. Ciliated trophozoite of *Balantidium coli*. Note the "U" shaped macronucleus. ×600.

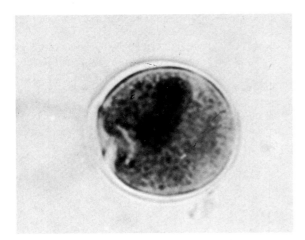

Figure 26.2. Cyst (i.e., the infectious stage) of *Balantidium coli*. ×600.

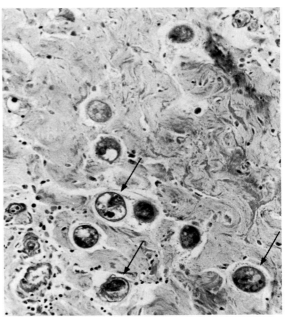

Figure 26.3. Trophozoites of *Balantidium coli (arrows)* in a lesion in the colon. ×150.

Pathogenesis

B. coli trophozoites burrow into the submucosa, ingesting host cells in the process. They also erode the muscularis, which can lead to bleeding. The mechanism by which this organism digests host tissues in unknown. However, balantidium is similar to the free-living ciliates, e.g., *Paramecium* sp. and *Tetrahymena* sp., in which phagolysosomes play a major part in digestion.

Grossly, the lesions consist of a circular, raised margin with dome-shaped necrotic center. Histologically, the ulcer resembles that caused by *E. histolytica* (Fig. 26.3). Some white cells are present, but there is no inflammatory response, unless the lesion is secondarily infected by bacteria.

Clinical Disease

Diarrhea is the most characteristic symptom, although few of the infected individuals are symptomatic; fewer still have dysentery. Fever, nausea, vomiting, and asthenia have been described.

E. histolytica, but, unlike the latter, *B. coli* rarely spreads by direct invasion or by the hematogenous route, and thus is usually limited to the bowel. Liver abscess has been described[3] and, rarely, the parasite has been found in the lungs and the heart.[4] Its trophozoites divide by binary fission, although in vitro they also undergo sexual conjugation. The trophozoites are shed into the lumen of colon, where they secrete a wall and encyst and are passed in the stools. The cyst stage survives in the environment. Pigs are the presumed reservoirs of this infection; human infection is very common in circumstances where man and pigs are closely associated.

Balantidium coli

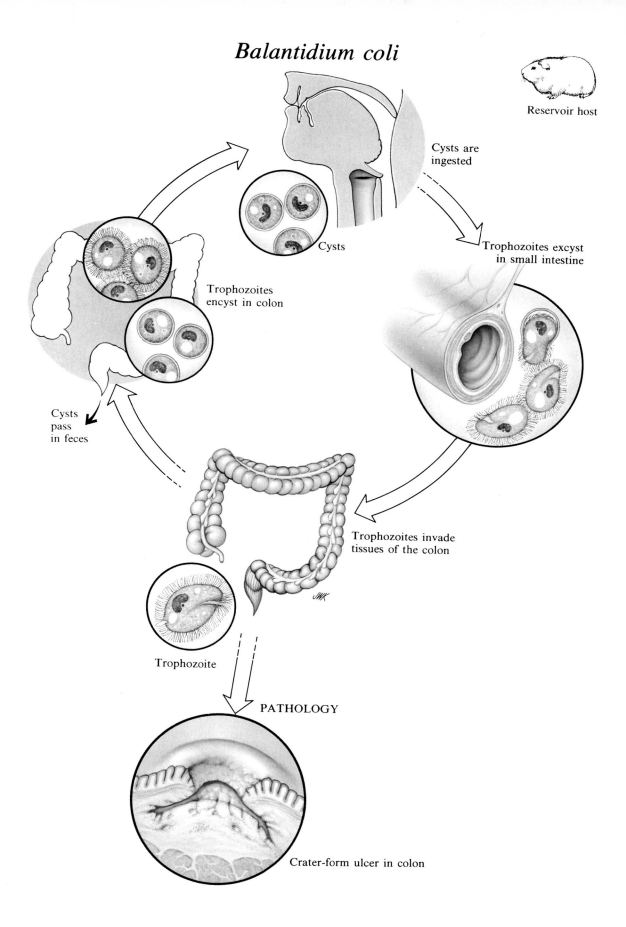

Reservoir host

Cysts are ingested

Cysts

Trophozoites encyst in colon

Trophozoites excyst in small intestine

Cysts pass in feces

Trophozoites invade tissues of the colon

Trophozoite

PATHOLOGY

Crater-form ulcer in colon

Diagnosis

Diagnosis is made by the identification of the organism, in the form of a trophozoite or a cyst (Figs. 26.1 and 26.2), in the stool of the patient. Stools negative by microscopic examination may be cultured on special media that support growth of this protozoan. There are no serological tests.

Treatment

The drug of choice is tetracycline, with iodoquinol as the alternative.

Prevention and Control

Spread from man to man may be controlled by proper disposal of feces. Prevention of contamination of the environment by pig feces, particularly in slaughterhouses, is important. In general, the same measures that limit spread of amebiasis and giardiasis also apply to balantidiasis.

References

1. Nuti M, De Comarmond C, De Dac C: An edemic focus of balantidiasis in the Seychelles Islands. In: Abstracts of the 10th International Congress of Tropical Medicine and Malaria, 1980, p 13
2. Malmsten PH: Infusorien als intestinal-Tiere beim Menschen. Arch Pathol Anat Physiol Klin Med (Virchow) 12:302–309, 1857
3. Wenger F: Abscesso hepatico producido por el *Balantidium coli*. Kasmera 2:433–435, 1967
4. Arean VM, Koppisch E: Balantidiasis: A review and report of cases. Am J Pathol 32: 1089–1117, 1956

27. *Toxoplasma gondii* (Nicolle and Manceaux 1908)

Toxoplasma gondii is an obligate intracellular protozoan parasite belonging to the subclass Coccidia. It has ubiquitous distribution and infects members of all age groups and both sexes. *T. gondii* is capable of infecting all mammals and is usually acquired by man through the ingestion of undercooked or raw meats. The cat, *Felis domestica,* and many other felines (e.g., lynx and bobcat), are the only hosts known to harbor the sexual stage of the parasite.

Infection of human adults is usually asymptomatic and only rarely causes a serious illness. Congenital infection, on the other hand, is serious and sometimes results in permanent damage to the fetus.

Historical Information

The organism was described, in 1908, by Nicolle and Manceaux,[1] working in North Africa on *Ctenodactylus gondi,* the so-called gondi, a desert rodent related to the gerbil, and by Splendore[2] in Brazil, working on rabbits. The publications appeared within 3 days of each other, but the investigators did not know of each other's work. The disease was described later, in 1923, by Janku,[3] who reported pathological findings of hydrocephalus and chorioretinitis in a case of congenital toxoplasmosis, but he did not isolate the organism. Wolf et al.[4], in 1939, reported three cases of congenital infection, thus confirming Janku's observations. They also showed that the lesions were caused by an agent transmissible to rabbits and mice. Acquired toxoplasmosis was identified, in 1941, by Pinkerton and Henderson[5] and by Sabin,[6] working independently. Sexual stages of the life cycle were discovered by Frenkel et al.[7], in 1970, who also recognized it as a coccidian parasite as did Hutchinson and colleagues in the same year.[8]

Life Cycle

Sexual Phase

The cat and related species of Felidae are the only known definitive hosts for *T. gondii.* Cats acquire the infection by ingesting oocysts or by consuming muscle or brain tissues of an intermediate host, usually a rodent, which harbors the asexual pseudocyst stage of the parasite (Fig. 27.1) containing hundreds of infectious units, the

Toxoplasma gondii

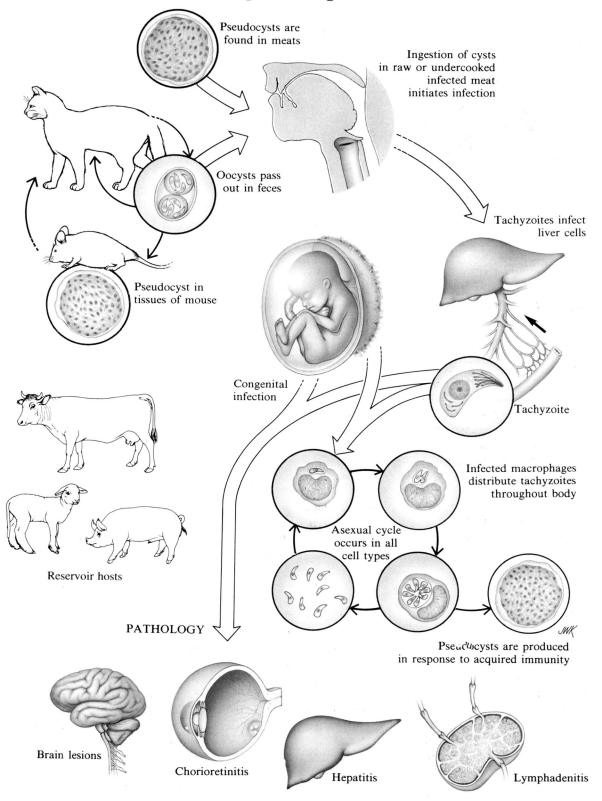

Pseudocysts are found in meats

Ingestion of cysts in raw or undercooked infected meat initiates infection

Oocysts pass out in feces

Pseudocyst in tissues of mouse

Tachyzoites infect liver cells

Reservoir hosts

Congenital infection

Tachyzoite

Infected macrophages distribute tachyzoites throughout body

Asexual cycle occurs in all cell types

PATHOLOGY

Pseudocysts are produced in response to acquired immunity

Brain lesions

Chorioretinitis

Hepatitis

Lymphadenitis

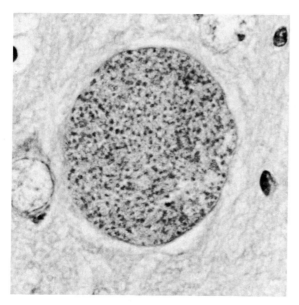

Figure 27.1. Pseudocyst of *Toxoplasma gondii* in mouse brain. × 1000.

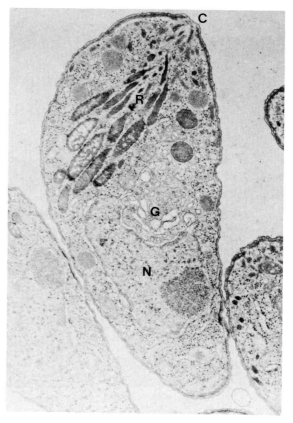

Figure 27.2. Transmission electron micrograph of a tachyzoite of *Toxoplasma gondii*. Various subcellular organelles are visible in this view. Nucleus (*N*), rhoptries (*R*), Golgi apparatus (*G*), conoid (*C*), × 26,000. (Courtesy of Dr. T Jones)

bradyzoites. The pseudocyst wall is digested in the cat's stomach. It ruptures in the small intestine and the bradyzoites are released in its lumen. They infect epithelial cells and transform into merozoites, divide many times, rupture the cell, and enter the lumen. Each merozoite can infect other epithelial cells, and thus perpetuate the infection. Some merozoites develop, instead, into gametocytes, and these sexual forms fuse to form the oocysts, which remain in the intestine, until they pass out with the stool. The oocysts contain the infectious sporozoites.

Asexual Phase

When an oocyst is ingested by a mammalian intermediate host, its wall becomes digested in the intestine, and the parasites (Fig. 27.2) are released. They rapidly penetrate the intestinal wall, are picked up by macrophages (Fig. 27.3 and 27.4), and spread throughout the body by the hematogenous route. Once in the macrophages the organisms are referred to as tachyzoites. The macrophages are unable to kill or digest the tachyzoites, because entry of the parasite into the vacuole in the cell does not initiate microbicidal mechanisms or fusion of the lysosomes with the vacuole containing the parasite. However, the macrophages can digest dead tachyzoites, even if they are phagocytized together with living organisms.

Virtually every type of cell in the mammalian host is susceptible to the infection. Thus, *Toxoplasma gondii* is the least host and tissue specific infectious agent known. Once within the cell, each sporozoite transforms into the tachyzoite stage and multiplies by binary fission to fill the cell, which eventually dies.

Host immune defenses, primarily those mediated by the T cells, eventually limit the rate of division of tachyzoites. As the result, pseudocysts containing large collections of infectious organisms develop within various cells and remain dormant for as long as host defenses remain active. Although all tissues can harbor such pseudocysts, the brain is an area of predilection and

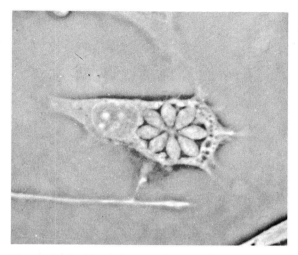

Figure 27.3. Macrophage infected with *Toxoplasma gondii*. Note how the tachyzoites form a rosette in the parasitophorous vacuole within the infected cell. ×450.

usually contains many cysts. When a cyst is eaten by the cat, the sexual development can begin and the life cycle is completed.

Intermediate hosts can also be infected by ingesting pseudocysts in the flesh of another inter-

mediate host. This route of transmission is most common among carnivores. In human populations, infection is usually acquired by ingestion of infected raw or insufficiently cooked meat of any animal. Congenital transmission occurs during infection of the mother when tachyzoites cross the placenta. Maternal antibodies acquired during an infection that occurred before pregnancy prevent fetal infection.

Pathogenesis

All tissues can become infected by toxoplasma. In congenital disease, the predominant lesions are in the central nervous system, although toxoplasmas can be widely disseminated in other vital tissues, such as the myocardium, the lungs, and the liver. Skeletal muscles also harbor the parasites. The host response is one of inflammation. The inflammatory lesions usually become necrotic and eventually calcify. Retinochoroiditis is a frequent lesion in congenital toxoplasmosis. The retina is inflamed and becomes necrotic. The pigmented layer becomes disrupted by infiltration of the inflammatory cells. Eventually, granulation tissue forms and invades the vitreous humor.

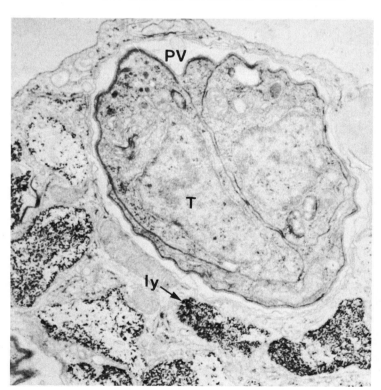

Figure 27.4. Transmission electron micrograph of a portion of macrophage infected with the tachyzoites of *Toxoplasma gondii (T)*. Although the lysosomes (*ly*) have taken up thorotrast, there is no evidence of fusion with the parasitophorous vacuole (*PV*). ×31,000. (Courtesy of Dr. T Jones)

In acquired toxoplasmosis, the lesions are less intense. There are foci of inflammation around the parasites in muscles and other tissues, such as spleen, liver, and lymph nodes, and there may be interstitial pneumonitis.

Clinical Disease

Congenital Toxoplasmosis

The spectrum of congenital infection varies from asymptomatic to one causing very severe damage to the central nervous system and stillbirth. Approximately 90% of infants born to mothers infected during pregnancy remain free of any disease; 7% have relatively minor abnormalities, but 3% have very severe damage that involves the vital tissues mentioned above. These frequencies are twice as high for those pregnancies in which the infection occurs during the first two trimesters.[9] Retinochoroiditis and cerebral calcifications are the most common abnormalities. Severely affected infants may have hepatosplenomegaly, liver failure, thrombocytopenia, convulsions, and hydrocephalus. Furthermore, in newborns who have acquired the infection congenitally, new lesions continue to develop, increasing the likelihood that severe impairment to the central nervous system will occur.[10]

Acquired Toxoplasmosis

The majority of acquired infections are asymptomatic. Those that are clinically apparent present usually as mild disease, characterized by generalized lymphadenopathy, with predominant enlargement of the cervical nodes, sometimes associated with a low-grade fever. In the main, the disease mimics infectious mononucleosis. Rarely, acquired toxoplasmosis can be quite severe, involving major vital organs and systems. Infected individuals may suffer myocarditis and encephalitis. In addition, some patients develop space-occupying lesions of the central nervous system, consisting of necrotic masses. Retinochoroiditis in acquired toxoplasmosis[11] is rare.

Recrudescent Toxoplasmosis

This form of toxoplasmosis is clinically identical to postnatal infection, but it usually occurs in immunosuppressed patients.[12] It can be distinguished from the acquired form only hypothetically, whenever it is possible to determine that the patient had positive serology *before* developing clinical manifestations. Toxoplasmic encephalitis is a major consequence of recrudescence, especially in immunologically impaired individuals.[13] The pseudocysts rupture, releasing organisms into the surrounding tissues.

Diagnosis

Specific diagnosis is made by serological tests and by demonstration of the organisms in tissues.

Serological tests depend on the identification of specific IgG, IgM, and complement fixing (CF) antibodies.[14] The commonly used tests measure IgG. These are either the Sabin-Feldman dye test or the indirect immunofluorescence test (IFA). The latter is easier to carry out, because it does not require live organisms; therefore, it is the more common test. Specific IFA test of the IgM is also available.

The IgM antibodies appear first a few days after the infection. Titers of IgM antibodies are usually elevated at a level greater than 1:80 during the first 2–3 months after infection and reach undetectable levels shortly thereafter. The IgG antibodies appear within 1–2 weeks after the infection and usually rise to titers above 1:1024; these antibodies are detectable for many years, perhaps indefinitely. CF antibodies first become detectable approximately 1 month after the infection, and the titer of 1:16 is considered significant in most laboratories. The CF antibodies are short-lived and parallel clinical disease. They may persist for several years, but eventually disappear completely.

Interpretation of serologic tests is fundamental to confirming the diagnosis. Significant rises in titers of IgG or CF antibodies between acute and convalescent serum specimens are best evidence of an acute infection. A single elevated IgM titer early in infection is also diagnostic. In congenital infections, presence of specific IgM antibodies in the infant's serum is diagnostic. In determining specific IgG titers, it is important to measure maternal antibodies simultaneously with those of the infant. If the titer in the infant's serum is significantly higher (a fourfold difference), the infant must be presumed to be infected. If the two titers are identical, it is necessary to repeat the test in the infant at 4 months of age. The infant must be presumed to have been infected if his titer has not decreased or has risen.

Histological examination of lymph node tissue obtained at biopsy may show the characteristic, but nonspecific, histiocytic hyperplasia (Fig. 27.5) consistent with toxoplasmosis.[15] Isolation of the organisms involves intraperitoneal inoculation of mice pretreated with corticosteroids. Smears of peritoneal fluid, or brain tissue of the mice, obtained 3–5 weeks later may reveal toxoplasma (Fig. 27.6). The test is laborious and can be carried out in only a few laboratories.

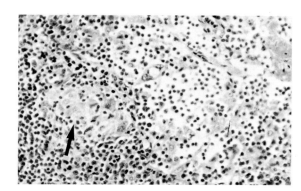

Figure 27.5. Cross section of a lymph node from an adult patient with lymphadenitis. Enlarged histiocytes, termed Piringa-Kuchenka cells (*arrow*), characteristic of infection with *Toxoplasma gondii* are seen in section. ×110.

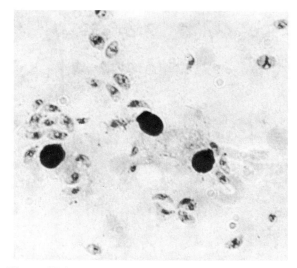

Figure 27.6. Impression smear of brain from mouse injected with a portion of a lymph node from a patient with suspected acquired toxoplasmosis. The patient was infected as seen by the presence of organisms in mouse brain cells. ×990.

Treatment

The infection must be treated with a combination of pyrimethamine and sulfadiazine for 4 weeks. Results can be difficult to evaluate because of the natural variability of the clinical disease. Congenital toxoplasmosis, severe acquired toxoplasmosis, and recrudescent infection in immunosuppressed patients must be treated. However, in the latter, rigorous treatment results in only a 50% cure rate.[16] Other forms of the infection require no therapy. Pyrimethamine is a folic acid antagonist. Therefore, it is necessary to monitor the patient's blood count for lymphocytopenia and thrombocytopenia. This undesirable effect of therapy can be prevented by administration of folinic acid.

Prevention and Control

Adult acquired toxoplasmosis can be prevented by avoiding consumption of uncooked or rare meat. However, this preventive measure often fails, because consumption of rare meat is common in many countries.

Prevention of infection from oocysts requires care in handling cat feces, especially during cleaning of litter boxes. This activity must be proscribed for pregnant women. Toxoplasmosis can also be acquired as the result of inhalation of dust containing oocysts.

References

1. Nicolle C, Manceaux LH: Sur une infection a coyes de Leishman (ou organismes voisins) du gondi. C R Hebdomad Seance Acad Sci 147:763–766, 1908
2. Splendore A: Un nuovo protozoa parassita dei conigli: Incontrato nelle lesioni anatomiche d'ua malttia che ricorda in molti punti il Kala-azar dell'uomo. Rev Soc Sci Sao Paulo 3:109–112, 1908
3. Janku J: Pathogenesis and pathologic anatomy of the ''congenital coloboma'' of the macula lutea in an eye of normal size, with microscopic detection of parasites in the retina. J Czech Phys 62:1021–1027, 1923
4. Wolf A, Cowen D, Paige BH: Human toxoplasmosis: Occurrence in infants as encephalomyelitis: Verification by transmission to animals. Science 89:226–277, 1939
5. Pinkerton H, Henderson RG: Adult toxoplasmosis: A previously unrecognized disease entity simulating

the typhus-spotted fever group. JAMA 116:807–814, 1941

6. Sabin AB: Toxoplasmic encephalitis in children. JAMA 116:801–807, 1941

7. Frenkel JK, Dubey JP, Miller NL: *Toxoplasma gondii* in cats: Fecal stages identified as coccidian oocysts. Science 167:893–896, 1970

8. Hutchinson WM, Dunachie JF, Sim JC et al.: Coccidian-like nature of *Toxoplasma gondii*. Br Med J 1:142–144, 1970

9. Desmonts G, Couvrer J: Congenital toxoplasmosis. A prospective study of 378 pregnancies. N Engl J Med 290:1110–1116, 1974

10. Koppe JG, Loewer-Sieger DH, Roever-Bonnet H: Results of 20-year follow-up of congenital toxoplasmosis. Lancet, 1:254–256, 1986

11. Masur H, Jones TC, Lempert JA, et al.: Outbreak of toxoplasmosis in a family and documentation of acquired retinochoroiditis. Am J Med 64:396–402, 1978

12. Ruskin J, Remington JS: Toxoplasmosis in the compromised host. Ann Intern Med 84:193–199, 1976

13. Wanke C, Tuazon CU, Kovacs A et al.: Toxoplasma encephalitis in patients with acquired immune deficiency syndrome: diagnosis and response to therapy. Am J Trop Med Hyg 36:509–516, 1987

14. Welch PC, Masur H, Jones TC, et al.: Serologic diagnosis of acute lymphadenopathic toxoplasmosis. J Infect Dis 142:256–264, 1980

15. Dorfman RF, Remington JS: Value of lymph-node biopsy in the diagnosis of acute acquired toxoplasmosis. N Engl J Med 289:878–881, 1973

16. Haverkos HW: Assessment of therapy for Toxoplasma encephalitis. Am J Med 72:907–914, 1987

28. *Cryptosporidium sp.*

Introduction

The genus Cryptosporidium constitutes a group of parasitic protozoans all of which can cause transient diarrhea in a wide variety of hosts, such as sheep, cattle, birds, rodents, and primates, including man.[1] Experimental evidence based on crossinfectivity of Cryptosporidium recovered from different hosts suggests that the number of species of this organism is quite limited.[2] It seems that many species of animals harboring Cryptosporidium act as reservoirs of the human infection. The organism is worldwide in distribution. It is considered a pathogen for all ages and both sexes of man, in whom it causes subclinical infection, or a mild diarrhea. In infants, immunodeficient adults, and AIDS patients it can cause severe diarrhea and even fatalities.[3]

Historical Information

Tyzzer, in 1907, provided a description of this organism based on histological sections of mouse intestine in which the parasites were observed attached to the epithelial cells. He originated the generic name Cryptosporidium.[4] The pathogenic characteristics of this protozoan were not recognized until much later when Slavin, in 1955, established that Cryptosporidium caused diarrhea in turkeys.[5] Human diarrheal disease due to Cryptosporidium was first described by Nime et al.[6] and Meisel et al[7], in 1976, who reported it in immunocompromised hosts.

Life Cycle

Most of the details of the life cycle of Cryptosporidium have been derived from experimental infections in mice and other rodents. Subsequently all of the stages have been demonstrated in man, as well.[8]

Infection begins when the host ingests the sporulated oocysts, each of which contains four sporozoites, which represent the infectious stage (Fig. 28.1). When the oocyst reaches the small intestine, the sporozoites excyst—by an unknown mechanism—and immediately attach to the epithelial surface of the mucosa. In response, the microvilli in the area immediately adjacent to the attachment fuse and elongate, and envelop the sporozoite. The parasite which is now intracellular, matures first into a trophozoite (Fig. 28.2)

Cryptosporidium

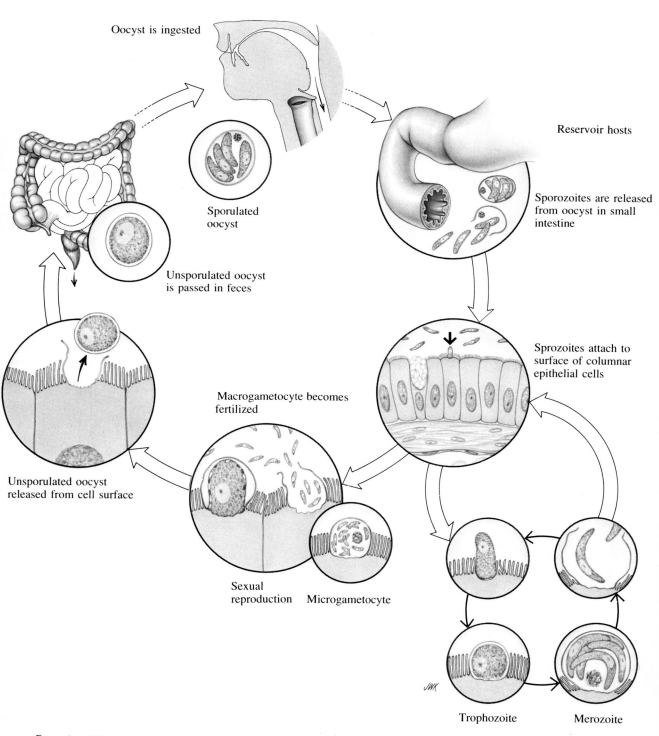

Oocyst is ingested

Sporulated oocyst

Unsporulated oocyst is passed in feces

Reservoir hosts

Sporozoites are released from oocyst in small intestine

Sprozoites attach to surface of columnar epithelial cells

Unsporulated oocyst released from cell surface

Macrogametocyte becomes fertilized

Sexual reproduction

Microgametocyte

Trophozoite

Merozoite

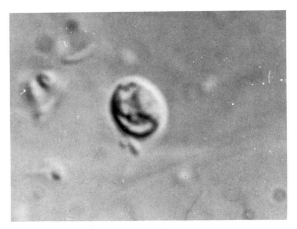

Figure 28.1 The unsporulated oocyst of *Cryptosporidium* Nomarski-phase interference photomicrograph. ×4,000.

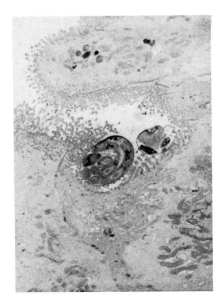

Figure 28.3 Merozoites of *Cryptosporidium sp*. Electron micrograph. Seven of the eight organisms can be seen in this view. × 4,000

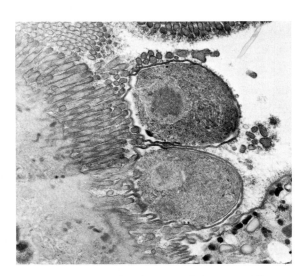

Figure 28.2 The trophozoite stage of *Cryptosporidium sp*. Electron micrograph. Note the host-derived limiting membrane surrounding the organisms .

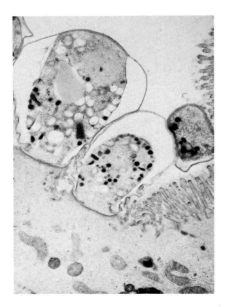

Figure 28.4 Macrogametocyte (♀) of *Cryptosporidium sp*. Electron micrograph.

and then into a schizont. The latter divides into eight first-generation merozoites (Fig. 28.3) which are released into the intestinal lumen as the infected cell ruptures. Each merozoite attaches to a new epithelial cell and division ensues once again, except that schizogony now results in only four merozoites. Second-generation merozoites attach to uninfected epithelial cells and transform into either male microgametocytes or female macrogametoctes (Fig. 28.4). The microgameto-

cytes undergo several divisions, producing microgametes capable of mating with macrogametocytes, the union producing a zygote. The zygote differentiates into an unsporulated oocyst, which detaches from the epithelium of the intestine and is shed in feces. The oocyst is infectious when shed. Each will sporulate upon being swallowed by a new host, or in the soil.

The mechanism of sexual differentiation of merozoites is not known, but it has been reproduced in vitro.[9] It appears therefore that a functioning immune system of the host does not play a role in determining the maturation of merozoites. It is known, however, that the life cycle of *Cryptosporidium* in immunocompromised hosts differs from that in the normal host. In patients with AIDS, for example, many more division cycles occur than in the normal host. In these patients, the entire surface of the small and large intestines (Fig. 28.5) can be infected with all stages of this protozoan.[10]

Pathogenesis

Infection with Cryptosporidium results in hypersecretion of intestinal fluid, which leads to loss of water and electrolytes, the mechanism of which is not known. Although the diarrhea resembles that of cholera, no toxin has been identified. Villous atrophy has been noted in patients with prolonged infection.[11] Ultrastructural studies[10] of the intestine of patients with AIDS have shown that infected epithelial cells have altered

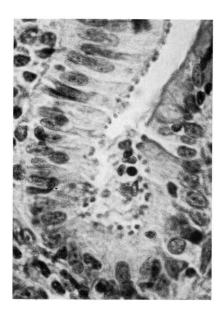

Figure 28.5 Histological section of small intestine from an AIDS patient who died as the result of infection with *Cryptosporidium sp*. Note the extent of the infection (arrows indicate individual organisms).

mitochondria, and myelin figures indicative of phagolysosomal activity. Whether these changes, limited as they are to this special group of patients, have any relationship to the pathophysiology of infection is uncertain.

Clinical Disease

Clinial manifestations of cryptosporidiosis vary from a subclinical infection or a mild diarrhea to fulminant watery diarrhea productive of loose stool, free of mucus and blood. There is associated upper abdominal cramping, anorexia, nausea, and vomiting.

The major factor in determining severity of the disease is immunocompetence. Normal individuals experience a self-limited disease lasting from several days—in the usual case—to one month. On the other hand in immunocompromised patients, cryptosporidiosis cases have a chronic course lasting for months and even years.[12,13] The disease assumes particular severity in patients with AIDS, who can lose some 3 liters of fluid per day.

Normal hosts recover from the infection with no untoward aftereffects. Immunocompromised hosts are in significant danger of dying; case fatality rate is 50%.[11] However, death is usually a result of associated conditions, such as malnutrition or superinfection with other pathogens. At post mortem examination, the organism has been confined to the gastrointestinal tract, within which is has been widely disseminated from the pharynx to the colon.

Diagnosis

There is no abnormality in any of the indirect tests, such as blood count and erythrocyte sedimentation rate. Diagnosis depends on the finding of oocysts in the stool (Fig. 28.1) or any of the stages of the organism on histological sections of the gut. Stool examination requires a special method of immersion of the specimen in a sucrose solution, which allows the oocysts to float to the surface.[14] They are then examined directly under phase contrast microscopy, or fixed and treated with a modified Kinyoun acid fast stain, which reveals them best, although they can also be examined using Giemsa, or hematoxylin-eosin stain. It is important to differentiate unsporulated oocysts from yeast.

Treatment

No therapy is required for normal patients with this infection, in whom it is self-limited. Immunocompromised hosts are treated with spiramycin, but fewer than half of the patients show any improvement. None of the usual antiprotozoal drugs is effective. Neither are any of the antidiarrheal agents, such as kaolin-pectin, diphenoxylate and opiates, or any dietary restrictions effective in alleviating the symptoms.[1]

Prevention and Control

Cryptosporidium is ubiquitous and therefore the infection it causes is difficult to prevent. There is insufficient information about its epidemiology to recommend any substantive preventive measures.

References

1. Navin, TR, Juranek DD: *Cryptosporidium:* Clinical, epidemiologic, and parasitologic review. Rev Inf Dis 6:313–327, 1984
2. Tzipori S, Angus TW, Grey EW et al.: Diarrhea in lambs experimentally infected with *Cryptosporidium* isolated from calves. Am J Vet Res 42:1400–1404, 1981.
3. Current WL, Reese NC, Ernst JV et al.: Human cryptosporidiosis in immunocompetent and immunodeficient persons. N Eng J Med 308:1252–1257, 1983
4. Tyzzer EE: A sporozoan found in the peptic glands of the common mouse. Proc Soc Exp Biol Med 5:12–13, 1907
5. Slavin D: *Cryptosporidium meleagridis* (Sp. nov.) J Comp Pathol 65:262–266, 1955
6. Nime FA, Burek JD, Page DL, et al.: Acute enterocolitis in a human being infected with the protozoan *Cryptosporidium.* Gasteroenterol 70:592–598, 1976
7. Meisel JE, Perera DR, Meloigro C, et al.: Overwhelming water diarrhea associated with *Cryptosporidium* in an immunosuppressed patient. Gastroenterol 70:1156–1160, 1976
8. Bird RG, Smith MD: Cryptosporidiosis in man. Parasite life cycle and fine structural pathology. J Pathol 132:217, 1980
9. Current WL, Haynes TB: Complete development of *Cryptosporidium* in cell culture. Science 224:603–605, 1984
10. Lefkowitch JH, Krumholtz S, Kuo-Ching F-C et al.: Crytosporidiosis of the human small intestine: A light and electron microscopic study. Hum Pathol 15:746–752, 1984
11. Stemmerman GN, Hayashi T, Glober GA, et al.: Crytosporidiosis: Report of a fatal case complicated by disseminated toxoplasmosis. Am J Trop Med Hyg 69:637–642, 1980
12. Slope KS, Dormashkin RR, Bird RB et al.: Chronic malabsorption due to crytosporidiosis in a child with immunoglobulin deficiency. Gut 23:80–82, 1982
13. Sloave R, Danne RL, Lonig Cl et al.: Crytosporidiosis in homosexual men. Ann Int Med 100:504–511, 1984
14. Ma P, Soave R: Three-step stool examination for cryptosporidiosis in 10 homosexual men with protracted watery diarrhea. J Inf Dis 147:824–829, 1983

29. The Malarias: *Plasmodium falciparum* (Welch 1898), *Plasmodium vivax* (Grassi and Filetti 1889), *Plasmodium ovale* (Stephens 1922), and *Plasmodium malariae* (Laveran 1881)

Malaria is a mosquito-borne infection caused by protozoa of the genus Plasmodium. Man is commonly infected by four species of the parasite, *Plasmodium falciparum, P. vivax, P. ovale,* and *P. malariae.* On rare occasions, certain species of Plasmodium of simian hosts also infect man.

Malaria is one of the most prevalent diseases in the world. More than 200 million cases and at least one million consequent deaths are estimated to occur annually. Over one-half of the world's population lives in areas where malaria is endemic. Although formerly found throughout much of the world, with seasonal outbreaks extending into temperate zones, malaria is now generally

Mosquito Cycle (Sporogany)

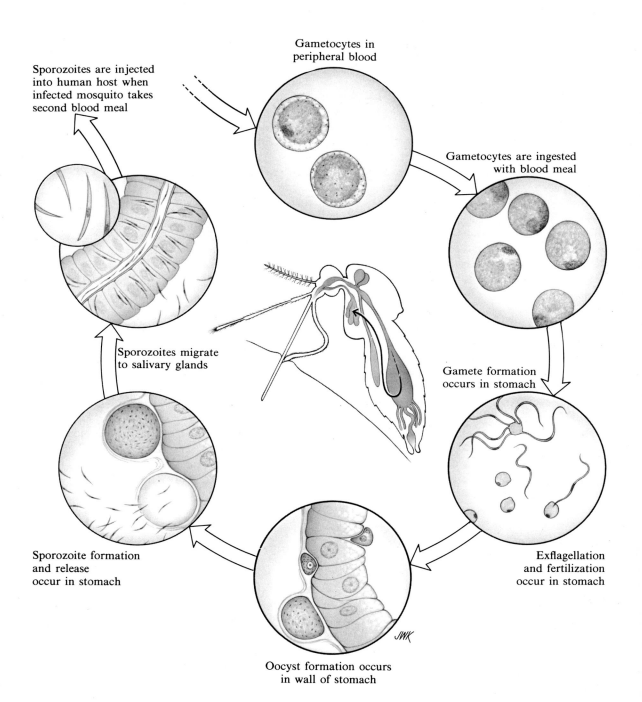

Gametocytes in
peripheral blood

Sporozoites are injected
into human host when
infected mosquito takes
second blood meal

Gametocytes are ingested
with blood meal

Sporozoites migrate
to salivary glands

Gamete formation
occurs in stomach

Sporozoite formation
and release
occur in stomach

Exflagellation
and fertilization
occur in stomach

Oocyst formation occurs
in wall of stomach

JWK

restricted to tropical and subtropical regions. However, travel and persistence of mosquito vectors continue to pose a threat of re-introduction of these parasites into non-immune populations.

Historical Information

Malaria most certainly afflicted man's ancestors. The earliest medical writers in China, Assyria, and India described malaria-like intermittent fevers, which they attributed to evil spirits. By the 5th century B.C., Hippocrates was able to differentiate quotidian, tertian, and quartan fevers and the clinical symptoms of the disease. At that time it was assumed that it was caused by vapors and mists arising from swamps and marshes. These theories persisted for more than 2000 years and were reinforced by repeated observations that the draining of swamps lead to reduction in the number of cases of malaria. Indeed, the names for this disease, "malaria" (*mal,* bad; *aria,* air) and "paludisme" (*palus,* marsh) reflect these beliefs.

All concepts of malaria changed within only 20 years following Laveran's description of the asexual stage of *P. falciparum* in 1880. The sexual cycle of the parasite was described by Mac-Callum in 1897. In 1898 Ross, using a species of bird malaria, and Grassi and colleagues, working with human malaria, showed that the parasite developed in the mosquito and was transmitted by the bite of the insect. Ultimately, Ross and Laveran were awarded Nobel prizes for their contributions.[1]

The basic life cycle of the malarial parasite was explained at the turn of this century. The scientific efforts then shifted to the attempts at control of the disease itself. In the main they were attempts to control the number of mosquitos. Another 30 years passed before the exoerythrocytic phase of malaria was described in birds; it was 20 years later that the analogous stages were discovered in the simian and human livers. The path taken by the malarial parasites after infection still remains obscure.

Chemotherapy of malaria preceded the description of the parasite by nearly 300 years. The Peruvian bark, cinchona, the so-called fever tree bark, was first used in the early part of the 17th century, but the details of its discovery and its introduction into Europe are unknown.[2] The alkaloids of the cinchona tree, quinine and cinchonine, were eventually isolated in 1820 by Pelletier and Caventou. Synthetic antimalarial compounds effective against various stages of the parasite were later developed in Germany (pamaquine, in 1924; mepacrine, in 1930; chloroquine, in 1934), in Britain (proquanil, in 1944), and in the United States (pyrimethamine and primaquine, in 1952).

The Greeks and Romans practiced the earliest forms of malaria control by draining swamps and marshes, albeit inadvertently, as their purpose was reclamation of land. These techniques were continued for centuries until the role of the mosquito as vector was discovered. Almost immediately, malaria control became synonymous with the control of mosquitoes. Destruction of breeding places by drainage and filling and killing of larvae by placing oil on the waters, and later by addition of the larvicide Paris Green, were the typical early attempts. With the development of DDT, a residual insecticide, large-scale control programs became possible. They culminated in 1957 in the launching by the World Health Organization of a worldwide eradication program.

Life Cycles

The biology of the four species of Plasmodium is generally similar and consists of two discrete stages, the sexual and the asexual. The asexual stage in man develops first in the liver and then in the circulating erythrocytes; the sexual stage develops in the mosquito.

Asexual Stages

Exoerythrocytic (Hepatic) Phase

When the infected female anopheles mosquito bites and sucks blood, she injects salivary fluids into the wound. These fluids contain sporozoites, small (10–15 μm long), spindle-shaped, motile forms of the parasite (Fig. 29.1), which initiate the infection. They are cleared from the circulation within an hour and eventually reach parenchymal cells of the liver (Fig. 29.2). The route that sporozoites follow to the liver has not been established beyond doubt and the hypotheses are

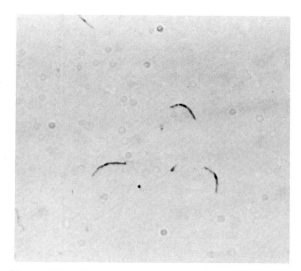

Figure 29.1. Sporozoite stage of malaria. ×990.

subjects of controversy. In vivo studies with the rodent malaria *P. berghei* suggest that circulating sporozoites are first taken up by the Küpffer cells and from there pass into hepatocytes.[3] In vitro experiments with a variety of malaria species, including *P. vivax*, *P. falciparum*, and *P. bergei* have shown direct invasion of a variety of cell types by sporozoites without the involvement of an intermediate step in Küpffer cells[4].

Once inside the liver cell, the parasites undergo asexual division (exoerythrocytic [EE] schizogony). The length of this EE phase and the number of progeny (merozoites) produced within each infected cell is a characteristic of the individual

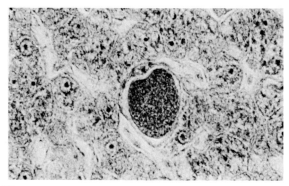

Figure 29.2. The liver parenchymal cell harbors the exoerythrocytic stages of the life cycle. Schizogony results in the production of hundreds of merozoites. ×690.

species of Plasmodium. *P. vivax* can mature within 6–8 days, and each of its sporozoites produces about 10,000 daughter parasites. For *P. ovale*, these values are 9 days and 15,000 merozoites; for *P. malariae*, 12–16 days and 2000 merozoites; and for *P. falciparum*, 5–7 days and 40,000 merozoites.

The phenomenon of a relapse in certain malarias, e.g. *P. vivax*, *P. ovale*, *P. cynomolgi*, has not been fully explained. By definition, a parasitological relapse in malaria is "the reappearance of parasitemia in sporozoite-induced infection, following adequate blood schizontocidal therapy."[5] It has been long accepted that the exoerythrocytic forms of relapsing malaria persisted in the liver as a result of cyclical development (i.e. rupture of infected cells, and invasion of new cells).[6] However, experimental evidence has lent support to a different hypothesis for the mechanism of relapse. It holds that some sporozoites fail to initiate immediate exoerythrocytic development in the liver and remain latent, as the so-called hypnozoites capable of delayed development and intitiation of relapse.[7]

In vivax and ovale malarias, eradication of parasites from the peripheral circulation with drugs aborts the acute infection. Subsequently a fresh wave of exoerythrocytic merozoites from the liver can reinitiate the infection. The dormant parasites, or hypnozoites can remain quiescent in the liver for up to five years. In order to achieve radical cure, it is necessary to destroy not only the circulating plasmodia, but also the hypnozoites. *P. falciparum* and *P. malariae* do not develop hypnozoites and therefore lack the capacity to relapse. Untreated *P. falciparum* can recrudesce for one to two years through the continuation of the erythrocytic cycle, which for periods of time remains at a subclinical, asymptomatic level; *P. malariae* can do so for up to 30 years. In both infections radical cure can be achieved by those drugs that eradicate only the parasites in the peripheral circulation.

Erythrocytic Phase

When merozoites are released from the liver schizonts, they invade red blood cells and initiate the erythrocytic phase of infection (Fig. 29.3). Invasion of the erythrocytes consists of a complex

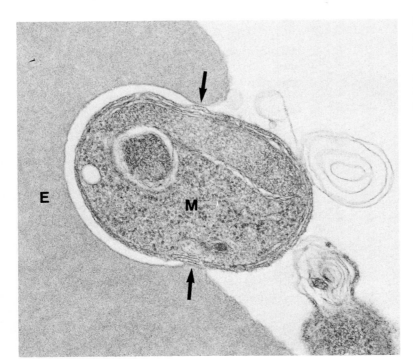

Figure 29.3. A merozoite of *Plasmodium falciparum* (*M*) in the process of entering an erythrocyte (*E*). The *arrows* indicate the points of contact between the parasite and the red cell membrane. ×47,000. (Courtesy of Dr. S. Langreth)

sequence of events beginning with contact between a free-floating merozoite and the red cell.[8] Attachment of the merozoite to the erythrocyte membrane involves an interaction with specific receptor sites. Thereafter, the erythrocyte undergoes rapid and marked deformation. The parasite enters by a localized endocytic invagination of the red cell membrane, utilizing a moving junction between the parasite and the host cell membrane.[9]

Once within the cell, the parasite begins to grow, first forming the ring-like early trophozoite (Fig. 29.4), then enlarging to fill the cell (Figs. 29.5 and 29.6). The organism then undergoes asexual division and becomes a schizont composed of merozoites. The parasites are nourished by the hemoglobin within the erythrocytes and produce a characteristic pigment, hemazoin. The erythrocytic cycle is completed when the red cell ruptures and releases merozoites, which proceed to invade other erythrocytes.

This cycle is characteristically synchronous and periodic. *P. falciparum*, *P. vivax*, and *P. ovale* complete the development from invasion by merozoites to the rupture of the erythrocyte within 48 h, thus exhibiting the so-called tertian periodicity.

P. malariae, the quartan malaria, requires 72 h to complete the cycle.

Infection with erythrocytic phase merozoites can also occur as a result of blood transfusion from an infected donor[10] or through a contaminated needle shared among drug addicts. Malaria acquired in this manner is referred to as induced malaria. Congenital malaria as a result of transplacental infection can develop.[11]

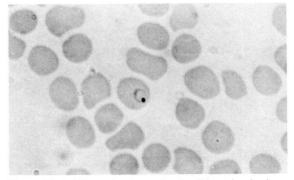

Figure 29.4. The early phase of red cell invasion is characterized by the "signet ring" stage of *Plasmodium* spp. ×1,140.

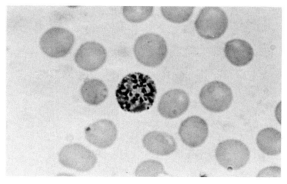

Figure 29.5. The end stage of trophozoite division called the schizont. ×1,140.

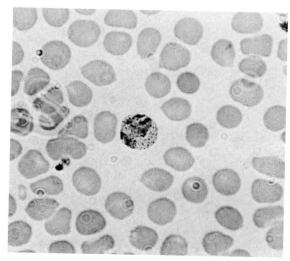

Figure 29.7. Macrogametocyte stage of *Plasmodium*. ×1,140.

Sexual Stages

Not all merozoites develop asexually. Some become differentiated into the sexual forms, the macrogametocytes (female) (Fig. 29.7) and microgametocytes (males) (Fig. 29.8), which can complete their development only within the gut of an appropriate mosquito vector. On entering the mosquito in the blood meal, the gametocytes shed their protective erythrocyte membrane in the gut of the vector. Male gametocytes initiate exflagellation (Fig. 29.9), a rapid process that produces up to eight active, sperm-like microgametes, which eventually fertilize the macrogametes. The resulting zygotes elongate into diploid vermiform

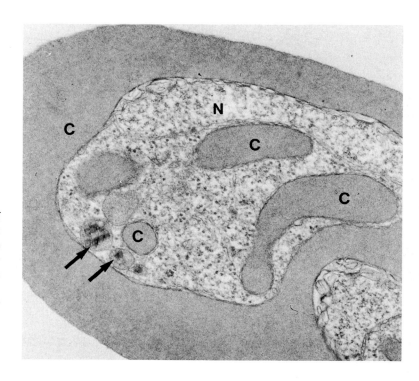

Figure 29.6. A young trophozoite of *Plasmodium falciparum* within an infected red cell. The food vacuoles (*arrows*) are filled with partially digested host cell cytoplasm and a breakdown product of hemoglobin. The nucleus (*N*) of the parasite is also seen, as well as an undigested portion of red cell cytoplasm (*C*). ×42,000. (Courtesy of Dr. S. Langreth)

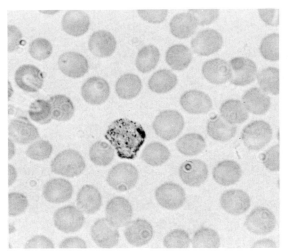

Figure 29.8. Microgametocyte stage of *Plasmodium.* × 1,140.

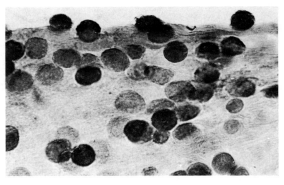

Figure 29.10. Oocysts on the stomach wall of an infected female anopheline mosquito. × 315.

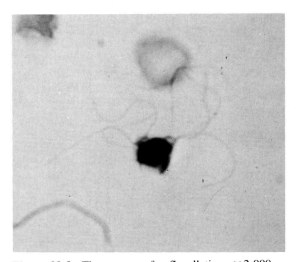

Figure 29.9. The process of exflagellation. × 2,000.

oökinetes, which penetrate the gut wall and come to lie under the basement membrane. The parasites then transform into oocysts (Fig. 29.10) within 24 h of ingestion of the blood meal. Development of sporozoites follows, leading to the production of thousands of these forms, which are now haploid. They mature within 10–14 days, escape from the oocyst, and invade the salivary glands. When the mosquito bites the human host again, a new cycle begins.

Although the four species have marked physiologic differences and some major differences in the pathologic course they pursue, they are best differentiated on the basis of their morphology. Thus the blood smear, fixed and stained with Giemsa or Wright solution, is the basis of the fundamental diagnostic test. Currently alternatives are being developed.

Plasmodium falciparum

Infection caused by *P. falciparum* produces a form of malaria historically referred to as aestivo-autumnal, malignant tertian, or simply falciparum malaria. This is the most pathogenic of the human malarias, accounts for most of the mortality caused by malaria, and is the most prevelant of the human malaria infections.

Falciparum malaria is now generally confined to tropical and subtropical regions and is the primary form of malaria in sub-Saharan Africa.

Identification of *P. falciparum* is usually based on the presence of small ring-stage parasites on blood smears (see Color Plate, Fig. 29.11). Infected erythrocytes are not enlarged, and multiple infections of a single erythrocyte are common. The rings often show two distinct chromatin dots.

As trophozoites mature, they become sequestered in the capillaries of internal organs, such as the heart, brain, spleen, skeletal muscles, the placenta, and others, where they complete their development. As a result of the sequestration, maturing parasites usually are not present in the peripheral circulation.

Appearance in the peripheral circulation of the mature asexual stages, i.e., larger trophozoites and schizonts, indicates an extreme severity of the disease.

Gametocytogenesis also proceeds in the sequestered erythrocytes and requires approximately 10 days. The falciparum gametocytes are characteristically crescent-, or banana-shaped. They remain infectious for mosquitoes for as long as 4 days.

Falciparum malaria does not relapse; i.e., the erythrocytes do not become reinfected from a persistent infection in the liver, once the parasites are cleared from the blood by drugs or by the immune response of the host. However, recrudescences, i.e., reinfections of the erythrocytes from the blood forms of the malaria maintained at very low levels, are common and can recur for about 2 years.

Plasmodium vivax

P. vivax infection is called benign tertian, or vivax malaria.

Red blood cells infected with P. vivax are enlarged and show stippling, known as Schüffner's dots, on the cell membrane (see Color Plate, Fig. 29.12). All stages of the parasite are present in the peripheral circulation. Single infections of invaded erythrocytes are characteristic. Gametocytes appear simultaneously with the first asexual parasites. The duration of their infectivity has not been determined.

P. vivax produces the classic relapsing malaria, initiated from hypnozoites in the liver, which have resumed development after a period of latency. Relapses can occur at periods ranging from every few weeks to a few months for up to 5 years following initial infection. The specific periodicity of the relapses is a characteristic of the geographic strain of the parasite. Vivax malaria also has recrudescences from the erythrocytic parasites.

Plasmodium ovale

P. ovale is the most recently described species of human malaria. Its distribution is limited to tropical Africa and to discrete areas of the Western Pacific. Ovale malaria (see Color Plate, Fig. 29.13) produces a tertian fever, clinically similar to that of vivax malaria, but somewhat less severe. It also exhibits relapses for as long as vivax malaria.

Plasmodium malariae

The disease caused by this species of the parasite (see Color Plate, Fig. 29.14) is known as quartan malaria. P. malariae has a wide, but spotty, distribution throughout the world. Development in the mosquito is slow and infection of man is not as intense as that due to the other Plasmodium species. Most current evidence indicates that P. malariae does not relapse. It does have recrudescences originating from chronic erythrocytic infections.

Simian Malarias That Infect Man

Some species of Plasmodium that are parasites of chimpanzees and monkeys occasionally infect

Plasmodium vivax

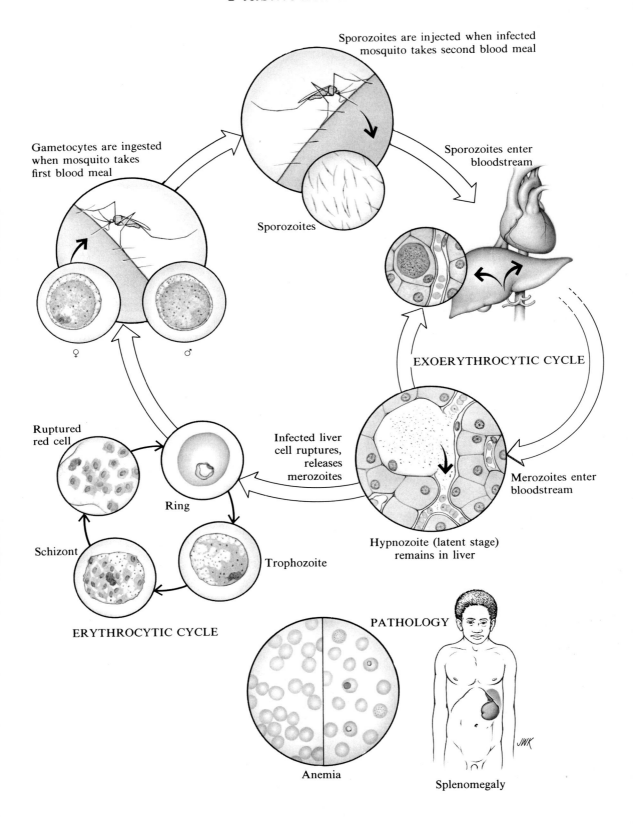

Sporozoites are injected when infected
mosquito takes second blood meal

Gametocytes are ingested
when mosquito takes
first blood meal

Sporozoites enter
bloodstream

Sporozoites

♀   ♂

EXOERYTHROCYTIC CYCLE

Ruptured
red cell

Infected liver
cell ruptures,
releases
merozoites

Ring

Merozoites enter
bloodstream

Schizont

Trophozoite

Hypnozoite (latent stage)
remains in liver

ERYTHROCYTIC CYCLE

PATHOLOGY

Anemia

Splenomegaly

JWK

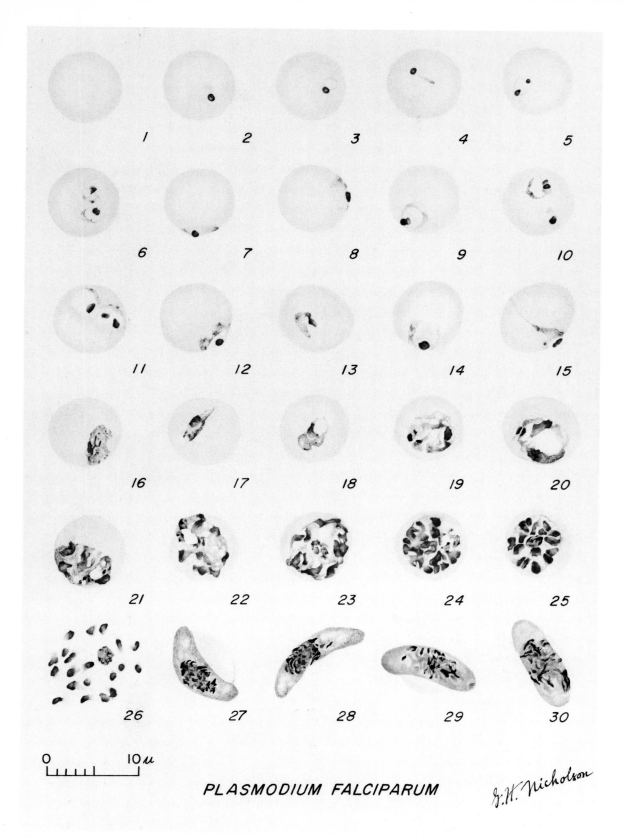

Figure 29.11. Erythrocytic stages of *Plasmodium falciparum*. Trophozoites (*1–18*); schizonts (*19–26*); macrogametocytes (*27, 28*); microgametocytes (*29, 30*).

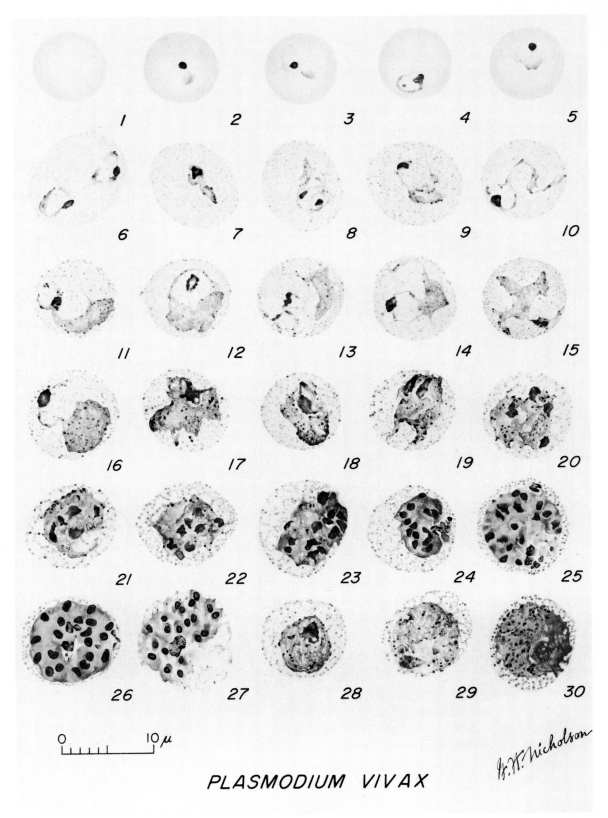

PLASMODIUM VIVAX

Figure 29.12. Erythrocytic stages of *Plasmodium vivax*. Trophozoites (*1–18*); schizonts (*19–27*); macrogametocytes (*28, 29*); microgametocyte (*30*).

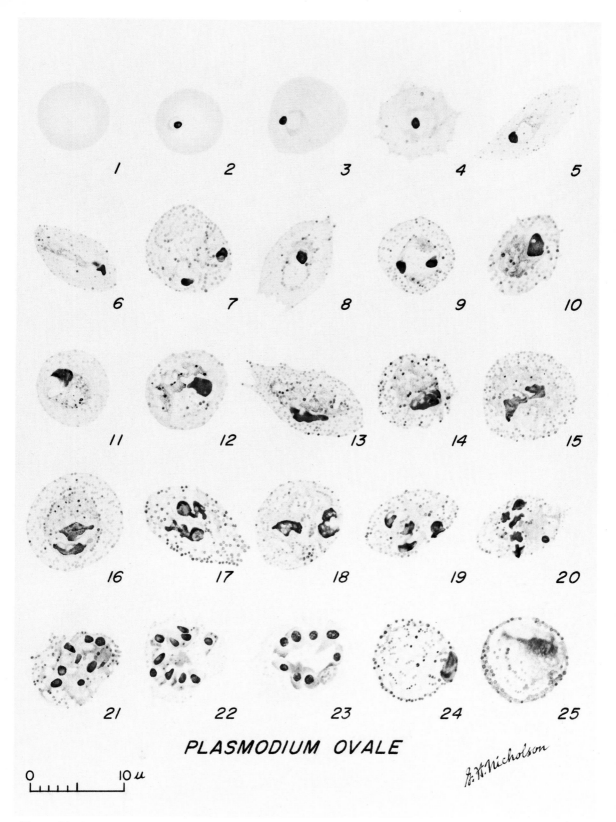

PLASMODIUM OVALE

0 � 10 μ

Ḟ.Ḣ.Nicholson

Figure 29.13. Erythrocytic cycle of *Plasmodium ovale*. Trophozoites (*1–15*); schizonts (*16–23*); macrogametocyte (*24*); microgametocyte (*25*).

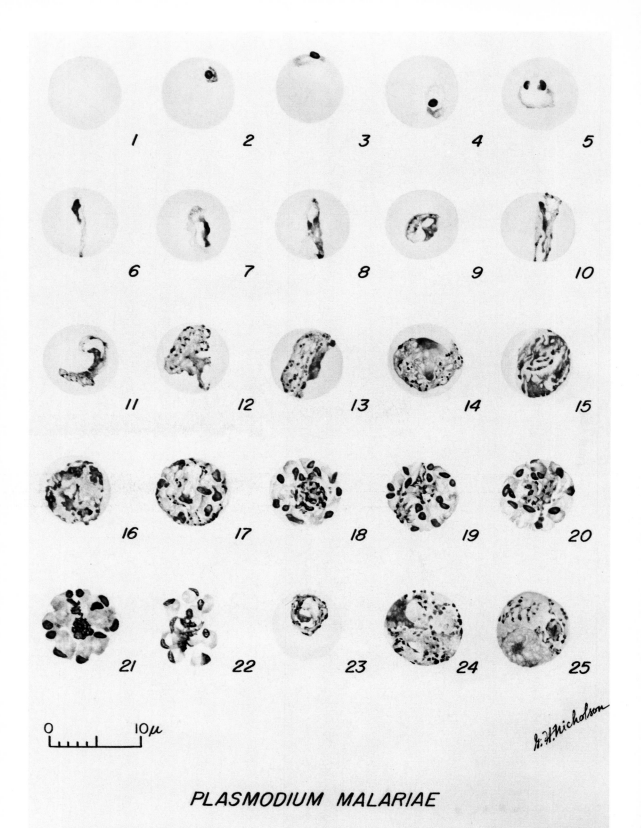

Figure 29.14. Erythrocytic stages of *Plasmodium malariae*. Trophozites (*2–13*); schizonts (*14–22*); macrogametocyte (*24*); microgametocyte (*25*).

man.[12] The disease they cause is relatively mild. Most notable is the quotidian fever (24-h cycle) caused by *P. knowlesi* and the vivax-like malaria caused by *P. cynomolgi*.

Pathogenesis

The rupture of erythrocytes and release of pyrogens cause fever and the consequent chills and sweating associated with malaria. Pathogenesis of general malaise, myalgia, and headache is not clear. The characteristic periodicity of the fever, based on synchronous infections, is not invariable. Early phases of all infections often are not synchronous. Some infections may be due to two or more broods of parasites, with the periodicity of one independent of that of the others. In severe falciparum malaria, the patient may feel febrile continually.[13]

Cerebral malaria (Fig. 29.15) is the most con-

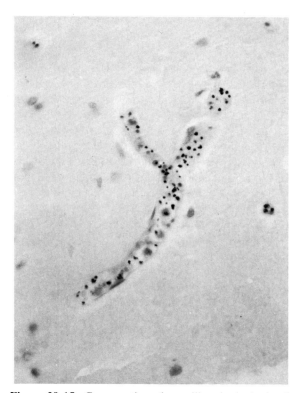

Figure 29.15. Cross-section of a capillary in the brain of a patient who died of cerebral malaria caused by *Plasmodium falciparum*. Note the malaria pigment in the infected red cells. × 126.

sequential manifestation of severe falciparum infection. It is caused by the blockage of the cerebral capillaries with infected erythrocytes, which adhere to the endothelium.[14] The mechanism of adherence is related to the presence of "knobs" on the surface of the infected red cells, and their subsequent attachment to appropriate receptors on the host endothelium. The knobs consist, in part, of a histidine-rich protein, and are induced by the parasites (Fig. 29.16). The nature of the receptors on endothelial cells is still unknown.[15]

In falciparum malaria, anemia caused by hemolysis can be quite severe. Damage to the erythrocytes by intravascular hemolysis often is greater than that caused by the rupture of the infected cells alone. Even uninfected cells have an increased osmotic fragility. Also present is bone marrow depression, which contributes to the anemia. Disseminated intravascular coagulopathy occurs in severely infected individuals.

The spleen plays a major role in host defense against malaria.[16] Parasitized cells accumulate in its capillaries and sinusoids, causing general congestion. Malarial pigment becomes concentrated in the spleen and is responsible for darkening of this organ. Chronic infection, particularly with *P. malariae,* often causes persistent splenomegaly and is responsible for the "big spleen disease," or tropical splenomegaly syndrome,[17] consisting also of hepatomegaly, portal hypertension, anemia, leukopenia, and thrombocytopenia. In vivax malaria, the spleen can become acutely enlarged and is susceptible to rupture. The liver is darkened by the accumulated malarial pigment and shows degeneration and necrosis of the centrilobular region. The gastrointestinal tract is also affected. There are focal hemorrhages, edema, and consequent malabsorption. The kidneys, particularly in severe falciparum malaria, show punctate hemorrhages and even tubular necrosis. Accumulation of hemoglobin in the tubules is responsible for hemoglobinuria, or "blackwater fever," which occurs after repeated attacks of falciparum malaria and is enhanced by therapy with quinine. It is a consequence of severe hemolysis, exacerbated by the host immune response against the intracellular parasites.

Chronic infections with *P. malariae* can lead to nephrotic syndrome, characterized by focal hyalinization of the tufts of glomeruli and by endothelial proliferation, apparently caused by the

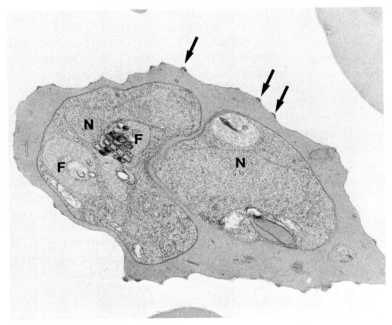

Figure 29.16. The outer surface of a red cell infected with *Plasmodium falciparum* showing the characteristic knobs (*arrows*) associated with the points of attachment to the endothelial cells of the capillaries. Nucleus (*N*), food vacuole (*F*). ×21,000. (Courtesy of Dr. S. Langreth)

deposition of immune complexes. In addition, recent evidence has suggested that an autoimmune process develops against glomerular basement membrane.

Congenital malaria can develop with any of the species of Plasmodium, although incidence of this complication is relatively low. The mechanism of the infection of the fetus is uncertain. Some investigators have postulated damage to the placenta as a prerequisite to congenital malaria, but it is also possible that the parasites can infect the fetus through an intact placenta, or at the time of birth. Placental insufficiency and consequent fetal wastage have also resulted from placental infection with Plasmodium.[18]

Malarial infections tend to suppress cell-mediated immune responses. It has been suggested that Burkitt lymphoma is caused by infection with the Epstein-Barr virus under the influence of immunosuppression by chronic falciparum malaria.[19]

Clinical Disease

The most pronounced clinical manifestations of malaria are periodic chills and fever, usually accompanied by frontal headache and myalgia. Fever can persist for several days before the typical periodicity develops. The initial appearance of symptoms of malaria usually occurs 10–15 days after the bite by the infected mosquito. Delays of up to several months, in the onset of symptoms and in the appearance of parasites in peripheral blood are common, particularly in some strains of *P. vivax* found in temperate zones. Patients undergoing chemoprophylaxis may not develop any symptoms until they stop taking the drug. The classic pattern of clinical disease consists of paroxysms of chills and fever, reaching 41°C and lasting for 6 h, followed by sweating and deffervescence. There are exceptions to this, however, as noted under Pathogenesis.

Additional symptoms in all malarias include malaise, nausea, anorexia, and abdominal pain. Vomiting can also develop and can be quite intense.

Initially, there can be mild anemia with an elevation of the reticulocyte count. Leukocyte count tends to be normal or even low; there is no eosinophilia.

All forms of untreated malaria tend to become chronic; repeated attacks are caused by recrudescence or relapses. Development of immunity eventually leads to spontaneous cure of falciparum malaria within 2 years and vivax and ovale malarias within 5 years. Infection with the quartan parasite can persist for 30 years or more.

Untreated falciparum malaria can be fatal during the initial attack. This is especially likely in young children.

Unexplained fever in patients who have received transfusions or who are drug addicts can indicate induced malaria. An infant who develops fever during the neonatal period should be suspected of malaria if his mother had been exposed to risk of this infection. Diagnostic tests for induced or congenital malaria are the same as for the conventional forms of the disease. It must be remembered that neither induced nor congenital malaria has an EE cycle in the liver; hence therapy directed against the liver cycle is inappropriate.

Innate resistance to malaria is mediated by factors other than immune mechanisms. *P. vivax* and *P. ovale* preferentially invade reticulocytes. In these infections, usually only about 2% of the red cells are parasitized and the clinical disease is relatively mild. On the other hand, *P. malariae* tends to invade older erythrocytes. Finally, *P. falciparum* attacks erythrocytes of all ages, producing high levels of parasitemia.

Possession of sickle-cell hemoglobin confers some protection against falciparum malaria. Individuals with sickle-cell trait (AS) have a selective advantage over those with either AA or SS genotype, because the heterozygotes are protected against the severity of malaria. The SS individuals are also protected, but their sickle-cell disease leads to an early death. This is an example of balanced polymorphism.[20,21,22,23]

The mechanism for the protection afforded by sickle hemoglobin has recently been studied in vivo. These results, if extrapolated to patients, suggest that the crystallizing hemoglobin S actually "stabs" the developing intracelluar parasites and kills them.[24] In a patient with the trait, the affected erythrocytes tend to lose potassium, which is required for ATPase activation; thus the parasites are deprived of nutrients by a reduced active transport system and die of starvation.[25,26]

Glucose-6-phosphate dehydrogenase deficiency and β-thalassemia have both been suggested as factors of innate resistance against *P. falciparum* infection, but convincing epidemiological evidence for these associations is lacking.

Duffy blood-type determinants are associated with receptor sites for *P. vivax* merozoites on the erythrocytes. Most West Africans are negative for the Duffy blood type and are insusceptible to infection with *P. vivax*.

Acquired immunity to malaria develops after long exposure and is characterized by low levels of parasitemia. Immune individuals have intermittent parasitemia, with only mild symptoms; this is referred to as premunition, in contrast with classic immunity, which prevents any degree of infection.

Diagnosis

Definitive diagnosis depends on the identification of the parasite on stained blood smears. Both thick and thin smears should be examined. When malaria is suspected and the initial blood smears are negative, new specimens should be examined at 6-h intervals.

Serological tests, such as direct fluorescent antibody test, radioimmunoassay, and others are useful for epidemiological studies, but do not detect the low antibody levels in the early phases of acute infections. Several new techniques are now being applied to the study of the epidemiology of malaria. Specific DNA probes will facilitate rapid diagnosis and identification of species.[27] Laborious microscopic examination of blood smears may become obsolete.[28] Species-specific monoclonal antibodies directed against the predominant surface antigens of the sporozoites are now being used in the radiometric (IRMA)[29] and ELISA[30] systems for detection of sporozoites in mosquito vectors. The capacity for rapid determination of the proportion of mosquito populations coming to feed that have infectious sporozoites in their salivary glands will allow for accurate assessment of the effects of intervention strategies in the control of malaria.

Treatment

An acute attack should be treated immediately with chloroquine phosphate, administered by mouth; the treatment should be repeated at a lower dose 6 h later and continued for two more doses at daily intervals. In case of infection with chloroquine-resistant *P. falciparum,* or with Plasmodium, whose resistance cannot be determined, the treatment consists of quinine sulfate, pyrimethamine, and sulfadiazine, administered immediately and continued for 3 days. As an alternative to pyrimethamine and sulfadiazine, quinine can be administered in conjunction with tetracycline. Strains resistant to all of these drugs have been reported.

As long as the geographic origin of falciparum infection is known, one can accordingly acquire susceptibility or resistance to chloroquine. If the origin of infection is unknown, as may be the case with induced malaria, one must treat as if the organisms were resistant. This course must also be taken with any case of falciparum malaria that does not respond promptly to chloroquine therapy, because it may be the first example of resistance from an area not previously known to harbor resistant parasites.

In patients who are too ill to take oral drugs, chloroquine hydrochloride must be administered intramuscularly. For resistant falciparum malaria, intravenous quinine dihydrochloride must be used. Intravenous administration of quinine is dangerous, because the drug can cause shock. It is mandatory to administer it slowly over a period of 1 h and to monitor the patient's vital signs.

Relapses due to *P. vivax* and *P. ovale* infections can be prevented by a course of primaquine. This need not be started immediately, but can be deferred until the patient has recovered from the acute attack. Primaquine tends to cause hemolysis in individuals deficient in glucose-6-phosphate dehydrogenase; therefore, the drug should not be administered until the proper test for this enzyme has been carried out. Patients who are deficient should be given an option of chloroquine prophylaxis for 5 years, or of treatment of each acute attack during the 5 years within which the infection is expected to relapse.

Prevention and Control

Although there are more than 300 species of Anopheles mosquito, only about 60 are considered important vectors of malaria. Some of the factors that influence efficiency of the insect are feeding habits, longevity, susceptibility to infection with the parasite, and size of the mosquito population.

Variability of the parasite plays an important role in pathogenicity of the disease. For example, geographic strains of *P. vivax* show markedly different patterns of incubation periods and of relapses, and *P. falciparum* shows considerable variability in its responses to antimalarial drugs.

Susceptibility of geographic strains of mosquitoes is also variable.

Malaria in the United States during the past 30 years has been of the imported variety. The wars in Korea and Vietnam wars increased the numbers of these imported cases, because of the returning service personnel. Refugees from endemic areas constitute the largest number of imported cases. In addition, there is a steady incidence of malaria among travelers returning from endemic areas. Autochthonous infections are rare in the United States, in spite of large persistent populations of anophelines vectors, *A. quadrimaculatus* and *A. freeborni*.

Travelers in endemic areas and short-term residents of such areas should take chloroquine at weekly intervals beginning 2 weeks before arrival in the malarial zone and continuing for 6 weeks after departure. Pyrimethamine and sulfadoxine, also given at weekly intervals, have been recommended as prophylactics against infection with chloroquine-resistant *P. falciparum*, although adverse reactions to this combination have been reported.[31] Resistance to these newer drugs has also been reported.

Furthermore, travelers should avoid, or minimize, contact with mosquitoes. Most anophelines bite at night; therefore, sleeping under netting and, if possible, in rooms fitted with window screens will be effective. Clothing that covers much of skin, and insect repellants, particularly those containing diethyltoluamide, are useful adjuncts to prevention. Individuals who reside permanently in endemic areas probably should not take drugs for prophylaxis. Frequent exposure to malaria will eventually render them immune and will protect them from severe clinical attacks.

Differential diagnosis of a febrile illness in travelers to endemic zones after they have returned home should include malaria. Delays in diagnosis, particularly of falciparum malaria, have resulted in death. Similarly, fevers in individuals who have received blood transfusions, or who are drug addicts, must also be evaluated for malaria.

The development of resistance of *P. falciparum* to chloroquine has been the most serious problem relating to malaria therapy. Multiple drug resistance is common in Southeast Asia and is rapidly spreading in the Asian subcontinent, in South America, and in Africa.

For wide-scale control of malaria, control of mosquitoes remains the only practical method.

Reduction in numbers of mosquitoes through drainage or modification of breeding sites, has been accomplished in some areas. Insecticides still offer the best means for reducing populations of mosquitoes. However, rising costs of these products, and development of resistance by the insects, have severely limited their application and usefulness. Wide-scale drug distribution or treatment programs have not been effective.

The development of a vaccine against malaria —subject of much research today—would provide a major addition to the currently available methods for the control of this disease.[32] Because of the complexity of the life cycle, with its distinctive morphological, physiological, and antigenic features of the various stages of this parasite, there could be several targets for the vaccine. Experimental vaccines directed against the sporozoites have shown promise for success,[33] and synthetic and genetically engineered peptides corresponding to the antigenically active sites on the sporozoites are being evaluated in clinical trials.[34,35]

However, there is a caveat to the development of a vaccine against the sporozoites, because if it is to succeed it must be effective absolutely. Even one sporozoite evading host defenses induced by the vaccine could initiate an infection.[36]

On the other hand, even partial immunity to the asexual stages of malarial parasites, which cause the clinical disease, would prevent, or at least attenuate morbidity. However, these asexual stages exhibit great antigenic diversity[36] and have the capacity to vary their antigenic nature under immune pressure.[37]

Ablation of the sexual cycle of malaria in the mosquito by induced antibodies from man would prevent the mosquitoes from becoming infected and from spreading malaria, although it would not protect the human host directly.[38]

The development of a malaria vaccine that would contain antigens representing the various vulnerable stages of the parasite has been proposed. Such a vaccine would accomplish all three purposes, i.e. it would prevent infection by the sporozoites, would prevent clinical expression of disease due to the merozoites, and would block transmission.

In spite of the experimental successes, a malaria vaccine available for wide application is still many years away. In the meantime, vector control and chemotherapy remain the primary strategies of control of malaria. However, effectiveness of these methods cannot be expected to last indefinitely because of the development of resistance to these chemicals. Novel approaches are needed to overcome these obstacles to control.

References

1. Harrison G: Mosquitoes, Malaria, and Man. New York, E P Dutton, 1978
2. Haggis AW: Fundamental errors in the early history of cinchona. Bull Hist Med 10:567–568, 1941
3. Meis JEGM, Verhave JP, Jap PHK, Meuwissen JHE Th: An ultrastructural study on the role of Küpffer cells in the process of infection by *Plasmodium berghei* sporozoites in rats. Parasitology 86:231–242, 1983
4. Hollingdale MR: Malaria and the liver. Hepatology 5:327–335, 1985
5. Coatney GR: Relapse in malaria–an enigma. J Parasitol 62:3–9, 1976
6. Schmidt LH: Compatibility of relapse patterns of *Plasmodium cynomolgi* infections in rhesus monkeys with continuous cyclical development and hypnozoite concepts of relapse. Am J Trop Med Hyg 35:1077–1099, 1986
7. Krotoski WA: Discovery of the hypozoite and a new theory of malarial relapse. Trans Roy Soc Trop Med Hyg 79:1–11, 1985
8. Dvorak, JSA, Miller LH, Whitehouse WC, et al.: Invasion of erythrocytes by malaria merozoites. Science 187:748–750, 1975
9. Aikawa M, Miller LH, Johnson J, et al.: Erythrocyte entry by malaria parasites, a moving junction between erythrocyte and parasite J. Cell Biol. 77:72–82, 1978
10. Garvey G, Neu HC, Katz M: Transfusion-induced malaria after open heart surgery. N.Y. State J. Med. 75:602–603, 1975
11. Covell G. Congential malaria Trop. Dis. Bull. 47:1147–1167 1950
12. Coatney GR, Collins WE, Warren N, et al.: The primate malarias. U.S. Department of Health, Education and Welfare, Bethesda, Maryland, 1971
13. World Health Organization: Severe and complicated Malaria. Trans Roy Soc Trop Med Hyg 80:(suppl) 1–50, 1986
14. MacPherson GG, Warrell MJ, White NJ et al. Human cerebral malaria: a quantitative ultrastructural analysis of parasitized erythrocyte sequestration. Am J Path 119:385–401, 1985
15. Udeinya I, Schmidt JA, Aikawa M, Miller LH, Green I: Falciparum malaria–infected erythrocytes bind to cultured human endothelial cells. Science 213:555–557, 1981

16. Looareesuwan S, Ho M, Wattanagoon Y, White NJ et al. Dynamic alteration in splenic function during acute falciparum malaria. N Eng J Med 317:675–679, 1987

17. Greenwood BM, Fakunle YM: The tropical splenomegaly syndrome. A review of its pathogenesis. In: The role of the spleen in the immunology of parasitic diseases. Tropical Disease Research Series. No. 1. Basel, Schwabe & Co., 1979, pp. 229–244

18. Bruce-Chwatt ZJ: Malaria. In: Jelliffe D.B., Stanfield JP (eds): Diseases of children in the subtropics and tropics, 3rd Edition, London. Edward Arnold, 1978, pp. 827–856.

19. Whittle HC, Brown J, Marsh K, Greenwood BM et al: T-cell control of Epstein-Barr virus-infected B cells is lost during *P. falciparum* malaria. Nature 312:449–450, 1984

20. Allison, AC: Protection afforded by sickle-cell trait against subtertion malarial infection. Br. Med. J. 1:290–294, 1954

21. Dean J, Schecter AN: Sickle-cell anemia: Molecular and cellular basis of therapeutic approaches (First of three parts) N Eng J Med 296:752–763, 1978

22. ———. (Second of three parts) 299:804–811, 1978

23. ———. (Third of three parts) 299:863–870, 1978

24. Friedman, MJ: Ultrastructural damage to the malaria parasite in the sickled cell. J. Protozool. 26:195–199, 1979.

25. Friedman MJ, Roth EF, Nagel RL, et al. *Plasmodium falciparum:* Physiological interactions with human sickle cells. Exp. Parasital. 47:73–80 1979

26. Bunn HF, Forget BG: In Hemoglobin: Molecular, Genetic, and Clinical Aspects. Philadelphia, W.B. Saunders Co., 1986 pp 690

27. Londner MV, Rosen G, Sintov A, Spira OT: The feasibility of a DOT enzyme-linked immunosorbent assay (DOT-ELISA) for the diagnosis of *Plasmodium falciparum* antigens and antibodies. Am J Trop Med Hyg 36:240–245, 1987

28. Collins FH, Zavala F, Graves PM, Cochrane AH, et al.: First field trial of an immuno-radiometric assay for the detection of malarial sporozoites in mosquitoes. Am J Trop Med Hyg 33:538–542, 1984

29. Beier JC, Perkens PV, Wirtz RA, Whitmire RE et al.: Field evaluation of an enzyme-linked immunosorbent assay (ELISA) for *Plasmodium falciparum* sporozoite detection in anopheline mosquitoes from Kenya. Am J Trop Med Hyg 36:459–468, 1987

30. Bruce-Chwatt LJ: From Laveran's discovery to DNA probes: New trends in diagnosis of malaria. Lancet 92:1509–1511, 1988

31. Miller KD, Lobel HO, Satriale RF, Kuritsky JN et al.: Severe cutaneous reactions among American travelers using Pyramethamine-Sulfadoxine (Fansidar®) for malaria prophylaxis Am J Trop Med Hyg 35:451–458, 1986

32. Miller LH, Howard RJ, Carter R, Good MF et al.: Research toward malaria vaccines. Science 234:1349–1356, 1986

33. Nussenzweig RS, Nussenzweig V: Development of a malaria vaccine based on the structure of the circumsporozoite protein. In: WA Siddiqui (ed) Proceedings of the Asia and Pacific Conference on Malaria: Practical Considerations on Malaria Vaccines and Clinical Trials. Honolulu, JA Burns School of Medicine, U of Hawaii, 1985. pp. 143–158

34. Ballow WR, Hoffman SL, Sherwood MR, Hollingdale MR et al.: Safety and efficacy of a recombinant DNA *Plasmodium falciparum* sporozoite vaccine. Lancet 1:1277–1281, 1987

35. Herrington DA, Clyde DF, Hosonsky M, Cortesia M et al.: Safety and immunogenicity in man of a synthetic peptide malaria vaccine against *Plasmodium falciparum* sporozoites. Nature 328:257–259, 1987

36. Marsh K, Howard RJ: Antigens induced on erythrocytes by *P. falciparum:* expression of diverse and converged determinants. Science 231:150–153, 1986

37. Howard RJ: Antigenic variation of bloodstage malaria parasites. Phil Trans Roy Soc London (B) 307:141–158, 1984

38. Carter R, Miller LH, Rener J, Kaushal DC et al.: Target antigens in malaria transmission blocking immunity. Phil Trans R Soc Lond (B) 307:201–213, 1984

30. *Trypanosoma cruzi* (Chagas 1909)

Infection with *Trypanosoma cruzi* is essentially limited to Central and South America. However, a few cases of *T. cruzi* have been diagnosed in the United States in California[1] and Texas.[2] The disease caused by this organism, Chagas disease, has a case fatality rate of about 5% in its acute phase;[3] the fatality rate in the chronic state is difficult to assess. It is estimated that between 10

Trypanosoma cruzi

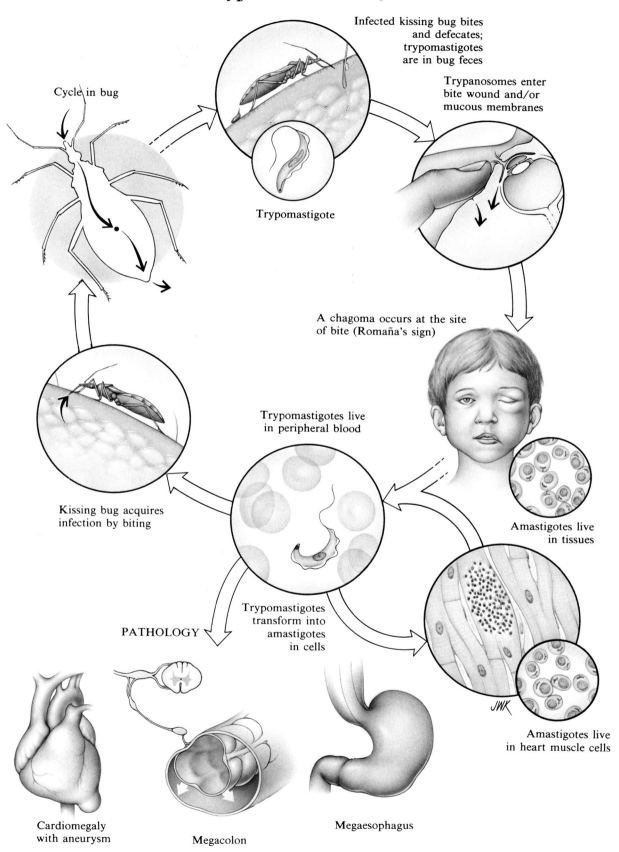

Infected kissing bug bites
and defecates;
trypomastigotes
are in bug feces

Trypanosomes enter
bite wound and/or
mucous membranes

Cycle in bug

Trypomastigote

A chagoma occurs at the site
of bite (Romaña's sign)

Kissing bug acquires
infection by biting

Trypomastigotes live
in peripheral blood

Amastigotes live
in tissues

PATHOLOGY

Trypomastigotes
transform into
amastigotes
in cells

Amastigotes live
in heart muscle cells

JWK

Cardiomegaly
with aneurysm

Megacolon

Megaesophagus

Reproduced from Despommier DD and Karapelou JW: Parasite Life Cycles. Copyright © Springer-Verlag, 1987.

and 12 million people at present are infected with *T. cruzi*.[4] *T. cruzi* is a flagellate, transmitted by vectors in the order Hemiptera, family Reduviidae, the subfamily Triatominae (see Chapter 38), which consists of nine genera, the most common of which are Panstrongylus and Rhodnius. In addition, the infection can be transmitted through blood transfusion.[5] In Mexico, 4.4% of the donated blood was found to be serologically positive for *T. cruzi*.[6] There are several important reservoir hosts, including rats, dogs, sloths, bats, and various nonhuman primates. Transmission takes place in both rural and urban settings. The incidence of this infection is highest in children.

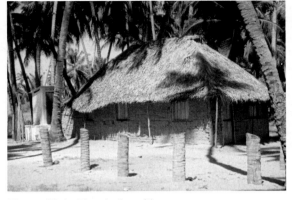

Figure 30.1. Thatched roof house.

Historical Information

Chagas, after whom the disease is named, discovered the infective stage of *T. cruzi*, in 1909, by chance while he was conducting a survey of vectors of malaria.[7] His discovery identified both the vector and the agent of a disease that was yet to be described in man. He inoculated many different species of mammals and learned that all of them became infected; some even died. He assumed that the infection affected man as well and embarked on a survey of rural Brazil, where he found both infected vectors and infected people. During the subsequent years, Chagas described the major clinical features of the disease as well as the morphology of the trypomastigote stage of the causative agent. He named the organism after his mentor, Oswaldo Cruz.

The complete life cycle of *T. cruzi* was described by Brumpt,[8] in 1912, and pathological changes caused by the organism by Vianna[9] in 1916.

Life Cycle

The infection is transmitted by a triatomid bug (Fig. 38.22), which characteristically feeds at night. The bug bites, near the mouth or eyes, ingests blood, and defecates immediately near the site of the bite. Its feces contain the parasite. The bite itself is painless, but subsequently the affected area begins to itch, causing the victim to rub the bug feces—and thus the protozoa—into the wound, or mucous membranes, in response to the itch. The infection can also occur without a direct contact with the bug. In rural Brazil, where houses with thatched roofs predominate, (Fig. 30.1) the triatomid bugs live in the roofs and their feces fall onto sleeping people, who can become infected by rubbing the parasites into the mucous membranes. Because triatomids feed on many mammals and the rural populations live in close proximity to their livestock, the probability of infection is quite high.

Immediately after introduction into the bite site, or the mucous membranes, the trypomastigotes (Fig. 30.2) penetrate a wide variety of cells and become transformed within these cells into amastigotes (Fig. 30.3). After several divisions, the parasites transform into trypomastigotes. The affected cells die and release the parasites, which reach the bloodstream and become distributed throughout the body. They infect many different tissues, including glial cells in the central nervous system, the heart muscle, the myenteric plexus in the gut, the urogenital tract, and reticuloendothelial system. In contrast with the African trypanosomes, *T. cruzi* is essentially an intracellular parasite.

The early lesion, usually on the face, is known as primary chagoma; it contains only the intracellular amastigotes. Triatomids become infected by feeding on the infected host. The trypomastigotes migrate to the midgut of the bug, where they transform into the epimastigote stage (Fig. 30.4) and then proceed to undergo many divisions. Thousands of organisms are produced within one bug without apparently affecting it.

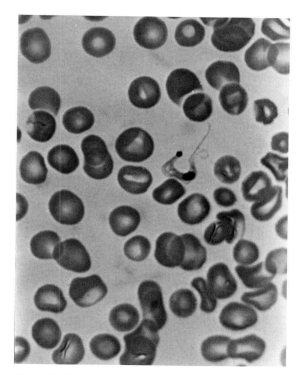

Figure 30.2. Trypomastigote stage of *Trypanosoma cruzi* in the blood of a patient in the acute phase of the infection. ×1,500.

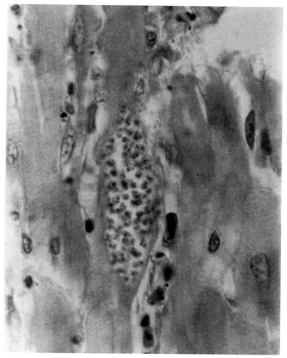

Figure 30.3. Amastigote stage (*arrows*) of *Trypanosoma cruzi* in the heart muscle cells. Hundreds of organisms fill the necrotic spaces in the cardiac muscle cells. ×976.

The triatomids remain infected for life, i.e., 1–2 years. The epimastigotes in the bug transform into metacyclic trypomastigotes and ultimately migrate to the hind gut, whence they are excreted with feces, following the bite.

In addition to these routes of infection, *T. cruzi* can be transmitted between partners during sexual intercourse and to the fetus across the placenta.

Pathogenesis

Chagas disease has two stages, the acute and the chronic. The acute stage is characterized by hematogenous spread of the parasite, leading to invasion of various tissues and organ systems. The invasion is accompanied by an intense inflammatory reaction, consisting of infiltration by mononuclear cells.

The chronic stage is a result of gradual tissue destruction. For example, in the heart, the my-

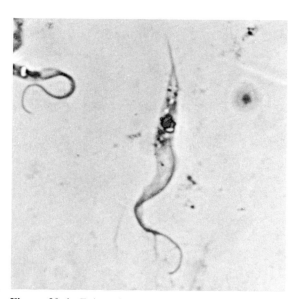

Figure 30.4. Epimastigote stage of *Trypanosoma cruzi*. ×2,900.

ofibrils and the Purkinje fibers are replaced by fibrous tissue. As a consequence, there are conduction defects, the heart enlarges (Fig. 30.5A), and on occasion develops a ventricular aneurysm (Fig. 30.5B). In the gut, the destruction of myenteric plexus is responsible for the development of megaesophagus and megacolon.

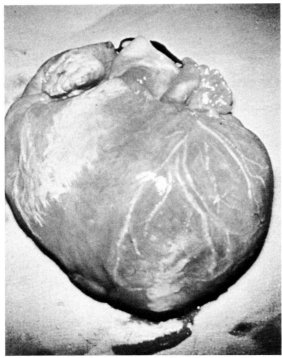

A

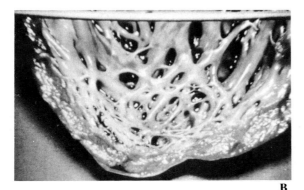

B

Figure 30.5. A. Gross specimen of an enlarged heart from a patient who died from chronic *Trypanosoma cruzi* infection. **B.** Section through the heart in **A** showing thinned wall of ventricle. (Courtesy of Dr. T. Jones)

Clinical Disease

The acute stage often is missed, because it can be asymptomatic or because the symptoms that do develop are protean and are often misdiagnosed. The infection usually occurs in early childhood and persists throughout life.

The incubation period is 4–12 days following the introduction of the organisms. The acute phase resulting from the insect bite on the face can be heralded by the unilateral appearance of edema and violaceous discoloration of the eyelids, the so-called Romaña sign. The swollen eyelids are firm to the touch. There can be an associated conjunctivitis. In addition there can be a nodule, known as chagoma, at the site of the bite. It is erythematous and brawny and firm to the touch. When it disappears after several weeks, it leaves an area of depigmentation.

An acutely infected patient can have systemic involvement including fever, lymphadenopathy, hepatomegaly, splenomegaly, and myocarditis. Some patients develop signs of meningoencephalitis. Rarely, a patient can have a morbilliform or urticarial rash.

The acute phase ends after approximately 2 months, on rare occasions lasting up to 4 months. Those who have recovered from the acute phase enter the chronic phase of the infection. However, many people, perhaps the majority, remain asymptomatic for the rest of their lives. Others remain well for many years before developing symptoms and signs of chronic disease, which mainly takes two forms, cardiac and gastrointestinal, the former predominating. At least half of the patients with Chagas disease have abnormal electrocardiograms.

The cardiac form can be silent and limited to electrocardiographic abnormalities, consisting of conduction defects, which at the extreme cause a complete heart block. Clinically, the patients experience extrasystoles, right ventricular enlargement, and eventually heart failure.

The gastrointestinal form includes development of megaesophagus and megacolon. The former is heralded by dysphagia and, later, regurgitation. The latter leads to constipation and fecal retention. Megaesophagus is the predominant abnormality of the digestive system; most patients with megacolon also have megaesophagus.

The disease is not limited to the heart and the

gut. Rarely, it leads also to megaureters, mega-bladder, megagallbladder, and bronchiectasis.

Involvement of the heart is the primary cause of death in Chagas disease.

Diagnosis

The diagnosis of the acute disease depends on discovery of trypomastigotes (Fig. 30.2) in the blood of the patient. If the direct examination of the blood smear fails to reveal the parasites, it may be possible to detect them in the buffy coat, after a blood sample has been centrifuged, or in the supernatant serum of a blood sample that has been left to clot. A further search for the para-sites can reveal their presence in a biopsy spec-imen obtained from a tender skeletal muscle, for example, the gastrocnemius. Other methods of search involve culturing blood on a medium, in-oculation of mice, and xenodiagnosis. The last involves placement of a reduviid bug that was reared in the laboratory, and is uninfected, on the skin of the patient. After the bug has taken a blood meal, it is maintained for 6 weeks and then killed to determine whether it has become infected.

There are also serological tests, variably useful. The indirect immunofluorescence test can detect the infected individual 2 weeks after in-fection. This serological test becomes positive earliest. The other tests detect precipitins and agglutinins. The complement fixation test be-comes positive 6 weeks after the infection.

In patients with the chronic infection, direct diagnosis is more difficult, because they have very few circulating trypomastigotes. Xenodi-agnosis is the most useful test, which will detect the infection in about half of the patients. In the others, it is necessary to rely on a positive ser-ological test together with symptoms and signs compatible with Chagas disease.

Treatment

Treatment is not completely satisfactory. Nifurti-mox appears to eradicate parasitemia during the acute phase of the infection and can effect radical cure. It has less effect in the chronic form of the disease. There is a differential susceptibility of the trypanosomes to nifurtimox; some appear to be relatively resistant.

Nifurtimox has serious side effects. It causes anorexia and vomiting, disorders of sleep, and polyneuritis. Another widely used drug throughout South and Central America is benznidazole. Like nifurtimox, it is effective in preventing spread of the parasites from tissue to tissue. However re-lapses are frequent after treatment with either drug, suggesting that the amastigotes in the tissue are not affected by these drugs.[10]

Chronic disease must be treated symptomati-cally with appropriate cardiac regimens. Mega-esophagus and megacolon are susceptible to sur-gical interventions.

Prevention and Control

Control of vectors is an effective method for re-ducing incidence of the infection. In Brazil, control efforts have been rewarded by considera-ble success. A massive seroepidemiological sur-vey provided accurate information about regional prevalence of Chagas' disease; the national prev-alence indicated about 6 million infected people. Spraying breeding sites in rural villages reduced the population of kissing bugs below the level required for transmission. This campaign led to a reduction of rate of infection from 20% to below 5% within a 2-year period.[11] Urbanization, with the attendant elimination of traditional huts, has also contributed to the reduction of this infection (see Chapter 38).

In addition, blood recipients can be protected from infection by treatment of donated blood with gentian violet (in a dilution of 1:4000), which kills trypomastigotes.[4]

There is no chemoprophylaxis. In the absence of an effective therapy a vaccine would be a major advance in dealing with this infection. However in spite of recent advances in identifi-cation and characterization of antigens that induce protection against *T. cruzi*, no effective vaccine has been developed.[12]

References

1. Schiffler RJ, Mansur GP, Navin TR et al.: Indig-enous Chagas' disease (American trypanosomiasis) in California. JAMA 251:2983–2984, 1984
2. Woody NC, Woody HB: American trypanosomiasis (Chagas' disease): First indigenous case in the U.S.A. JAMA 159:676, 1955

3. Koberle F: Chagas' disease and Chagas' syndromes: The pathology of American trypanosomiasis. In Dawes B (ed): Advances in Parasitology. New York, Academic Press, Vol 6. 1968, pp 63–116

4. Brener Z: Present status of chemotherapy and chemoprophylaxis of human trypanosomiasis in the western hemisphere. Pharmacol Ther 7:71–90, 1979

5. Schmuñis GA: Chagas' Disease and Blood Transfusion in: Infection, Immunity and Blood Transfusion. Alan R. Liss, Inc. pp. 127–145 1985.

6. Goldsmith RS, Zarte R, Kagan I, et al.: El potencial de la transmission en la enfermedad de Chagas por transfusion sanguinea: Hallazgoz serologicos entre donadores en el estade de Oaxaca. Sal Pub Mex 20:439–444, 1978

7. Chagas C: Nova trypanozomiaze humana. Estudos sobre a morfolojia e o ciclo evolutivo do *Schizotrypanum cruzi* n. gen, n. spec., ajente etiolojico de nova entidade morbida de homem. Memorias Inst Oswaldo Cruz 1:159–218, 1909

8. Brumpt AJE: Le *Trypanosoma cruzi* evolue chez *Conorhinus megistus. Cimex lectularius, Cimex boueti* et *Ornithodorus moubata.* Cycle evolutif de ce parasite. Bull Soc Pathol Exot 5:360–364, 1912

9. Vianna G: Contribuicao para o estudo da anatomia patolojica da "Moletia de Carlos Chagas" (Esquizotripanoze humana ou tireodite parazitaria). Memorias Inst Oswaldo Cruz 3:276–294, 1916

10. McGreevy PB, Marsden PD: American Trypanosomiasis and Leishmaniasis in: Chemotherapy of Parasitic diseases. (Campbell WC and Rew RS, eds) Plenum Press, New York and London. pp. 115–128, 1986

11. Dias JCP: Control of Chagas' disease in Brazil. Parasit Today 3:336–341, 1987

12. Brener Z: Why vaccines do not work in Chagas' Disease. Parasit Today 2:196–197, 1986

31. The African Trypanosomes: *Trypanosoma brucei gambiense* (Dutton 1902) and *Trypanosoma brucei rhodesiense* (Stephens and Fantham 1910)

Trypanosoma brucei gambiense and *T. b. rhodesiense,* two subspecies of hemoflagellates, are responsible for a disease commonly referred to as African trypanosomiasis. Both of these organisms are transmitted by the bite of various species of the tsetse fly of the genus Glossina (see Chapter 38) and infect human populations throughout equatorial Africa. *T. b. gambiense* is found mainly in western and central Africa (Senegambia, Guinea, Ivory Coast, Liberia, Ghana, Benin, Nigeria, Cameroon, Central African Republic, Zaire, Gabon, and Uganda), whereas *T. b. rhodesiense* is restricted to Zimbabwe, Zambia, Tanzania, Uganda, and Kenya in East Africa. There are no known reservoir hosts for *T. b. gambiense,* but many of the wild game animals of East Africa serve as reservoirs for *T. b. rhodesiense.* Trypanosomiasis is a serious problem in animal husbandry, because many species of the trypanosomes, related to those infecting man, cause severe disease in cattle.

Human trypanosomiasis is both epidemic and endemic. Untreated, it is almost universally fatal.

Historical Information

Sleeping sickness, the older name for African trypanosomiasis, was known to Europeans, at least, since 1742, when Atkins published his observations of this disease.[1] However, the association between the disease and its etiological agent was established much later. In 1895, Bruce[2] showed that a disease of cattle, nagana, was caused by a trypanosome transmitted by the tsetse fly. This disease, also called cattle trypanosomiasis, has prevented cattle ranching in tropical Africa and has been a major deterrent to economic growth of that vast region of the world.

A human equivalent of nagana, the disease caused by *T. b. gambiense,* was first described by Forde,[3] in 1902; *T. b. rhodesiense* was identified as a human pathogen by Stephens and Fantham,[4] in 1910.

Kinghorn and Yorke,[5] in 1912, proved by extensive, carefully conducted experiments that *T. b. rhodesiense* could be transmitted from man to animals by tsetse flies. Morever, they correctly concluded that game animals, such as waterbuck,

Trypanosoma gambiense

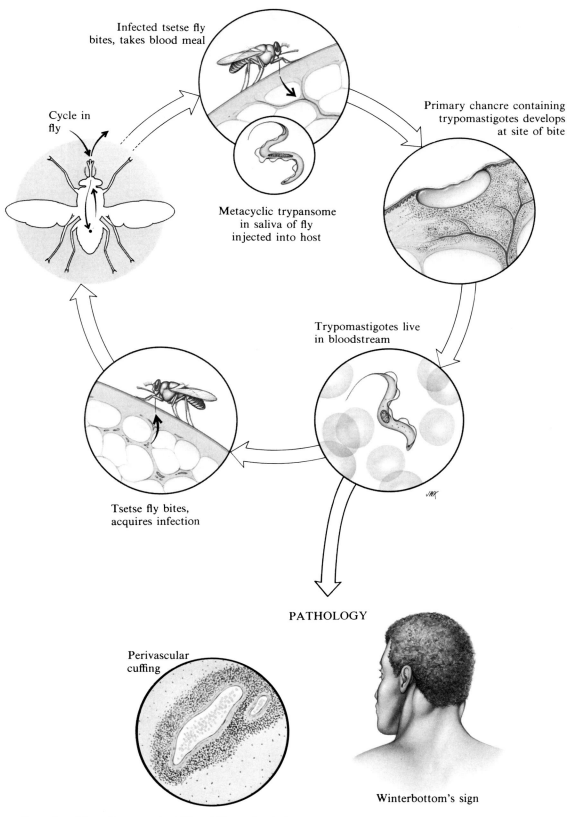

Infected tsetse fly bites, takes blood meal

Cycle in fly

Metacyclic trypansome in saliva of fly injected into host

Primary chancre containing trypomastigotes develops at site of bite

Trypomastigotes live in bloodstream

Tsetse fly bites, acquires infection

PATHOLOGY

Perivascular cuffing

Winterbottom's sign

hartebeest, impala, and warthog, could serve as reservoir hosts for this East African trypanosome.

Life Cycle

The patterns of development of *T. b. gambiense* and *T. b. rhodesiense* are very similar and the description that follows applies to both.

Six species of Glossina are the vectors of human African trypanosomiasis, and both sexes of the flies transmit the infection. The infective stage is the metatrypanosome (Fig. 31.1), injected intradermally by the fly. The metatrypanosomes rapidly transform into blood-form trypanosomes (Fig. 31.2A and B) which begin a series of divisions by binary fission at the site of the bite wound. This leads to the formation of the primary chancre.

The trypanosomes enter the bloodstream through the lymphatics and undergo more divisions, often reaching numbers in excess of 1500/mm^3. They are extracellular parasites inhabiting the bloodstream, cerebrospinal fluid, and the interstitial spaces.

The tsetse fly becomes infected by ingesting a blood meal from an infected host. In the midgut of the fly, the trypanosomes transform into pro-

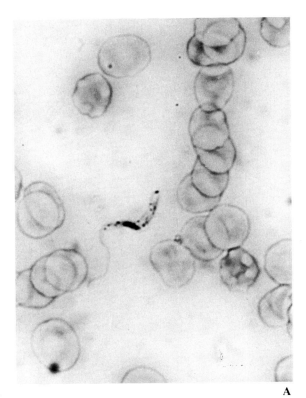

A

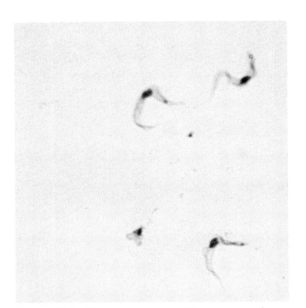

Figure 31.1. Metatrypanosome of *Trypanosoma b. rhodesiense*. This form lives in the salivary glands of the tsetse fly and is the infectious stage of the parasite. ×900. (Courtesy of Dr. I. Cunningham)

B

Figure 31.2. Trypomastigote stages of *Trypanosoma b. gambiense* (**A**) and *Trypanosoma b. rhodesiense* (**B**). A, ×1,575; **B**, ×1,500. (Courtesy of Dr. I. Cunningham)

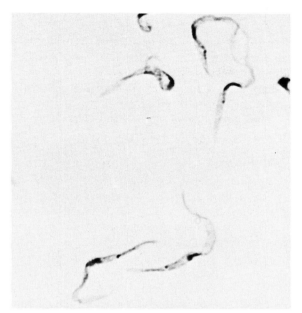

Figure 31.3. Procyclic trypomastigote stage of *Trypanosoma b. rhodesiense* from the midgut of *Glossina* sp. (tsetse fly). ×500. (Courtesy of Dr. I. Cunningham)

cyclic trypomastigotes (Fig. 31.3), which continue dividing for 10 days. When the divisions are completed, the organisms migrate to the salivary glands and transform into epimastigotes. These, in turn, divide and transform into metatrypanosomes, which are the stage infective for man and animals. The entire cycle in glossina lasts 25–50 days, depending on the species of the fly, the strain of the trypanosome, and the temperature of the environment.

Each fly remains infected for life (2–3 months) and is capable of delivering more than 40,000 metatrypanosomes whenever it feeds. The minimum infective dose for most hosts is 300–500 organisms.

It is possible that the infection can also be acquired through ingestion of raw meat from an infected carcass.[6] If this is an alternative mode of transmission, it may have a function of maintaining infection in the reservoir hosts among carnivores and may also play a role in transmission to man.

Pathogenesis

The host responds to the infection by producing antibodies of two classes. IgG antibodies seem to be directed mainly against cellular antigens, whereas the IgM antibodies are directed primarily against surface antigens. The surface antigenic determinants are glycoproteins in the coat of the trypanosomes.[7] The antibodies directed against them destroy, by agglutination and lysis, all antigenically identical organisms within a given population. A few trypanosomes with different surface antigens escape destruction. These variants multiply and replace those that were destroyed.[8] The host, again, responds by producing antibodies against the new antigenic variant. In turn a third variant arises. Thus yet another brood of trypanosomes takes over, the host responds once more, and this tug-of-war continues until the host is eventually overcome (Fig. 31.4).

Antigenic variation is based on rearrangements of genes encoding glycoproteins in the outer membrane of these protozoans.[9] Although the intent of some earlier studies was exploitation of the variant antigens of trypanosomes as candidates for vaccines, it seems unlikely now that host protection could be achieved by this method, because the repertoire of antigenic variants of the bloodstream trypomastigotes is very large. In the human disease, however, the ultimate number remains unknown.

Figure 31.4. Course of parasitemia in a patient with *Trypanosoma b. rhodesiense*. Each peak of parasitemia represents a new antigenic variant. (From Vickerman K, as redrawn from Ross and Thomson, Proc R Soc London [Biol] Sci 82:411–415, 1910.)

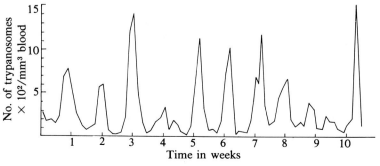

The predominant pathologic involvement is limited to the lymphatic and central nervous systems. All lymph nodes become enlarged, but posterior cervical ones do so earliest and most predominantly.[10] The nodes are hyperplastic and contain large numbers of the parasites.

In the natural course of the disease the trypanosomes enter the central nervous system and cause leptomeningitis, which eventually leads to the cerebral edema and encephalopathy that has given rise to the name sleeping sickness. The involved brain shows evidence of inflammation, with perivascular cuffing (Fig. 31.5), consisting of infiltrates of glial cells, lymphocytes, and plasma cells. There is also proliferation of astrocytes. Invasion of the central nervous system occurs much earlier in infections with *T. b. rhodesiense* than in those by other species.

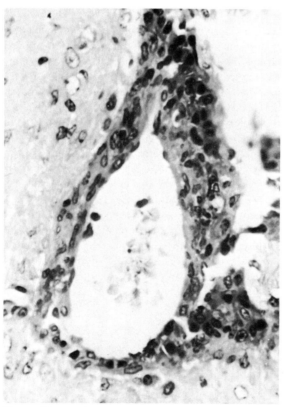

Figure 31.5. Cross-section of a vein in the brain of a patient who died from infection with *Trypanosoma b. rhodesiense*. Note perivascular cuffing with small lymphocytes. ×630.

Clinical Disease

Both trypanosomes cause the same type of clinical disease; only the time scale of its evolution differs. Infection with *T. b. rhodesiense* is more fulminant, has an incubation period of 2–3 weeks, and a course of several weeks, involving the brain after 3 or 4 weeks. The Gambian variety has an incubation period of several weeks to months and may not involve the brain for months and even years.

The first sign of either infection, occurring a few days after the bite, is a chancre at the site of the inoculation, where the organisms remain localized. When the incubation period is completed and the organisms have disseminated to the bloodstream, intermittent fever develops. Rashes, particularly erythema multiforme, occur in some patients. Lymphadenopathy, especially of the posterior cervical nodes, the so-called Winterbottom's sign, are characteristic, but not invariable.

Invasion of the central nervous system is heralded by headache, stiff neck, disturbance of sleep, and depression. Progressive mental deterioration follows and is associated with focal seizures, tremors, and palsies. Eventually, coma develops and the patient dies, usually of associated causes, such as pneumonia, inanition, or sepsis.

Diagnosis

History of travel in the endemic area and especially a bite by the tsetse fly—usually a remembered event, because the fly is large and the bite painful—and the presence of a chancre can steer the clinician to the correct diagnosis.

The definitive diagnosis depends on finding the trypanosomes in blood, cerebrospinal fluid, or aspirates of lymph nodes. It may be helpful to examine the buffy coat and the centrifuged sediment of the cerebrospinal fluid. If the direct examination fails to reveal the organism, it may be necessary to resort to in vitro culture and to inoculation of animals.

Current serological tests are unreliable for diagnosis of clinical disease, because of cross-reactions. An ELISA test[11] may become quite specific after technical refinements, including purification of antigens, have been achieved.

Differential diagnosis includes syphilis, leishmaniasis, and malaria. Indeed finding malarial parasites in the blood of a patient with trypanosomiasis can mislead the clinicians and divert their attention from the diagnosis of trypanosomiasis. Lymphoma must also be considered in any patient with protracted, unexplained fever.

Treatment

The most important principle of therapy is that it is best begun *before* the central nervous system is involved, because the most effective drug does not pass the blood-brain barrier. When properly treated, a patient free of central nervous system disease will usually recover without sequelae. Suramin administered intermittently, by intravenous infusion, is the drug of choice. It has a number of side effects, such as nausea, vomiting, pruritis, urticaria, paresthesias, hypesthesia, photophobia, and peripheral neuropathy. They are unpleasant, but not dangerous, and disappear several days after discontinuation of the therapy. Rarely, patients can develop renal damage. For that reason, it is important to ascertain the renal status of the patient before starting the therapy.

Pentamidine isethionate is an alternative, but it also has many side effects (see Chapter 35).

For patients whose central nervous system is affected, the therapy consists of melarsoprol. This drug is quite toxic and can cause myocarditis, renal damage, peripheral neuropathy, encephalopathy, and a Jarisch-Herxheimer type of reaction. It is possible to reduce these side effects, particularly the last, by pretreatment of the patient with suramin, but there may not be enough time to do this if the patient's central nervous system is severely affected. Five percent of patients die as the result of this treatment. Difluoromethylornithine (DMFO), an experimental non-toxic drug, effective in eliminating bloodstream forms of *T. b. rhodesiense* and *T. b. gambiense*,[12] has shown promising results in human trials.[13]

Prevention and Control

Attempts at prophylaxis with drugs have been largely unsuccessful. Although pentamidine isethionate can be used as a prophylactic, it is subject to the danger that a cryptic infection may develop. In addition, the drug is not free of side effects. Development of a vaccine has been hampered by the antigenic variation in the parasite.

In West Africa, the control of the vector has been effective, mainly because there are no reservoir hosts of *T. b. gambiense*. The main vectors in West Africa are riverine tsetse flies, *G. palpalis* being predominant. This vector has been successfully eradicated from certain areas through clearance of the vegetation along the rivers. This program takes advantage of the fact that the riverine flies are negatively phototropic and require a moist, shady environment to breed. Because the female fly lives only about 48 days and produces 2–4 eggs in its life time,[14] and because only 0.1% of flies become infected, a program of vector control has a potential for being effective. Nevertheless, clearance of vegetation has not been carried out consistently, and infection in West Africa persists.

The problem of control is much more complicated for *T. b. rhodesiense*, because this organism has many reservoir hosts and breeds in the savanna. The main vector in East Africa is *G. morsitans*. In some areas of East Africa, its distribution is less than one fly per square mile, and yet transmission continues to occur.

References

1. Atkins J: The Navy Surgeon, or Practical System of Surgery with a Dissertation on Cold and Hot Mineral Springs and Physical Observations on the Coast of Guiney. London, J Hodges, 1742
2. Bruce D: Preliminary Report of the Tsetse Fly Disease or Nagana in Zululand. Durban, Bennet and Davis, 1895
3. Forde RM: Some clinical notes on a European patient in whose blood a trypanosome was observed. J Trop Med 5:261–263, 1902
4. Stephens JWW, Fantham HB: On the peculiar morphology of a trypanosome from a case of sleeping sickness and the possibility of its being a new species (*T. rhodesiense*). Proc R Soc Lond S [Biol] 83:23–33, 1910
5. Kinghorn A, Yorke W: On the transmission of human trypanosomes by *Glossina morsitans* westw.; and on the occurrence of human trypanosomes in game. Ann Trop Med Parasitol 6:1–23, 1912

6. Bertram BCR: Sleeping sickness survey in the Serengeti Area (Tanzania) (1971). III. Discussion of the relevance of the trypanosome survey to the biology of the large mammals in the Serengeti. Acta Trop 30:36–48, 1973

7. Cross GAM: Identification, purification and properties of clone-specific glycoprotein antigens constituting the surface coat of *T. brucei*. Parasitology 71:393–417, 1975

8. Gray AR: Antigenic variation in a strain of *Trypanosoma brucei* transmitted by *Glossina morsitans* and *G. palpalis*. J Gen Microbiol 41:195–214, 1965

9. Buck GA, Eisen H: Regulation of the genes encoding variable surface antigens in African trypanosomes. ASM News 51:118–122, 1985

10. Winterbottom TM: An Account of the Native Africans in the Neighborhood of Sierra Leone, Vol. 2. London, J. Hatchard and J. Mawman, 1803

11. Voller A, Bidwell DE, Bartlett A, et al.: A comparison of isotopic and enzyme-immonoassays for tropical parasitic diseases. Trans R Soc Trop Med Hyg 71:431–437, 1977

12. Bocchi CJ, Nathan HC, Hutner SH, et al.: Polyamine metabolism: a potential therapeutic target in trypanosomes. Science 210:332–334, 1980

13. Schechter PJ, Sjoerdsma H: Difluoromethyloornithine in the treatment of African trypanosomiasis. Parasit Today 2:223–224, 1986

14. Phelps RJ, Vale GA: Studies on populations of *Glossina morsitans morsitans* and *G. pallidipe* (Diptera: Glossinidae) in Rhodesia. J Appl Ecol 15:743–760, 1978

32. *Leishmania tropica* (Wright 1903) and *Leishmania mexicana* (Biagi 1953)

The genus Leishmania has been the subject of much current taxonomic and clinical research. Through the use of DNA probes, ELISA tests, and differential respirometry, new species and subspecies of Leishmania have been identified and partially characterized.[1,2] Although taxonomy has introduced new species of this genus, from the clinical point of view only three major entities need to be discussed. They are cutaneous, muco-cutaneous, and visceral leishmaniases. Their severity varies with the geographic region and the strain of the parasite. The relative roles played by the host and the parsite in pathogenesis of this disease have not been defined. Table 32.1 provides a summary of the different Leishmaniae and the clinical manifestations attributed to them. Currently, precise speciation has only an epidemiological value, but offers no guidance to therapy, because regardless of the species or strain of Leishmania, only one drug is effective in treatment of these infections.

Cutaneous leishmaniasis is caused by an infection with either of two closely related species of protozoa, *Leishmania tropica* in the Old World, and *Leishmania mexicana* in the New World. Both organisms are transmitted by sandflies. Flies of the genus Phlebotomus are vectors of *L. tropica* throughout the Middle East, India, and Africa. Those belonging to genus Lutzomyia transmit *L. mexicana* in South and Central America. (Previous studies have suggested that what has been considered one genus, Lutzomyia, may in fact be composed of two genera, i.e., Lutzomyia and Psychodopygus.) Reservoir hosts include desert rodents and dogs for *L. tropica*, and armadillos, arboreal rodents, and dogs for *L. mexicana*.

Although it is known that the infection predominates among children and young adults, its prevalence has not been determined.

Historical Information

Russell[3] described cutaneous leishmaniasis as a clinical entity in 1856. It was Cunningham,[4] however, working in India, in 1885, who correctly described the leishmania organism he observed in a fixed section of a skin lesion. Finally Adler and Theodor[5] demonstrated that sandflies infected in the laboratory could transmit *L. tropica* to human volunteers.

Oriental sore had been well known among people living in the endemic area of the Middle East, India, and Africa. Indeed, a form of immunization was practiced in the Middle East, where it was known that persons once affected

Leishmania tropica

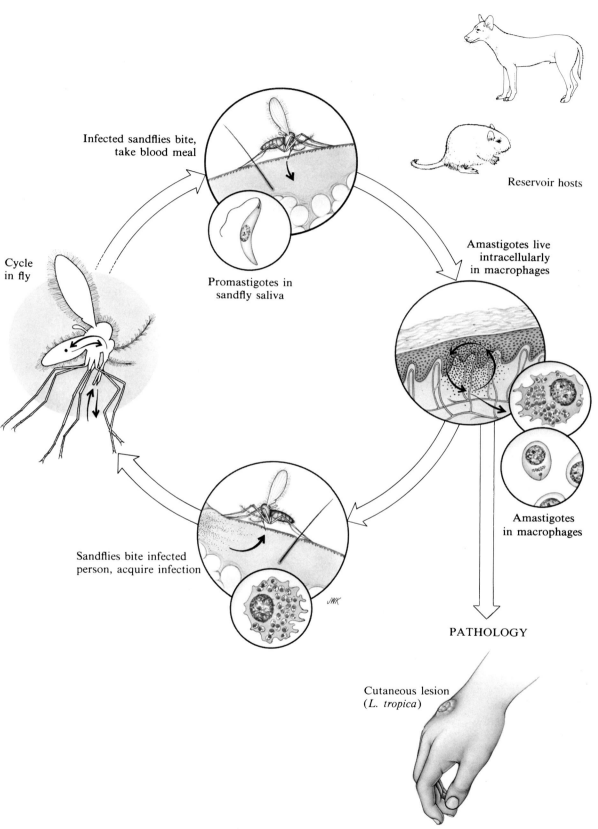

Infected sandflies bite, take blood meal

Promastigotes in sandfly saliva

Cycle in fly

Reservoir hosts

Amastigotes live intracellularly in macrophages

Amastigotes in macrophages

Sandflies bite infected person, acquire infection

PATHOLOGY

Cutaneous lesion (*L. tropica*)

TABLE 32.1* Clinical manifestations and geographic distribution of *Leishmania* sp.*

Parasite	Clinical Manifestation	Geographic Distribution
Leishmania tropica major	"wet" cutaneous leishmaniasis	Middle East, Mediterranean basin
L. tropica minor	"dry cutaneous" leishmaniasis	Asia, Middle East, Europe, North Africa, India
L. aethiopica	disseminated cutaneous leishmaniasis	East Africa
L. mexicana mexicana	cutaneous leishmaniasis	Mexico, Central America
L. mexicana amazonensis	cutaneous leishmaniasis	Amazon River Basin
L. mexicana pinfanoi	disseminated cutaneous leishmaniasis	
L. braziliensis braziliensis	mucocutaneous leishmaniasis	Central and South America
L. b. guyanensis	mucocutaneous leishmaniasis	Guyana
L. b. panamensis	metastatic cutaneous leishmaniasis (multiple lesions)	Panama
L. peruviana	non-metastatic cutaneous leishmaniasis (few lesions)	Peru
L. donovani	visceral leishmaniasis	Asia, Europe, Africa, South America

*(From Beaver PC, Jung RC, and Cupp EW (*Adapted from: Clinical Parasitology. Lea and Febiger, Phila. p65, 1984))

did not develop new lesions after the original ones had healed. Therefore, uninfected individuals were deliberately inoculated in areas other than the face with scrapings from the margins of active lesions. This resulted in a controlled infection and prevented disfiguring by the natural infection that might have affected the face.

Life Cycle

The sandfly is the vector of leishmaniasis. It is a small dipteran (see Fig. 38.5), whose flight range is very short. Only the adult females bite, and the blood they ingest is used in egg production.

Sandflies become infected by biting an infected individual. The amastigotes (1–3 μm in diameter), present in the macrophages (Fig. 33.1), are ingested by the fly and become disrupted in its stomach. Thus, the amastigotes are released and almost immediately become transformed into the promastigotes (Fig. 32.1). The promastigotes migrate to the gut and divide by binary fision. Ultimately, the promastigotes migrate to the proboscis and enter a new host when the insect bites.

On injection into man, the promastigotes are ingested by macrophages and other phagocytes, but remain intact intracellularly. The mechanism

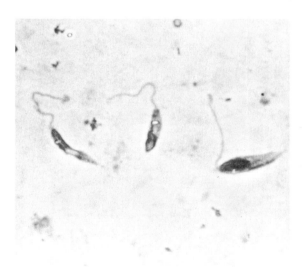

Figure 32.1. Promastigotes of *Leishmania tropica* cultured for 3 days in Schneider's medium. × 1,000. (Courtesy of Dr. S. Holmes-Giannini)

that protects them from digestion is unknown. Within these cells, the promastigotes are transformed into amastigotes and divide by binary fission. The infected host-cells lyse and release the organisms, now ready to infect new phagocytes.

The cutaneous lesion is caused by lysis of dermal cells. The organism, unlike *L. donovani* remains in the dermis and does not cause systemic infection. Most of the infected phagocytes remain in the immediate vicinity of the lesion; only rare ones stray any distance. Thus the fly, to become infected, must bite in the area where these cells have congregated.

Sandflies live approximately 2 weeks and take two or three meals during their lifetime. Once infected, the insects can transmit the infection until they die.

Pathogenesis

Following the bite, the individual develops a single nodule at the site of the bite. It may be either "dry" (Fig. 32.2) or "wet" (Fig. 32.3), and may remain quiescent for months or even years before becoming disseminated, although always remaining confined to the skin.

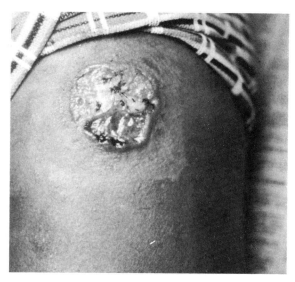

Figure 32.3. "Wet" lesion on skin of a patient infected with *Leishmania tropica*. Note the raised edge of the lesion and the shiny appearance of the necrotic center. (Courtesy of Dr. T. Jones)

The process of dissemination is aided by the development of anergy and, in this regard, resembles lepromatous leprosy. This often coincides with an intercurrent systemic illness and is associated with a negative reaction to intradermal in-

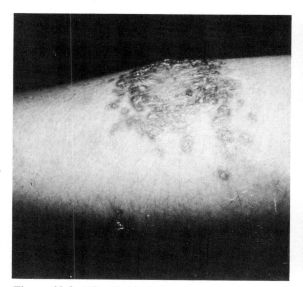

Figure 32.2. "Dry" skin lesion caused by *Leishmania tropica*. Note the secondary lesions and the crusty appearance of the primary lesion. (Courtesy of Drs. R. Armstrong and G. Zalar)

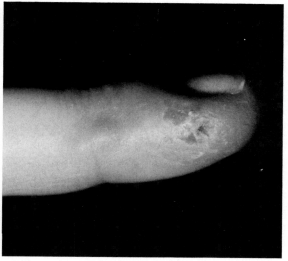

Figure 32.4. Cutaneous lesion caused by *Leishmania tropica*. Infection was acquired as the result of a laboratory accident. (Courtesy S. Mathews)

jection of leishmanin (a crude homogenate of the organisms). Ultimately, the patient develops immunity; the lesions become circumscribed and heal by forming scars (Fig. 32.4).

The single skin lesions can be differentiated from one another only by their clinical appearance; histologically they are indistinguishable. They result from rapid lysis of fixed and wandering phagocytes in the area of the bite. It had been postulated that a toxin is responsible for the lesion, but none has been identified.

Clinical Disease

The primary lesion is the small red papule appearing at the site of a bite after an incubation period of 2–8 weeks. It is an active lesion, progressing from a nodule of 1 cm in diameter to a much larger one by increasing centrifugally through the formation of satellite papules. It eventually ulcerates, becomes depressed, and heals through scarring. The patient then becomes immune for life. This type of disease is referred to as "urban."

The "rural" disease tends to be multifocal, but otherwise resembles the former pattern.

The diffuse, anergic cutaneous leishmaniasis begins as a single nodule on an exposed part of the skin, but it begins to grow and spread, eventually involving vast areas of the skin, so that the patient resembles one with lepromatous leprosy.

Diagnosis

This infection must be suspected in anyone with a chronic ulceration of the skin who resides in, or has visited, the endemic area. On clinical grounds alone, these lesions can be confused with those of leprosy and many fungal infections. The diagnosis is confirmed by the identification of organisms in the biopsy taken from the edge of the ulcer. A skin test with leishmanin, always positive by the time the ulcer has developed, remains negative during the initial stages of infection. Moreover, it does not help in an individual diagnosis in the endemic area, where a large segment of the population is positive. Patients with the anergic type of this disease have a negative skin test. There are no systemic manifestations and no abnormal blood tests.

If the organisms cannot be seen on a smear of the scrapings or on the histological section, they may appear in a culture of scrapings (Fig. 32.1) taken from the margin of the lesion and placed in a suitable medium.

Treatment

The disease tends to subside spontaneously, without complications. Therefore, therapy with the antimonial drugs, although effective, is not recommended because the drugs are toxic. However, if the lesion fails to heal in 6 months, or progresses in size, or invades mucous membranes—which implies that the infection is not cutaneous, but mucocutaneous—treatment with stibogluconate should be started. Bacterial infections of the leishmanial lesions, particularly the "wet" form, must be treated with antimicrobial agents, according to the sensitivity of the infecting organism.

Prevention and Control

Although control of vectors would prevent these infections, in practice such efforts have not been successful. Nevertheless, use of residual insecticides is helpful. This is particularly helpful in urban areas, in case of *L. tropica* infections in India and the Middle East. The sandflies are weak fliers and tend to rest periodically when hopping from place to place. Therefore, residual insecticides sprayed around windows and doors "catch" these insects as they alight inside the houses and rest.

Control of rodents and dogs has been effective in some urban communities. In rural communities, however, it has largely failed.

In Central and South America, people who work in the forests gathering chickle are at a high risk of infection as they travel to and from work at dawn and dusk, when the sandflies are most plentiful. Change of work schedule to avoid travel during the times when the flies bite would sharply reduce incidence of these infections.

Vaccination with promastigotes is a promising technique that has had some success in the southeastern part of the Soviet Union.[6]

On individual basis, insect repellents, nettings, and window screens offer some protection.

References

1. Wirth D, McMahon-Pratt D: Rapid identification of *Leishmania* species by specific hybridization of kinetoplast DNA in cutaneous lesions. Proc Nat Acad Sci USA 79:6999–7003, 1982
2. Pappas MG, Hajkowski R, Diggs CL, et al.: Disposable nitrocellular filtration plates simplify the Dot-ELISA for serodiagnosis of visceral leishmaniasis. Trans Roy Soc Trop Med Hyg 79:136, 1985
3. Russell A: Of the mal d'Aleppo. In Millar A (ed): Natural History of Aleppo and Parts Adjacent. London. 1856, pp 262–266
4. Cunningham DD: On the presence of peculiar parasitic organisms in the tissue of a specimen of Delhi boil. Sci Mem Med Officers Army India 1:21–31, 1885
5. Adler S, Theodor O: The transmission of *Leishmania tropica* from artificially infected sandflies to man. Ann Trop Med Parasitol 21:89–110, 1927
6. Sergeiev PG, Beislehem RI, Moshkovski SD, et al.: Massive vaccination against cutaneous leishmaniasis. Med Parasitol Parazit Bolezni 39:541–551, 1970

33. *Leishmania braziliensis* (Vianna 1911)

Leishmania braziliensis is the only causative agent of the mucocutaneous form of leishmaniasis. Its vectors are sandflies of the genus Lutzomyia. The infection is widely distributed throughout Central and South America. There are no data about its prevalence, but it appears to be less frequent than the cutaneous form of the infection. There is, however, a substantial coincidence of these two infections because the same vectors spread both diseases.

The reservoir hosts include the spiny rat, the opossum, and the sloth.

Historical Information

Carini,[1] in 1911, differentiated mucocutaneous lesions from the cutaneous types, thus establishing this infection as a separate nosological entity; the following year Vianna[2] identified and named *L. braziliensis* as the causative agent. Kligler[3] and Noguchi[4] finally identified this parasite serologically as a distinct species.

Life Cycle

In the sandfly, the life cycle of *L. braziliensis* resembles that of *L. mexicana.* In the mammalian host, however, it is different, because in addition to the skin it invades mucous membranes. The primary lesion in the skin resembles that due to *L. mexicana,* with the organisms residing in the phagocytic cells at the margins of the ulcer.

Secondary lesions develop by direct or hematogenous spread, in the latter case even many years after the healing of the original ulcer. These secondary lesions can appear at any mucocutaneous junction, such as the mouth, the anus, etc.

Pathogenesis

The lesions are characterized by massive necrotizing inflammation and are filled with a variety of cells, including lymphocytes, small histiocytes, and plasma cells. Skin (Fig. 33.1), mucous membranes, and cartilage can be involved. In the lesions of oral cavity, destruction of the soft palate, nasal septum, and invasion of the larynx can occur (Fig. 33.2). These lesions contain few parasites. After healing, the ulcers become replaced by fibrous tissue.

Clinical Disease

This form of leishmaniasis develops as the cutaneous variety, but the skin lesions are followed a short time (a few weeks) or a long time (many years) later by lesions of the mucocutaneous border of the mouth, nose, or—more rarely—of the soft palate, the larynx, the conjunctiva, the anus, and the extemal genitalia. These lesions can be quite disfiguring, often becoming large granulomas that heal slowly, scar, and eventually deform the tissues in which they are found.

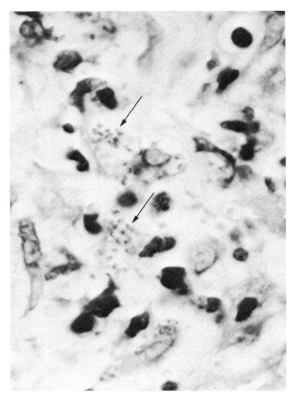

Figure 33.1. Section of skin infected with *Leishmania braziliensis (arrows)*. This section was taken from the margin of a lesion and shows the organisms present in skin macrophages. ×1,250. (Courtesy of Dr. T. Jones)

Diagnosis

Identification of the organisms in histological sections of the ulcer provides the definitive means of diagnosis. However, the organisms in this form of leishmaniasis are rare, and therefore a culture of the affected tissue is more likely to yield the diagnosis. Two media are available for culture. The newer, Schneider's medium, has the advantage of rapid results, because the promastigotes develop within 3 days of inoculation (Fig. 33.3). This is in contrast with the older method, which often required weeks. A skin test employing killed promastigotes that have been cultured in vitro can be helpful, but it becomes positive only after the initial lesion has healed, i.e., after several months of the infection. None of the available serological tests is completely satisfactory, but a direct agglutination test using promastigotes is likely to become the most useful for all forms of leishmaniasis.

Treatment

Treatment with the antimonial drugs, as indicated under kala-azar (Chapter 34), is recommended. The diffuse disease will respond initially, but in cases of relapse may be resistant to therapy, in which event amphotericin B should be used.

Prevention and Control

See Chapter 32.

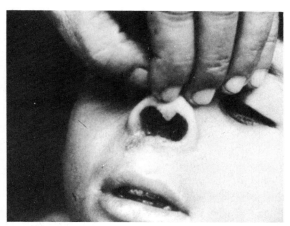

Figure 33.2. Erosion of the nasal septum caused by infection with *Leishmania braziliensis*. (Courtesy of Drs. T. Jones and P. Marsden)

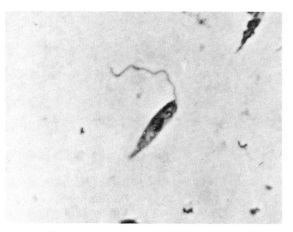

Figure 33.3. Promastigotes of *Leishmania braziliensis* grown in culture (Schneider's medium) ×1,000.

Leishmania braziliensis

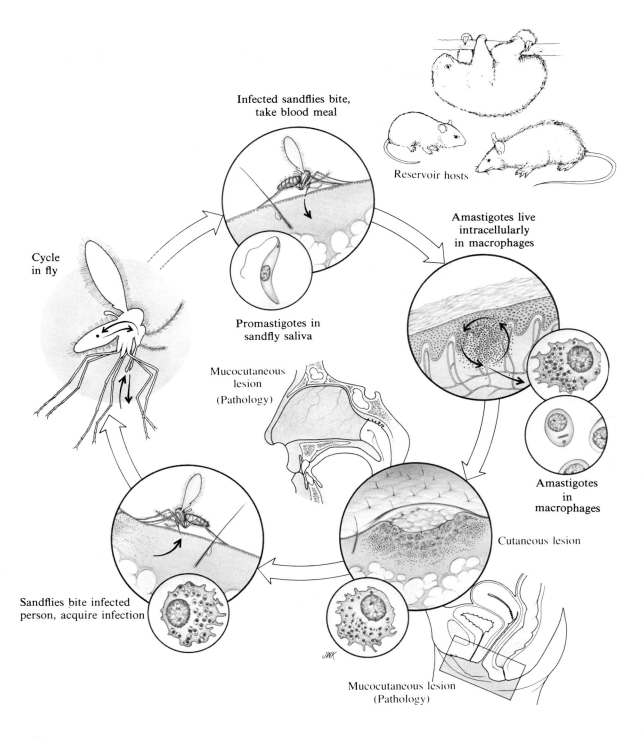

Infected sandflies bite,
take blood meal

Reservoir hosts

Promastigotes in
sandfly saliva

Cycle
in fly

Amastigotes live
intracellularly
in macrophages

Amastigotes
in
macrophages

Mucocutaneous
lesion
(Pathology)

Cutaneous lesion

Sandflies bite infected
person, acquire infection

Mucocutaneous lesion
(Pathology)

JWK

References

1. Carini A: Leishmaniose de la muqueuse rhino-buccopharyngee. Bull Soc Pathol Exot 4:289–291, 1911
2. Vianna G: Tratamento da leishmaniose tegumentar por injecoes intravenososas de tartaro emetico. Ann do 7 Congresso Brasileiro de Medicina e Cirurgia. 4:426–428, 1912
3. Kligler IJ: The cultural and serological relationship of leishmania. Trans R Soc Trop Med Hyg 19:330–335, 1916
4. Noguchi H: Comparative studies on herpetomonads and leishmaniasis. II. Differentiation of the organisms by serological reactions and fermentation tests. J Exp Med 44:305–314, 1929

34. *Leishmania donovani* (Ross 1903)

Visceral leishmaniasis, also known as kala-azar, or black fever, has a wide distribution in tropical and subtropical Africa, South America, and Asia. In addition, it is seen in the temperate zones of Asia and in endemic foci in the Mediterranean region. No accurate estimate of its prevalence is currently available. The infection is caused by a protozoan, *Leishmania donovani*, and spread by a vector, the sandfly. *Phlebotomus* sp. transmit it in Europe, Africa, and Asia; *Lutzomyia* sp. are its vectors in South America. Various species of mammals, including dogs, cats, foxes, gerbils, hamsters, ground squirrels, and monkeys act as reservoirs.

Historical Information

The causative agent of visceral leishmaniasis was discovered simultaneously, in 1903, by two physicians, Leishman[1] and Donovan,[2] while both were working in India, Leishman in the British Army and Donovan in the Indian Medical Service. Sir Ronald Ross named the genus and species after them in recognition of their landmark discovery. The morphology of the newly named species *L. donovani* was so similar to an organism described by Cunningham[3] in 1885—later to be named *L. tropica*—that it was often referred to as the Cunningham-Leishman-Donovan body when seen in histological sections of infected tissues.

Nicolle,[4] in 1908, discovered that other mammals, particularly the dog, could serve as reservoir hosts for the parasite. Swaminath and colleagues,[5] working in India, in 1942, proved in human volunteers that the infection was transmitted by the phlebotomus flies. (It is worth noting that the ethical standards under which human investigation is conducted today would not permit this type of an experiment, because there was no effective drug against this potentially lethal pathogen. This study violated another ethical standard, i.e. the names of the volunteers were listed in the publication.)

Life Cycle

Human infection begins with a bite of an infected sandfly (Fig. 38.5). The promastigotes (Fig. 34.1) enter the bite wound and are quickly taken up by the macrophages. Rapidly, within the phagocytic vacuole, the promastigotes become transformed into the amastigotes (Fig. 34.2A and B). Although lysosomes fuse with the vacuole containing the parasite and release acid hydrolases, the leishmania resists destruction by these enzymes. The mechanism of this resistance is unknown. The parasites divide within the macrophage and eventually fill the cytoplasm. The infected cell dies and releases the amastigotes, which are taken up by new macrophages. This cycle is repeated many times throughout the body. Eventually, all organs containing macrophages or fixed phagocytes become infected. The spleen, liver, and bone marrow are the most seriously affected organs.

The cycle is completed when an infected man is bitten by an uninfected sandfly, which ingests macrophages containing the amastigotes. These forms are released in the fly's stomach by digestion, reach the midgut, and quickly transform into promastigotes. After many divisions, they migrate into the anterior region of the fly's gut, ready for injection into a new host. The duration of the cycle within the fly is approximately 10 days.

Leishmania donovani

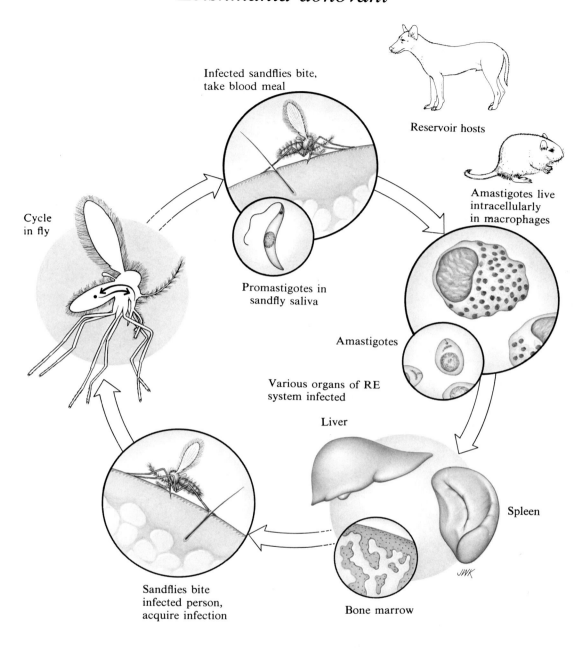

Infected sandflies bite, take blood meal

Reservoir hosts

Amastigotes live intracellularly in macrophages

Cycle in fly

Promastigotes in sandfly saliva

Amastigotes

Various organs of RE system infected

Liver

Spleen

Bone marrow

Sandflies bite infected person, acquire infection

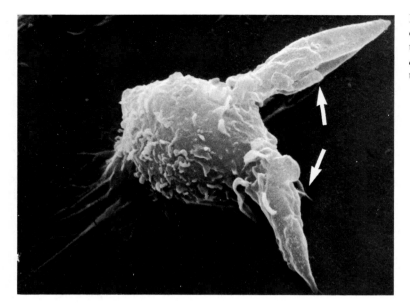

Figure 34.1. Scanning electron micrograph of a macrophage engulfing two promastigotes of *Leishmania donovani (arrows).* ×2,500. (Courtesy of Dr. K.-P. Chang)

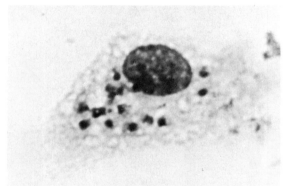

A

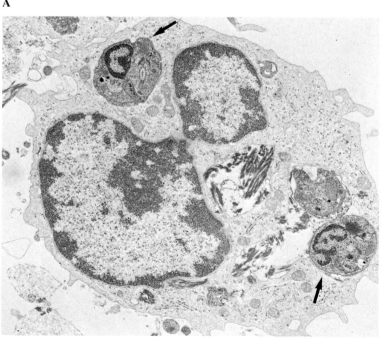

B

Figure 34.2. A. Light micrograph of a macrophage infected with amastigotes of *Leishmania donovani.* **B.** Transmission electron micrograph of macrophage with amastigotes of *Leishmania donovani.* **A,** ×2,000; **B,** ×15,300. (**A:** Courtesy of Dr. H. Murray; **B:** Courtesy of Dr. K.-P. Chang)

Pathogenesis

The infection and subsequent destruction of histiocytes and macrophages, both fixed and wandering, is the underlying cause of all pathological changes in this disease. The organisms replicate in the spleen (Fig. 34.3), liver (Fig. 34.4), and bone marrow (Fig. 34.5). Splenomegaly and hypersplenism develop. There is an accelerated production of macrophages, which potentiate the disease by providing a substrate for the replication of the parasites. Skin histiocytes also harbor the organisms, as do any skin lesions that may appear after therapy.

Clinical Disease

Kala-azar

The majority of cases have an incubation period of 3–6 months. Longer incubation periods have been reported, but they may have been spurious, because the time of the infection could not be determined with certainty. In experimental dis-

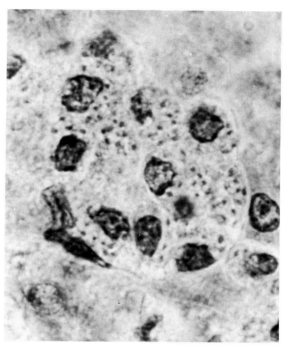

Figure 34.4. Section of liver showing amastigotes of *Leishmania donovani*. ×1,575.

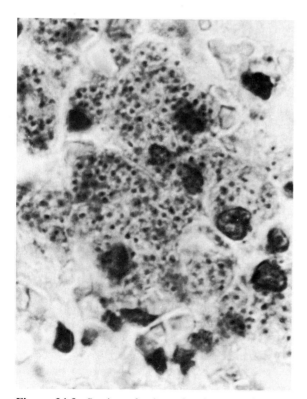

Figure 34.3. Section of spleen showing amastigotes of *Leishmania donovani*. ×1,575.

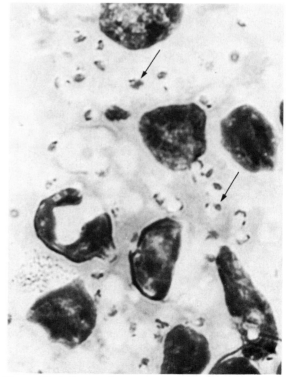

Figure 34.5. Impression smear from liver tissue infected with amastigotes (*arrows*) of *Leishmania donovani*. ×2,000.

ease, the incubation period varies between several days and 10 months. The onset can be either gradual or sudden. In the former, the initial symptoms can be nonspecific, often relating to the enlarging spleen. The clinical diagnosis is often missed or is discovered inadvertently when patients present with some other acute illness, such as a respiratory or gastrointestinal infection.[6] In the latter, the onset is heralded by high fever, which is sometimes intermittent, giving rise to the classic, but by no means invariable, "dromedary" fever, with a double daily spike. Periods of fever tend to subside for days, or even several weeks, only to return. Thus they resemble undulant fever. Splenomegaly evolves, and in a patient ill for several weeks, the spleen tends to be large enough to occupy most of the left side of the abdomen.

The patient, although weak, does not feel very ill and withstands periods of fever without malaise or apathy. This is an important clinical differential diagnostic point, distinguishing patients with kala-azar from those with typhoid fever or malaria. Indeed, it may be said that the clinical disease is more apparent to the objective observer than to the patient himself. Generalized lymphadenopathy and, later, also hepatomegaly eventually develop.

Periodicity of fever and afebrile state can continue for weeks, or even months, while the patient becomes increasingly emaciated and weak. Many patients die *with* kala-azar, rather than *of* kala-azar, because of an intercurrent acute infection superimposed on this subacute disease. Throughout this period, the patients become anemic and develop hypersplenism with the leukocyte counts of 3000/mm^3, or even lower. There is also thrombocytopenia. The patients, particularly those in late stages, have a high concentration of serum protein approaching 10 g/100 ml. This is almost exclusively due to rise in IgG.

The disease has certain regional differences. For example, in Africa, there may be a primary cutaneous nodule preceding systemic symptoms by several months. In the Mediterranean countries, in Africa, and in China, the generalized lymphadenopathy is more intense than in other parts of the world. Hyperpigmentation of hands, feet, and abdomen is not as apparent in Africans, because of their dark skin, as it is in Indians of lighter skin coloration. On the other hand, warty eruptions and ulcers appear in the skins of the Africans. Among Indians whose disease has been treated or who recovered spontaneously, about 20% of patients develop a skin rash 1–2 years later. This rash is characterized by hypopigmented or erythematous macules, which eventually become papular and nodular. They are particularly prominent on the face and the upper parts of the body, resembling those of lepromatous leprosy. These lesions are filled with histiocytes containing leishmaniae and serve as sources of infection for the sandflies. Among the African patients, only 2% of those who recover develop such skin lesions.

Diagnosis

Diagnosis of kala-azar must be suspected in anyone with protracted fever and splenomegaly who has lived in, or visited, an endemic area. Granulocytopenia, anemia, and elevation of γ-globulins strongly support the diagnosis.

Definitive diagnosis depends on isolation of the parasite. This can be accomplished by aspiration of bone marrow (Fig. 34.5), spleen, a lymph node, or liver. Because of the relative safety, bone marrow aspiration is the preferred method for obtaining the parasites. These organisms can usually be seen in the specimen stained with Giemsa solution. Although the organisms are present in the macrophages, these cells tend to rupture in the preparation of the specimen and therefore free parasites are seen in the smear. In addition, the parasites can be cultured (see Fig. 33.3).

Immunodiagnosis is also possible. Antibodies to the leishmania can be demonstrated by indirect immunofluorescence in about 90% of the infected patients. The leishmanin skin test is usually negative in patients with active infection, but becomes positive after successful therapy.

Treatment

The drug of choice is pentavalent antimony, presented as sodium stibogluconate, administered by injections over a period of several days. Side effects characteristic of antimonial drugs do occur. They include nausea, vomiting, skin reactions, and interference with the cardiac rhythm. This therapy is usually quite effective, although in the East African and Mediterranean varieties of the disease there are occasional failures. They may be treated with the alternative drug, pentamidine isethionate. It must be remembered that leishmaniasis is a subacute or chronic disease and that the response will be gradual. Clinical signs will also be slow to recede; in particular, splenomegaly may never disappear completely. Because of the slow convalescence, it is essential to provide the patient with good nursing care and nutritional support. The ultimate proof of a cure is a negative bone marrow culture 1 year after completion of therapy. Absence of humoral antibodies after cure has also been reported. Relapses are quite rare and can be retreated in the same fashion as the original infection.

Prevention and Control

L. donovani infections can be reduced or eliminated by control of the vector, as outlined in Chapter 32. This was partially achieved in the Mediterranean as a byproduct of malaria eradication programs, which reduced *Phlebotomus* sp. when insecticides were applied against mosquitoes. Now that malaria has been controlled and insecticides are no longer used, sandflies have returned and with them kala-azar.

References

1. Leishman WB: On the possibility of occurrence of trypanosomiasis in India. Br Med J 1:1252–1254, 1903
2. Donovan C: On the possibility of occurrence of trypanosomiasis in India. Br Med J 2:79, 1903
3. Cunningham DD: On the presence of peculiar parasitic organisms in the tissue of a specimen of Delhi boil. Sci Mem Med Officers Army India 1:21–31, 1885
4. Nicolle C: Nouvelles acquisitions sur Kala-azar: Cultures; inoculation au chien; etiologie. CR Hebdom Sci 146:498–499, 1908
5. Swaminath CS, Shortt HE, Anderson LAP: Transmission of Indian kala-azar to man by the bites of *Phlebotomus argentipes*. Ann Brun Indian J Med Res 30:473–477, 1942
6. Badaro R, Jones TC, Cawalho EM, et al.: New perspectives on a subclinical form of visceral leishmaniasis. J Infect Dis 154:1003–1011, 1986

35. *Pneumocystis carinii* (Delanoë and Delanoë 1912)

Pneumocystis carinii is an extracellular ameboid organism with three developmental forms, defined only on the basis of their morphology. It is ubiquitous and affects all age groups and both sexes.

Immunocompromised individuals tend to develop *P. carinii* pneumonia. Among them patients with AIDS, with lymphoma and leukemia in remission, as well as those immunosuppressed for organ transplantation, and malnourished infants are the most common victims.[1]

In patients with AIDS, treatment has been effective in delaying death, as has been prophylactic medication, especially by inhalation.

Historical Information

P. carinii was originally described by Chagas[2] in 1909, although he assumed it to be a developmental stage of the trypanosome. In 1912, Delanoë and Delanoë[3] observed it in the lungs of rats that were free of trypanosomes, defined it as a distinct organism, and gave it its current name.

Life Cycle

The life cycle of *P. carinii* is not known. The largest forms of this organism are "cysts," spheres, or crescents 5 μm in diameter, which contain 8 oval structures, the "sporozoites," 1–2 μm in diameter. In addition, there may be sickle-shaped structures, 2–5 μm in diameter, not contained within the cysts and referred to as "trophozoites" (Fig. 35.1A and B). There is much controversy about the classification of this organism, but it is probably a protozoan.[4] It is an eukaryote, and its cytoplasm possesses rough endoplasmic reticulum and mitochondria.[5] It is sensitive to antiprotozoan drugs. On the other hand, its staining characteristics with periodic acid-Schiff's reagent and silver methenamine resemble those of fungi.[6]

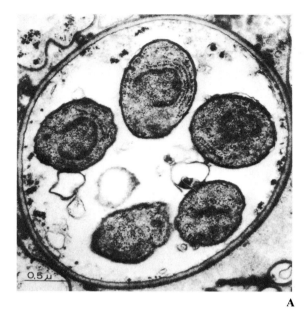

A

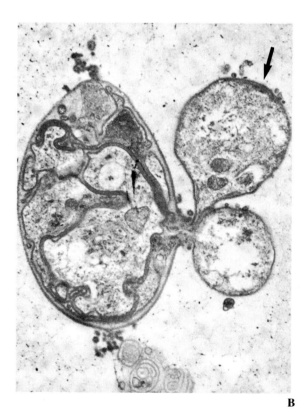

B

The nutritional requirements of pneumocystis have not been investigated, but the organism is probably a commensal that becomes an opportunistic parasite.

It has been possible to propagate the organism in vitro, in primary chicken lung epithelial cells.[7] In this system, trophozoites attach to the cell surfaces, then, after detaching themselves from the cells, change into cysts within 90 min, the entire cycle being completed in 4–6 h. It is probable that the cycle in vivo is similar and that encystation and excystation occur in the alveolar spaces.

Pathogenesis

In a patient with pneumonia due to pneumocystis, the alveolar spaces in the lungs are distended and filled with a frothy honeycombed material (Fig. 35.2). These secretions contain numerous cysts and trophozoites best seen stained with silver methenamine, which provides contrast with the

Figure 35.1. A. Transmission electron micrograph of a cyst of *Pneumocystis carinii.* Five of the eight trophozoites are visible in this view. **B.** Transmission electron micrograph of an excysting trophozoite *(arrow)* of *Pneumocystis carinii.* **A,** ×5,000; **B,** ×7,500. (**A:** courtesy of Drs. M. Vossen and P. Beckers; **B:** courtesy of Dr. T. Jones)

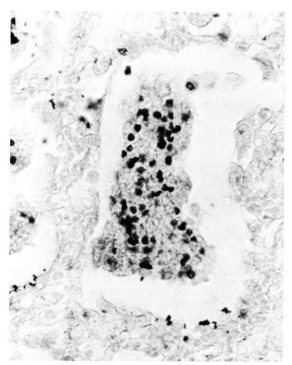

Figure 35.2. Cross-section of a portion of lung biopsied from an adult infected with *Pneumocystis carinii.* The silver methenamine stain highlights the outer cyst wall as a dark ovoid object. ×500.

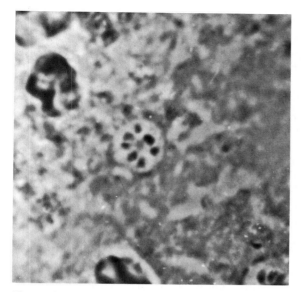

Figure 35.3. The cyst stage of *Pneumocystis carinii* as seen on an impression smear made from a lung biopsy specimen. Eight trophozoites within the cyst are visible in this Giemsa-stained preparation. ×2,100.

cyst wall and often shows the eight trophozoites within it (Fig. 35.3). The interstitial septa are infiltrated with plasma cells.

The immunosuppressed or immunoincompetent individuals are the prime targets of this infection. Failure of humoral immunity, especially depression of IgG,[8] appears to be the predisposing factor in children with congenital immunodeficiency. This is apparently in contrast to patients with malignancies, who develop this infection in the presence of normal or high levels of IgG.[9] In malnourished infants, elevations of IgM have been reported with the infection, followed by permanent immunity in the survivors, who show rises in serum IgG concentration 4–6 weeks after the onset of the infection.[10]

Clinical Disease

Clinical disease has no unique characteristics. It resembles a number of severe pneumonias caused by opportunists in susceptible subjects. The mode of onset can be either insidious or fulminating. In debilitated, malnourished infants, the onset tends to be insidious, with progressively increasing respiratory distress. In the immunoincompetent patients, the onset is usually abrupt, with dyspnea

and tachypnea at rest being common features. Physical examination reveals nasal flaring and intercostal retractions. The patient is hypoxic, may be cyanotic, and is usually ashen. The respirations are shallow and rapid, and there are scattered rhonchi and rales. Fever is not frequent; indeed, when it occurs, it is likely to have a cause other than the pneumocystis infection. The chest radiogram is not characteristic either, although most patients with pneumocystis pneumonia tend to have diffuse interstitial infiltrates. Untreated, the disease has a virtually 100% case fatality rate. In patients with AIDS, the organism becomes disseminated throughout the body, probably transported by the macrophages.[1,2]

Diagnosis

In view of the great danger it poses for the patient, pneumocystis infection must be diagnosed swiftly. It must be suspected on clinical grounds in a patient known to be at risk. Unfortunately, the only reliable diagnostic methods are invasive. Transbronchial, or open lung biopsy, is most precise; bronchopulmonary lavage, or endobronchial brush biopsy, is also reliable, although providing a lower yield. No dependable serological test is available.

Treatment

Treatment with trimethoprim sulfamethoxazole is effective.[13] Because it is relatively free of side effects, this drug has often been prescribed in the absence of a definitive diagnosis. Trimethoprim sulfamethoxazole has also been used in prophylaxis against pneumocystis in patients at risk.[14] Pentamidine isethionate is an alternative therapy. It is more toxic, causing hypotension, hypoglycemia, blood dyscrasias, vomiting, renal damage, and local pain at the site of injection. In the United States, this drug must be obtained from the Centers for Disease Control.

Prevention and Control

The mode of spread of this infection is unknown; hence no preventive or control methods can be suggested, except the above-mentioned prophylaxis with trimethoprim sulfamethoxazole.

References

1. Dutz W: *Pneumocystis carinii* pneumonia. Pathol Annu 5:309–341, 1970
2. Chagas C: Novo trypanomaiazaia human. Mem Inst Oswaldo Cruz 1:159, 1909
3. Delanoë P, Delanoë M: Sur les rapports des kystes de carinii du pneumon des rats avec le trypanosoma Lewisii. C R Acad Sci 155:658, 1912
4. Vossen MEMH, Beckers PJA, Meuwissen JHETh, et al: Developmental biology of *Pneumocystis carinii*, an alternative view on the life cycle of the parasite. Z Parasitenkd 55:101–118, 1978
5. Masur H, Jones TC: The interaction in vitro of *Pneumocystis carinii* with macrophages and L-cells. J Exp Med 147:157–170, 1978
6. Varva JK, Kucera K: *Pneumocystis carinii* Delanoë, its ultrastructure and intrastructural affinities. J Protozool 17:463–483, 1970
7. Pifer LL, Hughes WT, Murphy MJ Jr: Propagation of *Pneumocystis carinii* in vitro. Pediatr Res 11:305–316, 1977
8. Walzer PD, Schultz MG, Western KA, et al.: *Pneumocystis carinii* pneumonia and primary immunodeficiency diseases of infancy and childhood. J Pediatr 82:416–422, 1973
9. Brazinsky JH, Phillips JE: Pneumocystis pneumonia transmission between patients with lymphoma. JAMA 209:1527–1529, 1969
10. Koltay M, Illyes M: A study of immunoglobulin in the blood serum of infants with interstitial plasma cellular pneumonia. Acta Paediat Scand 55:489–496, 1969
11. Grimes MM, La Pook JD, Bar MH, et al.: Disseminated *Pneumocystis carinii* infection in a patient with aquired immunodeficiency syndrome. Human Path 18:307–308, 1987
12. Schinella RA, Breda SD, Hammerschlag PE: Otic infection due to *Pneumocystis carinii* in an apparently healthy man with antibody to the human immunodeficiency virus. Assoc Int Med 106:399–400, 1987
13. Wharton JM, Coleman DL, Wolfsy CB, et al.: Trimethoprim sulfamethoxazole or pentamidine for *Pneumocystis carinii* pneumonia in the acquired immunodeficiency syndrome Ann Int Med 105:37–44, 1986
14. Hughs WT, Rivera GK, Schell MJ et al.: Successful intermittent chemoprophylaxis for *Pneumocystis carinii* pneumonitis. N Eng J Med 316:1627–1632, 1987

36. Protozoans of Minor Medical Importance

Babesia spp.

Babesiosis, or piroplasmosis, in man is a rare, zoonotic, protozoan infection transmitted by ticks. Infections can also be acquired by blood transfusion.[1] The parasite infects erythrocytes and the disease that results is similar to malaria, although it has been confused with Rocky Mountain spotted fever. It has two clinical patterns. Patients without spleens are likely to have fatal infections caused by species of babesia associated with cattle: *Babesia bigemina*, *B. divergens*, and *B. bovis*. Normal individuals, who develop a self-limited disease, tend to be infected by a parasite of rodents, *B. microti*, the most common species of babesia infecting man in the United States.

B. bigemina, the cause of red water fever in cattle, was the first organism shown to be transmitted by the bite of an arthropod vector[2] and served as a model for the more dramatic studies of mosquitoes as vectors of malaria and yellow fever. Although long recognized as an important infection of wild and domestic animals, particularly cattle, babesiosis as a human disease received little attention. The first attribution of a human infection to babesiosis was incorrect when, at the beginning of this century Rocky Mountain spotted fever was thought to be caused by, or at least associated with, *"Piroplasmosis hominis."*[3] The first case of babesiosis in man was identified in 1957.[4]

Babesia infects erythrocytes, proceeds through stages of development within them and multiplies by budding. Neither exoerythrocytic nor sexual stages have been described. The parasite is transmitted by the bite of blood-feeding hard ticks of the family Ixodidae (see Chapter 39). In some tick species, the parasite may be passed from stage to stage as the tick molts (transstadial transmission), or it may be transmitted from female tick by the egg to the offspring (transovarial transmission). After several cycles of multiplication within the tick, the parasite enters the salivary glands and infects the vertebrate host when the tick attaches and feeds.

The disease appears to be the consequence of hemolysis caused by the parasite. In contrast with plasmodium, babesia does not produce any pigment within the red cells. Nothing is known about exoerythrocytic sites or about specific involvement of any organs. Postmortem examinations reveal nonspecific hyperemia of most organs and scattered hemorrhages, particularly in the liver. Liver and spleen are enlarged, and many tissues show capillaries blocked by the parasitized cells. Renal tubular damage, due to intravascular hemolysis, has also been described. Parasitemia is prolonged, except in individuals who lack the spleen, in whom the disease usually is rapidly fatal.[5] This, coupled with experimental studies in the hamster, has suggested that the spleen is the major site of host defense.

Babesiosis in man is a malaria-like disease characterized by fever, chills, headache, lethargy, and myalgia. Physical examination reveals hepatomegaly and splenomegaly. Fever is irregular and lacks periodicity. There are no specific clinical symptoms. Hemolytic anemia and hemoglobinuria are characteristic and may be severe. Individuals with intact spleens infected with *B. microti* usually recover spontaneously without treatment, although the course of the infection may be protracted.

The disease should be suspected in any individual with an illness resembling malaria who recently resided in areas where babesia is endemic. Microscopic examination of thin blood smears stained with Giemsa or Wright's solution reveals erythrocytes containing small parasites, although in some cases the parasitemia may be so low that it is difficult to detect. The small rings of babesia are superficially similar to the early rings of *Plasmodium falciparum,* and careful differentiation is critical (Fig. 36.1). Absence of pigment (hemozoin) in red cells parasitized by babesia is a helpful criterion in differentiating infection with this parasite from that due to *P. falciparum.* However, it is also absent in red cells containing *young* rings of the malarial parasites, and this may make early differentiation

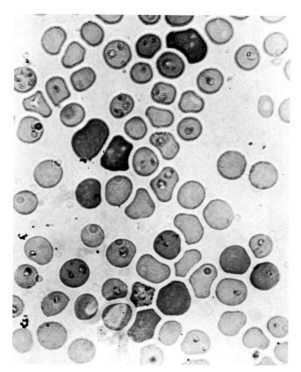

Figure 36.1. Red blood cells infected with *Babesia microti.* × 1,000.

difficult. A white vacuole is present in some of the larger rings of babesia.[6]

B. microti, grows well in hamsters. Thus multiplication of the parasite after subinoculation into these animals can serve as a confirmatory test. *B. divergens,* which infects cattle in Europe, replicates in gerbils.[7] Serologic tests for babesia are possible early in the infection.[8] Experimental evidence suggests that the indirect immunofluorescence test may be useful in diagnosing babesiosis.[9]

No satisfactory drugs are available for treatment of babesiosis, although a number of compounds have been tested.[10] Chloroquine seems to relieve the symptoms, but does not reduce parasitemia. Pentamidine has also been used, but its effects have not been evaluated adequately. Analgesics and antipyretics provide symptomatic relief.

Patients lacking spleens who are infected with babesia of cattle and have a potentially life-threatening disease should be treated aggressively with antitrypanosome drugs such as pentamidine and a veterinary compound of diminazene aceturate and antipyrine known as Berenil; quinine sulfate has been reported effective in one asplenic patient.[11] Exchange transfusions have been useful for reducing parasitemia in patients with fulminant infections.[12]

Because babesia and *P. falciparum* can be initially confused, chloroquine therapy may be initiated until a definitive diagnosis is made.

Seven cases of babesiosis in the Old World, caused by *B. bovis* or *B. divergens*, have been recorded in patients without spleens, and five of these were fatal. All but one of the cases were clearly associated with cattle and the tick vector was *Ixodes ricinus*.[6,12] Six cases of babesiosis probably of bovine origin have been reported from the New World (Mexico, three; California, two; and Georgia, one). Only the California cases involved patients without spleens; none was fatal.[12]

A major focus of human babesiosis has been reported from the northeastern United States. Ninety-nine cases, most of them from islands off Massachusetts and New York, have been recorded. The majority of the patients had intact spleens. Three cases were transmitted by transfusions and one of these was fatal.[12]

Babesiosis in the eastern United States is caused by *B. microti*, a parasite of meadow voles and field mice.[13] Man becomes infected by the bite of nymphs of the hard tick *I. dammini* (Fig. 39.6).[14,15] Ticks are infected as larvae when they feed on rodent reservoirs of the parasite. The parasite is passed transstadially with the molt from the larval to the nymphal stage. Nymphs feed on rodents, deer (which support both nymphal and adult ticks), and occasionally on man. It is the infected nymphal ticks that transmit the parasite to rodents or man. There is no evidence for transovarial transmission of babesia. Nymphs feed from May through September and human infections usually become patent 1–3 weeks after the bite of an infectious tick.

No extraordinary control measures are recommended because babesiosis is a rare disease. Avoidance of areas infested with ticks will minimize contact with the vectors. Individuals frequenting areas where ticks are common may use repellants containing diethyltolumide (DEET) and should check carefully for the presence of ticks on the body at regular intervals (see Chapter 39, for general discussion of tick removal).

Dientamoeba fragilis (Jepps and Dobell 1918)

Infection with *D. fragilis*, an ubiquitous enteric protozoan, often results in mild diarrhea, but only rarely in dysentery.[16] No fatalities have been reported. The organism is binucleate and ameboid in shape (Fig. 36.2), measuring 6–9 μm in diameter. Its name is misleading, because *D. fragilis* is more closely related structurally and antigenically to the flagellates (trichomonads)[17] than to the amebae. Moreover, in contrast with amebae, it does not form cysts. Therefore, it probably is a trichomonad that has lost its flagella. *D. fragilis* lives in the large intestine. Pathogenesis of the disease it causes is unknown; the organism does not invade tissues. Diagnosis is established by microscopic examination of stool. Therapy consists of administration of iodoquinol.

Transmission of this infection probably occurs through the oro-fecal route.

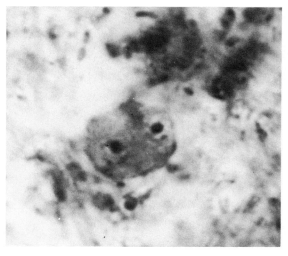

Figure 36.2. Trophozoite of *Dientamoeba fragilis*. ×2,500.

Naegleria fowleri, Acanthamoeba castellani, and Blastocystis hominis

Naegleria spp.[18] and *Acanthamoeba* spp.[19] (sometimes referred to as Hartmanella-Acanthamoeba), two genera of free-living amebae found throughout the world, are capable of causing meningoencephalitis. The acanthamebae (Fig. 36.3) were discovered by accident, when cerebrospinal fluid was inoculated into a tissue culture of fibroblasts in an attempt to demonstrate a viral etiology. The monolayer of the cells was destroyed, which suggested a cytopathic effect of a virus. Further examination revealed the amebae.

N. fowleri (Fig. 36.4) is a common inhabitant of freshwater, and is usually present in low numbers. However, when the water temperature exceeds 35°C, the ameba begins to reproduce, rapidly expanding its population. It has both trophozoite and cyst stages. *N. fowleri* apparently infects by entering the central nervous system through the cribriform plate. It invades the cerebral cortex (Fig. 36.5) and causes a fulminating disease that is invariably fatal. There is no evidence of any innate predisposition to this infection. The only common factor is swimming in, and especially diving into, stagnant warm waters.

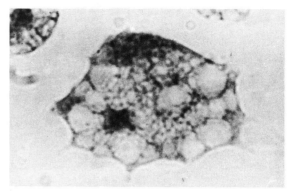

Figure 36.4. *Naegleria fowleri* trophozoite. × 1,575.

Diagnosis is made by demonstration of the amebae in the cerebrospinal fluid by direct examination.

No treatment is effective, although amphotericin B has been used experimentally.[20]

A. castellanii is found in soil contaminated by human feces, where it grows and reproduces as a free-living organism. The exact route of infection in man is not known, but it is possible that cysts may be contaminants of the conjunctivae or the skin, and individuals with an underlying severe, debilitating disease, such as a malignancy, or those who are immunosuppressed are subject to an opportunistic infection.

The disease has a variable clinical pattern. After inducing granulomatous lesions in the skin or mucous membranes, the amebae gain access to

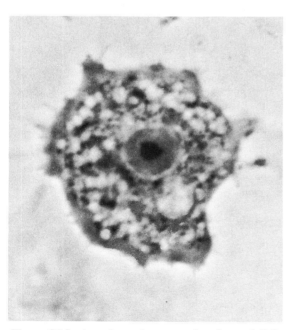

Figure 36.3. *Acanthamoeba* sp. trophozoite. × 1,950.

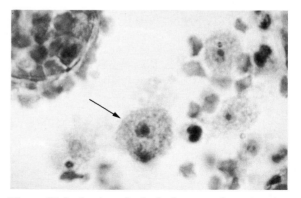

Figure 36.5. Section of a brain from a patient who died of primary amebic meningoencephalitis. The *arrow* indicates an amoeba. × 390. (Courtesy of Dr. R. Hays)

the viscera and may produce granulomatous abscesses in the kidneys, adrenal glands, the pancreas, and the central nervous system. The disease caused by acanthamoeba is less severe than that due to *N. fowleri*, and some patients have recovered from the infection, perhaps as the result of the treatment. Keratitis caused by acanthamoeba in patients with no apparent immune failure, who had either surgery or trauma to the eye, has been reported.[21] Moreover, wearers of soft contact lenses have become infected with *A. castellani*.[22] A common source of the infection has been homemade saline solutions used to wash and store the lenses. Such an infection has also resulted from swimming in waters contaminated with the ameba, while wearing the lenses.

Diagnosis follows the pattern described for *N. fowleri*.

Treatment consists of administration of amphotericin B.[3] Infections with these organisms have a more protracted course than those due to *N. fowleri*. It is appropriate to start therapy with amphotericin on suspicion of the diagnosis and continue it if the diagnosis is established.

Prevention of infection with *N. fowleri* involves avoidance of swimming in warm stagnant waters, particularly if their temperatures exceed 30°C. Methods of prevention of infection with *A. castellani* are still not available, since the precise mode of transmission remains unknown.

Blastocystis hominis is an anaerobic protozoan of uncertain classification. Some clinical studies have suggested that it is an etiologic agent of diarrhea.[23,24] However simultaneous presence of known enteric pathogens in many patients infected with *B. hominis* makes specific attribution of cause of the diarrhea uncertain.[25] No specific treatment has been effective in eradicating this protozoan.

References

1. Smith RP, Evans AT, Popovsky M, et al.: Transfusion-acquired babesiosis and failure of antibiotic treatment. JAMA 256:2726–2727, 1986
2. Smith T, Kilbourne FL: Investigations into the nature, causation and prevention of Texas or south cattle fever. USDA Bureau Anim Indust Bull 1:1–301, 1893
3. Skrabalo Z, Deanovic Z: Piroplasmosis in man. Documenta Med Geogr Trop 9:11–16, 1957
4. Garnham PCC: Human babesiosis: European aspects. Trans R Soc Trop Med Hyg 74: 153–156, 1980
5. Hoare CA: Comparative aspects of human babesiosis. Trans R Soc Trop Med Hyg 74:143–148, 1980
6. Williams H: Human babesiosis. Trans R Soc Trop Med Hyg 74:157–158, 1980
7. Ruebush TK II: Human babesiosis in North America. Trans R Soc Trop Med Hyg 74:149–152, 1980
8. Chisolm ES, Ruebush TK II, Sulzer AJ, et al.: *Babesia microti* infections in man: Evaluation of indirect immunofluorescent antibody test. Am J Trop Med Hyg 27:14–19, 1978
9. Miller LH, Neva FA, Gill F: Failure of chloroquine in human babesiosis (*Babesia microti*). Ann Intern Med 88:200–202, 1978
10. Brendt AB, Weinstein WM, Cohen S: Treatment of babesiosis in asplenic patients. JAMA 245: 1938–1939, 1981
11. Dammin GJ, Spielman A, Benach JL, et al.: The rising incidence of clinical *Babesia microti* infection. Hum Pathol 12:398–400, 1981
12. Healy GR, Spielman A, Gleason N: Human babesiosis: Reservoir of infection on Nantucket Island. Science 192:479–480, 1976
13. Spielman A: Human babesiosis on Nantucket Island: Transmission by nymphal Ixodes ticks. Am J Trop Med Hyg 25:784–787, 1976
14. Spielman A, Clifford C, Piesman J, et al.: Human babesiosis on Nantucket Island, U.S.A.: Description of the vector *Ixodes (Ixodes) dammini*, n. sp. (Acarina: Ixodidae). J Med Entomol 15:218–234, 1979
15. Spencer MJ, Garcia LS, Chapin MR: *Dientamoeba fragilis* an intestinal pathogen in children? Am J Dis Child 133:390–393, 1979
16. Dwyer DM: Analysis of the antigenic relationships among Trichomonas, Histomonas, Dientamoeba, and Entamoeba: I. Quantitative fluorescent antibody methods. J Protozool 19:316–325, 1972
17. Carter RF: Primary amoebic meningoencephalitis: Clinical, pathological, and epidemiological features of six fatal cases. J Pathol Bacteriol 96:1–25, 1968
18. Culbertson CG: The pathogenicity of soil amebas. Annu Rev Microbiol 25:231–254, 1971
19. Carter RF: Primary amoebic meningo-encephalitis—an appraisal of present knowledge. Trans R Soc Trop Med Hyg 66:193–213, 1972
21. Ma P, Willaert K, Juechter KB, et al.: A case of keratitis due to *Acanthamoeba* in New York, New York and features of 10 cases. J Infect Dis 143:662–667, 1981
22. Stehr-Green JK, Bailey TM, Brandt FH, et al.: Acanthamoeba keratitis in soft contact lens wearers. A case control study. JAMA 258:57–60, 1987

23. Zierdt, CH: *Blastocystis hominis,* a protozoan parasite and intestinal pathogen of human beings. Coin Micro Newsletter 5:57–59, 1983

24. Vanaratta B, Adamson D, Mullican K: *Blastocystis hominis* infection presenting as recurring diarrhea. Ann Int Med 102:495–496, 1986

25. Markell EK, Udkow MP: *Blastocystis Hominis:* Pathogen or fellow traveler? Am J Trop Med Hyg 35:1023–1026, 1986

37. Nonpathogenic Protozoa

Many species of protozoa can infect man, but most are commensals and cause no diseases. Their presence in the stool, however, is an important indicator that the patient had ingested some fecal matter, and therefore identification of them has diagnostic value. In addition, it is important for the clinician to recognize these organisms as commensals rather than, in ignorance, to treat the patients unnecessarily.

Commensal Flagellates

Tables 37.1 and 37.2 list and describe, respectively, the five nonpathogenic flagellates and the six commensal species of amebae commonly found in human stool.

Two species of trichomonas, *T. tenax* (Fig. 37.1) and *T. hominis,* are found in the mouth and gastrointestinal tract, respectively. Both are anaerobes. Neither organism forms cysts, and therefore infection of man with the first requires mouth-to-mouth contact; the latter is transmitted through food or water freshly contaminated with feces. In some cases, *T. hominis* has been found in pleural fluid. This is usually a result of perforation of a viscus and seepage of the fluid into the pleural cavity. There is no evidence that in such cases trichomonas acts as a pathogen.[1]

Enteromonas hominis, Retortamonas intestinalis (Fig. 37.2), and *Chilomastix mesnili* (Fig. 37.3A and B) have not been implicated in any human disease. All three produce cysts and, like pathogenic amebae, are transmitted by contaminated food or water. It is important therefore in patients suspected of amebiasis in whom these nonpatho-

Table 37.1. Commensal Flagellates

Name of Organism	Location in Body	Mode of Transmission	Morphological Characteristics	
Trichomonas tenax	Oral cavity, between gingival flaps	Oral–oral route	Trophozoite: 7 μm × 3 μm	
Trichomonas hominis	Lumens of small and large intestine	Fecal–oral route	Trophozoite: 10 μm × 8 μm	
Enteromonas hominis	Lumens of small and large intestine	Fecal–oral route	Trophozoite: 7 μm × 4 μm	Cyst: 7 μm × 5 μm
Retortamonas intestinalis	Lumens of small and large intestine	Fecal–oral route	Trophozoite: 7 μm × 4 μm	Cyst: 6 μm × 4 μm
Chilomastix mesnili	Lumen of large intestine	Fecal–oral route	Trophozoite: 15–20 μm × 8 μm	Cyst: 9 μm × 5 μm

gens are found to continue searching for the pathogenic amebae

Commensal Amebae

There are six commensal species of amebae capable of infecting man (Table 37.2). *Entamoeba gingivalis* (Fig. 37.4) is the only ameba found in the mouth. It is an anaerobe and lives at the in-terface between gingiva and the tooth. This entameba does not produce cysts and therefore can be transmitted only directly. It is often found in patients with periodontal disease, but there is no evidence that is has an etiological relationship to the disease. It is possible, however, that the disease of the gums provides an expanded niche of anaerobiasis and promotes growth of the ameba.

Entamoeba coli (Figs. 37.5 and 37.6A–D), *Endolimax nana* (Fig. 37.7A and B), and *Ioda-*

Table 37.2. Commensal Amebae

Name of Organism	Location in Body	Mode of Transmission	Morphological Characteristics	
Entamoeba gingivalis	Oral cavity, under gingival flaps	Oral–oral route	Trophozoite: 10–20 μm	
Entamoeba coli	Lumen of large intestine	Fecal–oral route	Trophozoite: 15–50 μm	
			Cyst: 10–30 μm	
Entamoeba hartmanni	Lumen of large intestine	Fecal–oral route	Trophozoite: 5–15 μm	
			Cyst: 5–10 μm	
Entamoeba polecki	Lumen of large intestine	Fecal–oral route	Trophozoite: 12 μm	
			Cyst: 5–15 μm	
Endolimax nana	Lumen of large intestine	Fecal–oral route	Trophozoite: 5–25 μm	
			Cyst: 5–15 μm	
Iodamoeba buetschlii	Lumen of large intestine	Fecal–oral route	Trophozoite: 5–25 μm	
			Cyst: 5–15 μm	

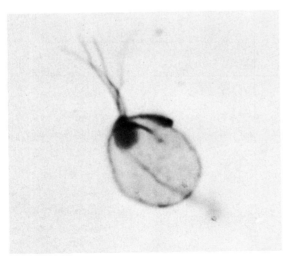

Figure 37.1. Trophozoite of *Trichomonas tenax*. ×2,800. (Courtesy of Dr. B. Honigberg)

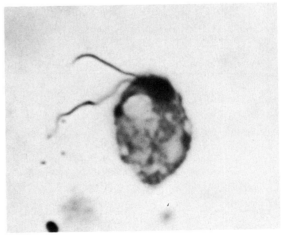

Figure 37.2. Trophozoite of *Retortamonas intestinalis*. All members of this genus are similar in morphology. ×2,500. (Courtesy of Dr. B. Honigberg)

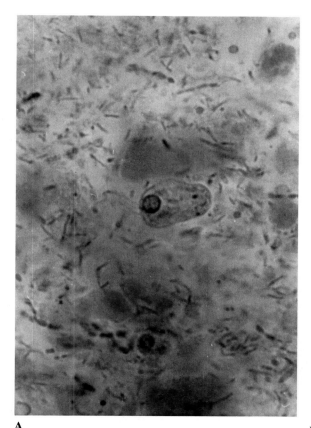

A

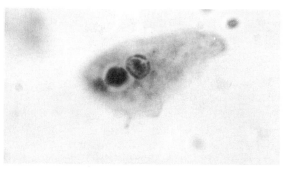

Figure 37.4. Trophozoite of *Entamoeba gingivalis.* ×750.

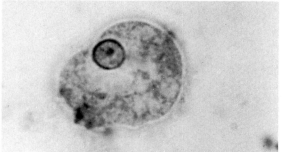

Figure 37.5. Trophozoite of *Entamoeba coli.* Note the eccentric karysome, which differentiates this ameba from the trophozoite of *Entamoeba histolytica* (see Fig. 25.1A). ×700.

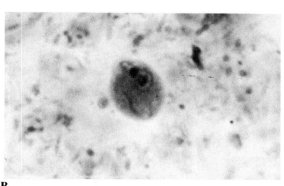

B

Figure 37.3. Trophozoite (**A**) and cyst (**B**) of *Chilomastix mesnili.* **A,** ×1,700; **B,** ×2,250.

moeba buetschlii (Fig. 37.8A and B) are three nonpathogenic amebae found in human colon. They form cysts and are transmitted in the same manner as the pathogenic amebae.

E. coli is the ameba most frequently mistaken for *E. histolytica,* because the nuclear structures its trophozoite can be difficult to distinguish from those of *E. histolytica.* The karyosome of *E. coli* is eccentric, in contrast with a central karyosome of *E. histolytica.* In addition, its cytoplasm differs from that of the pathogenic ameba. It is frothy, often includes bacteria, but rarely contains any red blood cells. Treatment directed against *E. histolytica* does not eradicate *E. coli.*

E. polecki, occasionally found in human stools, is a parasite of pigs and monkeys. *E. hartmanni* (Fig. 37.9), now considered a nonpathogen, was for many years classified as "small race" of *E. histolytica.* Epidemiologic and experimental evidence indicates that it causes no disease.

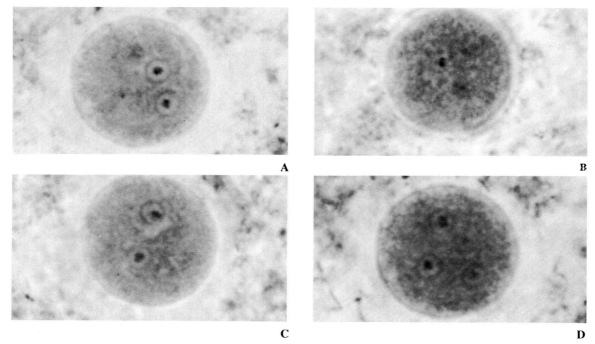

A

B

C

D

Figure 37.6. A–D Cyst stage of *Entamoeba coli*. Eight nuclei are seen in this through-focus series of photomicrographs. ×500.

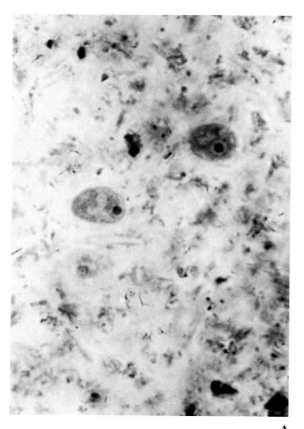

A

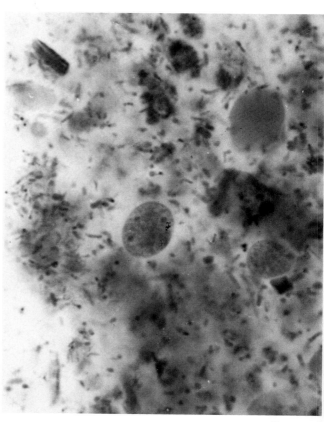

B

Figure 37.7. A. Trophozoite stage of *Endolimax nana*.

B. Cyst stage of *Endolimax nana* possesses four nuclei. **A,** ×1,350; **B,** ×1,550.

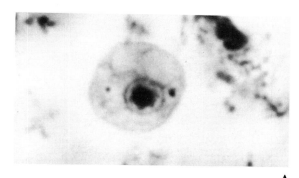

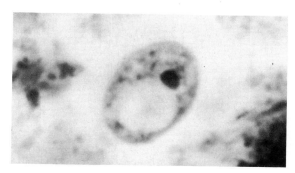

A

B

Figure 37.8. Trophozoites **(A)** and cysts **(B)** of *Iodamoeba buetschlii* possess a single nucleus. The cyst also has a prominent vacuole that is filled with starch. **A** and **B**, × 1,500.

Commensal Sporozoa

Two species of sporozoa, *Isospora belli* and *I. hominis,* have been found in human small intestine. Both organisms are intracellular within the columnar epithelium. During the early phase of the infection they may cause a mild diarrhea, which rarely lasts longer than 2 days. Treatment is symptomatic.

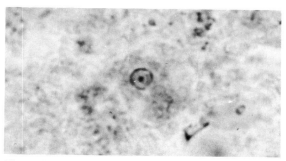

Figure 37.9. Trophozoite stage of *Entamoeba hartmanni.* The nucleus resembles that of *Entamoeba histolytica* (Fig. 25.1A), except that it is smaller. × 1,660.

Reference

1. Honigberg BM: Trichomonads of importance in human medicine. In Kreier JP (ed): Parasitic Protozoa, Vol 2. New York, Academic Press, 1978, pp 275–454

V
The Arthropods

Introduction

Arthropods influence human well being not only as hosts of parasitic organisms and vectors of a wide variety of pathogens but also as direct causes of tissue damage and disease. They also affect human health by reducing the availability of food. Insects destroy an estimated 20% of all food crops; this destruction continues despite the increasing use of pesticides in the fields and storage areas. Livestock are also affected by arthropod-borne infections. Vast areas of Africa are short of protein foods, because cattle suffer trypanosomiasis transmitted by tsetse flies and a variety of tick-borne diseases.

Although the pathogenic effects of arthropods are most pronounced in the tropics, they are by no means negligible in the United States and other temperate areas.

Lyme disease and babesiosis, transmitted by ticks, has rapidly spread throughout the northeastern U.S.[1] *Aedes albopictus,* the Asian Tiger mosquito has been introduced in shipments of used automobile tires into the southern U.S. and has spread as far north as central Ohio, Indiana, and Illinois and the introduced strain of the mosquito apparently can overwinter in the egg stage in temperate climates.[2] *A. albopictus* is an efficient vector of dengue.

Although fear has been expressed that blood-feeding arthropods, especially mosquitoes, could transmit AIDS, no evidence implicating arthropods has been presented. On the contrary, epidemiological evidence, most impressive in Africa, does not support the hypothesis that AIDS can be transmitted by arthropods.[3]

Even as arthropods cause problems for man and livestock, they are also beneficial as pollinators, producers of honey, natural regulators of harmful insects, and as essential members of food chains. Indiscriminate destruction of arthropods in programs designed to control pests can result in serious modification of the environments with deleterious consequences far worse than the original problem.

The phylum Arthropoda contains an enormous diversity of members, with the number of species exceeding that of all other phyla combined. The arthropods share a number of characteristics that distinguish them from all other animal groups. Some of these features are absent in a parular species or group at some period of development. Nevertheless, all species in the phylum are identifiable as members of the phylum. Among the morphological characteristics are bilateral symmetry, a hard exoskeleton, segmented body, and paired, jointed appendages. The term arthropod, derived from Greek, means jointed foot.

Growth by metamorphosis is another characteristic of the arthropods. In some groups, growth is gradual, each change from a stage to the next one, known as a molt, giving rise to a stage somewhat larger but morphologically similar to its predecessor. Among the spiders, eight or nine immature stages can precede the final molt to the sexually mature adult.

38. The Insects

The insects have two distinct types of development. The more primitive insect orders pass through a series of stages by incomplete metamorphosis (Fig. 38.1). A typical life cycle involves the egg, a usually fixed number of immature nymphal stages, and the mature adult stage. The insect molts between stages, sheds its old exoskeleton, and reveals a new skin within. Nymphs appear similar to the adult but lack wings and are sexually immature.

In contrast, complete metamorphosis is characteristic of some of the more advanced insect orders including the Diptera (Fig. 38.2) and the Siphonaptera (Fig. 38.3). The life cycle of an insect exhibiting complete metamorphosis includes the egg, a fixed number of larval stages, a single pupal stage, and the adult stage.

Table 38.1 lists arthropods of importance to human health, the pathogens they harbor and transmit, and the diseases they cause. The methods by which the arthropod vectors transmit pathogens vary. Some pathogens, unchanged by any interaction with the vector, are transmitted mechanically from one host to another on contaminated legs or mouthparts of the arthropod, or in its feces. Other pathogens require passage through the arthropod as part of their life cycle. In such cases the pathogens undergo specific developmental changes, which usually include multiplication, in the arthropod.

Arthropods can also be pathogens themselves. They can infest the host and cause mechanical injury through bites, chemical injury through the injection of toxins, and allergic reactions to the materials they transmit by the bite.[4]

Entomophobia and arachnophobia, inordinate fears of insects and arachnids, particularly spiders, are not uncommon psychological conditions.[5]

The Flies: Diptera

No single group of insects has so affected human evolution, development, or history as the Diptera, the order of insects comprising the flies. Malaria, yellow fever, elephantiasis, sleeping sickness, dengue, and river blindness are among the more serious diseases carried by members of this large order.

Notorious as vectors of pathogenic organisms of man and animals, dipterans are also important for the mechanical damage (i.e., myiasis) caused by the larvae of some species and the allergic responses caused by the bites of others.

Flies develop by complete metamorphosis and thus have distinct larval, pupal, and adult forms (Fig. 38.2). Larvae are usually vermiform, often living in water or damp places, or developing in living or dead tissue. Pupae represent a nonfeeding transitional stage. Adult dipterans, which possess wings, have only one pair (*diptera,* two wings). The mouthparts of the adults may be adapted for biting, piercing of flesh, and sucking of blood, or only for sucking of fluids.

Diptera is a large order, divided into three suborders containing over 100 families. Only nine families are of medical concern. The most primitive suborder, the Nematocera, contains four medically important families: the Psychodidae, the Ceratopogonidae, the Simuliidae, and the Culicidae. In the suborder Brachycera, only the Tabanidae are of any medical significance; in the third suborder, Cyclorrhapha, the Muscidae, Gasterophilidae, Cuterebridae, and Oestridae are of major concern.

The Biting Midges: Ceratopogonidae

Ceratopogonids, commonly called punkies, noseeums, sandflies, or midges, are minute (0.4–5 mm long), slender, blood-sucking dipterans, which constitute a serious pest problem in many areas of the tropics, the temperate zones, and in the arctic. Most of the species that affect man belong to two genera, Culicoides and Leptoconops, which act as vectors of several filarids infecting man in Africa and the New World. Species of Culicoides may also serve as vectors of filarids and viruses infecting animals.

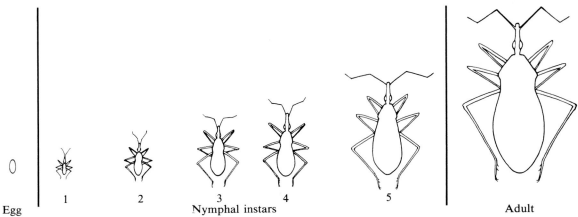

Egg 1 2 3 4 5 Adult
Nymphal instars

Figure 38.1. Incomplete metamorphosis in insects. Typical example of incomplete metamorphosis is the kissing bug, *Rhodnius prolixus*. Immature stages are wingless, smaller versions of the winged adult. All stages, except the egg, have 3 pairs of legs. The number of lymphal stages varies with the species.

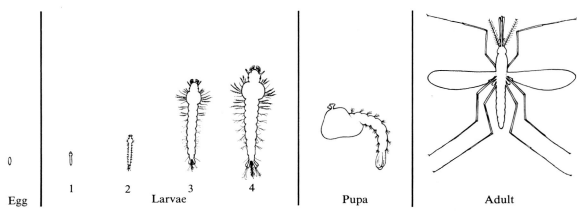

Egg 1 2 3 4 Pupa Adult
Larvae

Figure 38.2. Complete metamorphosis in insects: Aquatic. Typical example of complete metamorphosis in an insect with aquatic immature stages is the Anopheles mosquito, which begins as an egg laid on the surface of water and develops through four larval stages and a single pupal stage to a sexually mature, winged adult.

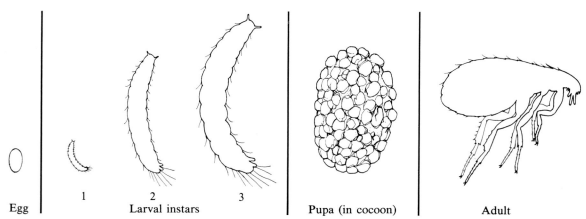

Egg 1 2 3 Pupa (in cocoon) Adult
Larval instars

Figure 38.3. Complete metamorphosis in insects: Terrestrial. Typical example of complete metamorphosis in an insect with terrestrial immature stages is the flea, which begins as an egg laid on the fur of the host or in the nest area. Several maggot-like larval stages are followed by a single pupal stage, encased in a sand-covered cocoon, from which a wingless, sexually mature adult flea emerges.

Table 38.1. Arthropods of Medical Importance and the Pathology They Cause

Order and Representative Species	Common Name	Geographical Distribution	Effects on Man
INSECTA			
Anoplura (sucking lice)			
Pediculus humanus humanus	Body louse	Worldwide	Skin reactions to bites, vectors of rickettsiae and spirochetes
P. humanus capitis	Head louse	Worldwide	Skin reaction to bites
Phthirus pubis	Crab louse	Worldwide	Skin reaction to bites
Heteroptera (true bugs)			
Cimex lectularius	Bedbug	Worldwide	Skin reaction to bites
C. hemipterus	Tropical bedbug	Tropical and subtropical	
Triatoma infestans *Rhodnius prolixus* *Panstrongylus megistus*	Kissing bug, cone-nosed bug	Tropical and sub-tropical regions of the New World	Skin reaction to bites, vectors of *Trypanosoma cruzi*, the cause of Chagas disease
Hymenoptera (bees, wasps, ants)			
Apis mellifera	Honeybee	Worldwide	Painful sting, potential anaphylaxis
Bombus spp.	Bumblebee	Worldwide	Painful sting, potential anaphylaxis
Various genera and species of the family Vespidae	Wasps, hornets, yellow jackets	Worldwide	Painful sting, potential anaphylaxis
Solenopsis spp.	Fire ant	Tropical America, southeastern United States	Painful bite and multiple stings, potential anaphylaxis
Diptera (flies, mosquitoes and their relatives)			
Ceratopogonidae			
Culicoides spp. *Leptoconops* spp.	No-see-ums, sandfly	Worldwide	Serious biting pest, skin reaction to bites, vectors of several filarid nematodes
Psychodidae			
Phlebotomus spp. *Lutzomyia* spp.	Sandfly	Worldwide	Skin reaction to bites, vectors of leishmania, Pappataci fever, and Carrion's disease
Simuliidae			
Simulium spp.	Blackfly, buffalo gnat	Worldwide	Serious biting pests, skin reaction to bites, vectors of Onchocerca and Mansonella
Culicidae			
Aedes spp. *Anopheles* spp. *Culex* spp. *Culiseta* spp. *Mansonia* spp.	Mosquito	Worldwide	Serious biting pests, skin reaction to bites, vectors of viruses protozoa, and filaria

Table 38.1. *(Continued)*

Order and Representative Species	Common Name	Geographical Distribution	Effects on Man
Tabanidae			
Tabanus spp.	Horsefly	Worldwide	Biting pests, painful bite followed by skin reaction
Chrysops spp.	Deerfly	Worldwide	Biting pests, vectors of tuleremia and *Loa loa.*
Muscidae			
Musca domestica	Housefly	Worldwide	Mechanical disseminator of pathogens
Stomoxys calcitrans	Stablefly	Worldwide	Serious biting pest
Glossina spp.	Tsetse fly	Africa	Vector of trypanosomes of man and animals
Calliphoridae Cuterebridae Sarcophagidae			
larvae of various genera and species	Maggots	Worldwide	Myiasis, accidental or obligate development of larval flies in human tissue
Siphonaptera (flea)			
Xenopsylla cheopis	Oriental rat flea	Worldwide	Vector of bubonic plague
Ctenocephalides felis	Cat flea	Worldwide	Biting pest
C. canis	Dog flea		
Pulex irritans	Human flea	Worldwide	Biting pest, plague vector
Tunga penetrans	Chigoe flea	Africa and South America	Infestation of toes, feet and legs, causing severe pain and secondary infection

Life Cycle

Ceratopogonid larvae develop in aquatic or semiaquatic habitats, often in freshwater, but usually in brackish water or tidal flats. Some important species are associated with the highly polluted runoff from livestock holding areas. Larval stages are long, slender, and maggot-like and in some species may undergo diapause, a state of arrested development, for as long as 3 years, while awaiting optimal environmental conditions. Adult female ceratopogonids (Fig. 38.4) require blood for the production of eggs. They typically feed at dusk and may attack in large numbers.[6]

Pathogenesis

The mouthparts of ceratopogonids are short and lancet-like, producing a painful bite.[7] Because of their large numbers, they can be important pests, particularly in beach and resort areas near salt

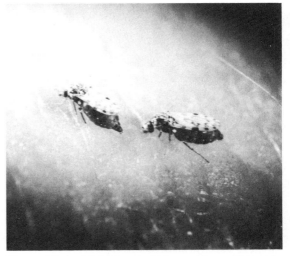

Figure 38.4. Adult female biting midges, *Culicoides variipennis,* feeding on blood. ×5. (Courtesy of Dr. J. Linley)

marshes. Bites can produce local lesions that persist for hours or days. Sensitized individuals develop allergic reactions.[8]

Midges of the genus Culicoides are the main vectors of the filarid nematodes, *Dipetalonema perstans* and *D. streptocerca* in Africa and *Mansonella ozzardi* in the New World tropics (see Chapter 12).

Control

Ceratopogonids develop in a wide range of habitats and each species presents its own special problems with respect to control. Salt marsh habitats can be drained or channeled and other breeding sites modified, but treatment of breeding sites with insecticides remains the most effective short-term control measure. Window screens are ineffective unless they are treated with insecticides, because they allow an easy entry by these minute insects. Commercial mosquito repellents containing diethyltoluamide (DEET) may be useful against some of the common species of pests.[9]

Psychodidae: The Moth Flies or Sand Flies

A single subfamily of the Psychodidae, the Phlebotominae of tropical, subtropical, and temperature regions, contains members that suck blood. Phlebotomine sand flies are small (1–3 mm), hairy, delicate, weakly flying insects that feed on a wide range of cold- and warm-blooded animals and transmit a number of viral, bacterial, and protozoan infections. Flies of the genus Phlebotomus and Lutzomyia are most important as vectors of the leishmaniae (see Chapters 32–34).

Historical Information

The role of phlebotomine flies in the transmission of leishmaniasis was suggested in 1912 (see Chapter 34).[10]

Life Cycle

Phlebotomine larvae develop in nonaquatic habitats such as moist soil, animal burrows, termite nests, loose masonry, stone walls, or rubbish heaps. The four larval stages are completed within 2–6 weeks; the pupal stage may last 8–14 days. The adults (Fig. 38.5) are weak fliers, exhibiting a hopping movement rather than a sustained flight. Only female phlebotomines require blood, feeding usually at night. Some species prefer to feed on man, but none are exclusively anthropophilic and also feed on dogs and rodents.[11]

Pathogenesis

The mouthparts of the female phlebotomine are short and adapted for piercing and sucking. The bite may be painful, producing a local lesion that itches. Sensitized individuals can show severe allergic reactions.

Although phlebotomines cause problems in some areas as pests, they are of particular concern as vectors of a number of diseases. Bartonellosis, also called Carrión's disease, Oroya fever, or verruga peruana, is a South American disease transmitted from man to man by *Phlebotomus verrucarum* and related species. It is caused by a bacterium, *Bartonella bacilliformis*, which invades erythrocytes and reticuloendothelial cells. The organism can produce a severe febrile illness, complicated by profound anemia. Un-

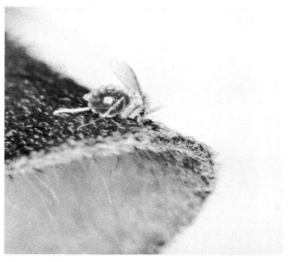

Figure 38.5. Adult female phlebotomine sand fly, *Lutzomyia anthophora,* feeding on the ear of a rodent reservoir host of leishmaniasis. ×6. (Courtesy of Dr. R. Endris)

treated, bartonellosis is fatal in 50% of cases. There is no known animal reservoir.

Sand fly, or papatasi, fever is a viral disease occurring in the Mediterranean, central Asia, Sri Lanka, India, and China. *P. papatasii* is the main vector of this acute febrile disease characterized by severe frontal headaches, malaise, retroorbital pain, anorexia, and nausea. Female flies become infected when they feed on viremic individuals. After an incubation period of 7–10 days, the flies become infective and remain so for the rest of their lives.

Leishmaniasis (see Chapters 32–34) is transmitted by a number of phlebotomine species. Flies initially pick up the parasite while feeding on infected man or animals. In the fly, the parasite undergoes asexual multiplication, eventually accumulating in the mouthparts, whence it is transmitted to the host when the insect feeds.

Control

Phlebotomine sand flies are particularly sensitive to insecticides, and the use of DDT in campaigns against malaria coincidentally controlled these flies and virtually eliminated sand fly-borne diseases in many regions. In the areas where malaria has been eliminated, or where malaria control programs have been abandoned, the phlebotomine flies have become reestablished and the sand fly-borne diseases have returned.

Sand flies may be controlled with residual or short-lived insecticides applied to breeding sites or houses. Treatment of window screens with insecticides may also be effective. Mosquito repellents can be used to reduce the frequency of sand fly bites.

The Black Flies: Simuliidae

Members of the family Simuliidae, commonly called black flies, buffalo gnats, or turkey gnats, are small (1–5 mm long), hump-backed, bloodsucking dipterans usually breeding in fast-flowing streams and rivers. Simulids are important as vectors of *Onchocerca volvulus,* the causative agent of onchocerciasis (see Chapter 8). In addition, they present a serious pest problem in many temperate and arctic areas. Black flies may also serve as vectors of bovine onchocerciasis and protozoan parasites of various species of birds.

within a cocoon. Adult female simulids require blood for egg production. They feed primarily during daylight hours. Male simulids do not feed on blood.[14]

Adult black flies in temperate areas may emerge synchronously in large numbers. Their bites cause serious damage to man and animals. Black flies often reach such high population densities that they can actually kill livestock and wild animals, torment campers and fishermen, and render large areas uninhabitable by man for long periods of time.

Historical Information

Black flies first stimulated medical interest in 1910, when they were incorrectly considered vectors of pellagra.[12] Their role in the transmission of onchocerca was demonstrated in 1926.[13]

Life Cycle

Adult female simulids lay eggs at or below the surface of moving, well oxygenated water. Larvae and pupae, equipped with gills for respiration, remain attached to objects below the surface. Larvae are nourished by food filtered from the passing water. They undergo development in five stages. The nonfeeding pupae gradually assume adult characteristics while they are enclosed

Pathogenesis

The bite of the female simulid is particularly painful. The insect's mouthparts consist of six blades in the shape of lancets, which tear the skin surface to induce bleeding. The fly feeds from the resulting pool of blood, and the bite wound continues to bleed for some time after the fly has departed. Simulid bites leave a characteristic point of dried blood at the wound site. The extreme pain of the initial bite is followed by itching and swelling due to reactions to the injected salivary secretions. Blood loss from multiple bites can be considerable. Allergic reactions in previously sensitized individuals are common and sometimes can reach serious levels, including anaphylaxis.

Control

Control of black flies is most effectively achieved by slow dripping of insecticides into rivers or streams. Mass control programs using insecticides applied by fixed-wing aircrafts and helicopters have been successful in West Africa. Clearing debris from stream beds can also reduce breeding. Repellents are not effective.

The Mosquitoes: Culicidae

Mosquitoes constitute one of the largest dipteran families and are of major significance both as vectors of disease and as biting pests. Their economic, cultural, and evolutionary impact has been devastating.[15,16] Mosquitoes develop in a wide range of aquatic larval habitats and in all climates from the arctic to the tropics. Adult mosquitoes are generally similar in appearance. They are usually small, have delicate legs, a single pair of wings, long antennae, and elongated mouthparts capable of piercing flesh and sucking blood. Larvae and pupae are aquatic and their development proceeds through complete metamorphosis (see Fig. 38.2).

Historical Information

The association between mosquitoes and various tropical fevers had been suggested by various writers in the past. Formal recognition of the association of these fevers with mosquitoes was finally given in the 19th century. The actual proof that mosquitoes could transmit diseases was provided by Manson, in 1878, when he showed that mosquitoes were intermediate hosts of *Wuchereria bancrofti* (see Chapter 7).

Transmission of malaria by mosquitoes was suggested by Manson as early as 1884, but Ross and Italian investigators under the direction of Grassi were the first to prove that mosquitoes transmitted malaria.[17] The incrimination of *Aedes aegypti* in the transmission of yellow fever was suggested by Finlay in 1880, and proved by Reed and his co-workers in 1900.[18]

Life Cycle

Both major subfamilies of the Culicidae, the Anophelinae and the Culicinae, are involved in transmission of diseases. Members of these subfamilies share a number of basic similarities in their life cycles and development. They lay eggs on or near water, or on surfaces that become flooded. Their larvae are always aquatic. The four larval stages are elongate, active "wigglers," which feed by filtering particulate matter from water and must remain in contact with the surface for respiration. The pupae, known as "tumblers," shaped like commas, are also aquatic. They remain at the surface unless disturbed. Adult mosquitoes of most species are good fliers. Males and females feed on nectars and sugars but females of most species, in addition, feed on blood. They require a blood meal for each clutch of eggs, which may contain 100–200 eggs. A female may produce six or more clutches during her lifetime. Eggs require 48–72 h to develop within the female. They are deposited almost as soon as they mature. Consequently, a female may take a blood meal every 2–4 days and contact a number of hosts during that period, thus providing an excellent opportunity for the dissemination of pathogens.[19]

Subfamily Anophelinae

The genus Anopheles contains the species responsible for the transmission of human malarias (see Chapter 28). The anopheline female lays eggs singly, usually on the surface of water. The eggs are equipped with floats and the patterns of

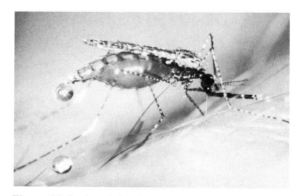

Figure 38.6. *Anopheles dirus*, one of the major malaria vectors in Southeast Asia, feeding on blood from a human host. ×5.

the egg shells and the floats are characteristic for a given species. Eggs hatch 2–4 days after they are laid. The aquatic larvae attach to the surface and assume a horizontal position. The larval period may last 1–3 weeks, depending on environmental temperature. Anopheline pupae are superficially similar to the pupae of other mosquitoes. The pupal stage lasts 1–3 days. Adult anophelines are delicate, long-legged mosquitoes (Fig. 38.6). Although some species are capable of extended flight and dispersion from breeding sites, typically anophelines remain close to their food supplies and breeding habitats.

Most anophelines are night feeders, with peaks of biting activity characteristic for each species. Some species are exclusively zoophilic, some are anthropophilic, and others are nonspecific biters. The feeding habits also vary. Certain species readily enter houses and feed on sleeping individuals; others feed only outdoors.

In temperate areas, anophelines spend the winter as inseminated adult females; in the tropics, these mosquitoes breed continually, although their population levels may fluctuate drastically in relation to rainfall and dry seasons.[20]

Approximately 300 species of Anopheles mosquitoes have been described. However, within any geographic area only a small number of species are important as malaria vectors (e.g., An. gambiae and An. funestus in sub-Saharan Africa, An. culicifacies and An. stephensi on the Indian subcontinent, and An. quadrimaculatus and An. freeborni in North America). Moreover, within any species, populations vary in their competence as vectors and capacity for transmission.

Intense study has led to the division of several old, well-established species of vectors into morphologically similar but genetically distinct groups or complexes of species. The important vector of malaria in Africa, An. gambiae, consists of at least six discrete but cryptic species, most of which are not major vectors. Similar revision of species has resulted in a clearer definition of the members of the European An. maculipennis complex and the southeast Asian An. balabacensis group. It appears that reexamination of most of the anopheline species that occupy large or ecologically diverse geographic areas will lead to the description of closely related but genetically divergent species.

Anophelines also play an important role as vectors of filarial nematodes (See Chapter 7). An. gambiae and An. funestus are the main vectors of Wuchereria bancrofti in Africa, and An. hyrcanus in China and An. barbirostris in southeast Asia are vectors of both W. bancrofti and Brugia malayi. Anophelines sometimes transmit certain viral pathogens. Although anophelines are not usually involved in the transmission of viruses, An. gambiae and An. funestus are the vectors of O'-nyong-nyong fever.

Subfamily Culicinae

The subfamily Culicinae consists of more than 1500 species, distributed among 20 genera, five of which, Mansonia, Psorophora, Culiseta, Aedes, and Culex, are of major importance to human health.

Culicine mosquitoes are primary vectors of a number of viruses and filariae, and pose a serious problem as pest insects in many parts of the world.

Species belonging to the genus Aedes, the largest of the culicine genera, are found in `all habitats ranging from the tropics to the Arctic. The typical aedine mosquito is robust, a strong flier, and usually a vicious biter. Its eggs are laid singly, without floats, on or near the surface of water, or in areas likely to be flooded periodically. Unlike the eggs of anopheles or culex mosquitoes, which usually hatch within a few days of deposition, aedine eggs have the capacity for an extended period of dormancy. This dormancy allows the eggs to survive the winter or to delay hatching until conditions are ideal for development. Aedine mosquitoes occupy salt marsh habitats, flood plains, tree holes, irrigated pasture lands, and man-made containers.

Aedine larvae are nourished by food filtered from water. They develop and feed while suspended from the surface of water by a breathing tube. Larvae develop by progressing through four stages within 4–6 days. Aedine pupae are typical of those of most mosquitoes. This stage usually lasts for less than 3 days. Adults usually emerge from breeding sites synchronously. This is followed by mass migrations of females in search of blood.

Aedine species may develop overwhelming populations in salt marsh, tundra, pasture, and flood water, and have a severe impact on wildlife, livestock, and man. If left uncontrolled, the salt-marsh mosquitoes of the east coast of the United States, *Ae. sollicitans* and *Ae. taeniorhynchus,* could deny vast areas of seashore to development and tourism. The flood water mosquito, *Ae. vexans,* develops after spring rain and flooding; the Arctic species begin hatching with the first melting snows. Populations of Arctic *Aedes* at times become so great that man and larger mammals do not venture into the tundra areas.

Aedines, breeding in treeholes in the populated areas of temperate zones, such as *Ae. triseriatus,* seldom produce large populations but can become local pests and important vectors of various viral infections.

In tropical regions, populations of aedine mosquitoes are usually much smaller than in the Arctic. *Ae. aegypti,* the yellow fever mosquito, occurs alongside man throughout the tropics and subtropics. *Ae. aegypti* usually breeds in man-made containers such as discarded auto tires, flower pots, blocked gutters, water jugs, rain barrels, cemetery urns, and tin cans. The mosquito lays eggs above the water line in these containers and the eggs remain dormant there, often as long as 6 months, until the container becomes filled with water. Because this mosquito is closely associated with man and is almost exclusively anthropophilic, it has most of the characteristics of a good vector. Indeed, *Ae. aegypti* (Fig. 38.7) is the primary vector of yellow fever and dengue in urban environments throughout the world.[21]

In the South Pacific, container-breeding members of the *Ae. scutellaris* complex are vectors of certain viruses and *W. bancrofti.*

The genus Culex is the second largest group in the subfamily, best represented by *Cu. pipiens pipiens,* the northern house mosquito found in temperate areas, and *Cu. pipiens quinquefasciatus* (formerly known as *Cu. fatigans*), the southern house mosquito found throughout the subtropics and tropics.

Culex mosquitoes deposit their eggs in rafts usually containing 50–200 eggs cemented together. The eggs float perpendicular to the water surface and hatch within 2–3 days. The four larval stages develop and feed on nutrients in the water, much like aedine mosquitoes. The siphon in the culex mosquito is usually longer and more slender than that of aedines. The larval period lasts less than 2 weeks and the pupal stage less than 2 days. Adults usually feed at night. Many show a preference for avian blood, but most members will also feed on man or other mammals. *Cu. p. quinquefasciatus* is the major vector of *W. bancrofti* (see Chapter 7) throughout the tropics. The species is particularly well adapted to development in polluted waters, breeding in or near population centers and readily biting man.

The genus Mansonia includes a number of species important as vectors of Malayan filariasis (see Chapter 7). This genus differs in its development from most mosquitoes in that its larvae and pupae affix themselves below the surface of water to the stems and roots of aquatic plants and derive oxygen from these plants.

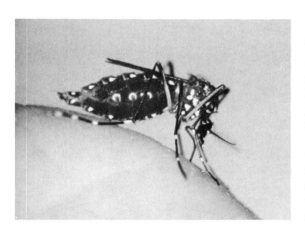

Figure 38.7. The yellow fever mosquito, *Aedes aegypti,* in typical feeding position. ×5.

Pathogenesis of the Mosquito Bite

The mouthparts of the adult female mosquito are adapted for piercing flesh and sucking the blood needed by the female for the production of eggs. In the act of feeding, the female repeatedly injects saliva, which produces the reaction that follows the bite.[22]

Although the mechanical damage induced by the feeding mosquito can cause pain and irritation, the immediate and delayed immune reactions are of greater concern. Individuals with no previous exposure to mosquitoes show neither immediate nor delayed reactions. However, after sensitization, a bite is followed by a small flat wheal surrounded by a red flare, which appears within a few minutes and lasts about 1 h. This reaction is mediated by antibodies. The delayed reaction consists of itching, swelling, and reddening of the wound region. It can persist for days. Repeated exposure can lead to loss of the delayed reaction and perhaps eventual desensitization. Desensitization to one species does not necessarily extend to other members of the same genus and usually does not include protection against the bites of mosquitoes of other genera.[23–25] The intense itching, primarily associated with the delayed reaction, encourages scratching and secondary infection of the wound site.

Treatment

Local anesthetics are useful in treating reactions to mosquito bites.

Mosquito-borne Viral Diseases

Yellow fever is a severe, hemorrhagic disease characterized by high fever, jaundice, and prostration. Case fatality during epidemics can exceed 10%. The yellow fever virus naturally infects monkeys and is maintained in a monkey-to-monkey sylvatic cycle by forest-dwelling mosquitoes. When the sylvatic cycle is disturbed, by, for example, wood cutters, man can be bitten by one of these monkey-feeding vectors. When this individual returns to his village and becomes viremic, the ubiquitous *Ae. aegypti* is available to initiate the urban cycle of transmission from man to man. An effective vaccine for yellow fever is available and recommended for travelers to endemic areas.

Dengue is an acute, nonfatal viral disease characterized by high fever, severe headache, backache, and arthralgia, hence the common name "breakbone fever." A hemorrhagic form of dengue occurs in southeast Asia and Oceania; it is frequently fatal. *Ae. aegypti* is the usual vector of both the typical and hemorrhagic forms of dengue, although other aedine mosquitoes may transmit the organism. There is no verified animal reservoir for dengue and no vaccine is available.

The mosquito-borne viral encephalitides include, in the United States, St. Louis encephalitis (SLE), eastern equine encephalitis (EEE), and western equine encephalitis (WEE). These are viral diseases of wild birds transmitted by mosquitoes. Under certain conditions, normally ornithophilic mosquito species that had previously fed on viremic birds will feed on man or other mammals.

SLE may be transmitted by members of the *Cu. pipiens* complex in urban areas, *Cu. tarsalis* in rural areas in the western states, and by *Cu. nigripalpus* in Florida. *Cu. tarsalis* is the main vector of WEE in the West and *Culiseta melanura* is one of the main vectors of EEE in the East.

In the Orient, Japanese B encephalitis is transmitted by *Cu. tritaniorhynchus* and *Ae. togoi*. In Australia and New Guinea, Murrey Valley encephalitis is transmitted by various Culex species.

Rift Valley fever (RVF), an East African disease usually associated with wild animals and livestock, caused a serious epidemic in Egypt in 1977–78, infecting millions. The viral agent of RVF has been assigned to the sand fly fever group of viruses and is probably transmitted in Egypt by *Cu. pipiens* and by other Culex and Aedes mosquitoes throughout the rest of Africa.

California group viruses, including LaCrosse virus, rarely cause epidemics. They are transmitted by tree-hole breeding *Ae. triseriatus* in the midwestern United States.

Mosquito Control

The most effective method of mosquito control is reduction of the source, i.e., the elimination or modification of the aquatic sites in which the mosquitoes breed. This can take the form of drainage, impoundment, or level control of large bodies of water, the clearing or filling of ditches, or the elimination of manmade containers. Methodology must be tailored to the specific breeding requirements of the species. Chemical insecticides may be required where reduction at the source is inadequate. Larvicides can be applied to breeding sites. Under extreme conditions, pesticides can be directed against adult mosquitoes.

The most common and effective method of malaria control employs insecticides applied to the walls of houses. Anopheline malaria vectors tend to rest on walls after feeding. They come in contact with the residual insecticide and die.

Consequently, insecticides applied to the insides of walls affect only those mosquitoes that have fed on man and are potentially infected. This scheme does little to reduce mosquito populations and usually has little environmental impact, but reduces malaria by interrupting transmission of the disease.[26]

A number of effective mosquito repellents are available as sprays or lotions. When applied according to direction they can reduce the annoyance caused by the insects. The most effective repellents usually contain DEET.

The Horse and Deer Flies: Tabanidae

The Tabanidae are a large family of blood-sucking dipterans with a cosmopolitan distribution. These are robust flies, ranging in size from 7 mm to 30 mm in length and locally referred to as horse flies, deer flies, mango flies, or greenheads. Tabanids are strong fliers, capable of inflicting painful bites, and in some areas of the world are considered serious pests of man and animals. Flies of the genus Chrysops act as vectors of the filarial eye worm, *Loa loa* (see Chapter 9) in Africa, and can be involved in the mechanical transmission of anthrax, tuleremia, and *Trypanosoma evansi*.

Historical Information

Tabanids were implicated in the transmission of anthrax as early as 1874 and of *T. evansi* in 1913. The role of tabanids as intermediate hosts and vectors of *Loa loa* was verified, in 1914, by Leiper.[27]

Life Cycle

Tabanids usually lay eggs on vegetation near moist areas. Their larvae develop in water or wet earth and pass through four to nine stages. In some species the larvae remain dormant during the winter. Pupation occurs in dry earth and the quiescent pupal stage may last 2–3 weeks. Adult females feed on blood, the males on plant juices.

Pathogenesis

Tabanid mouthparts are short and blade-like. In the act of biting, the insect inflicts a deep, pain-ful wound causing blood to flow. The fly then laps up blood from the freshly formed pool. Individuals can become sensitized to tabanid bites and suffer severe allergic reactions after attack.

Tabanids act as efficient mechanical vectors of several pathogens. They are easily disturbed during feeding. They fly to another host, and begin the process anew. Consequently, the fly's mouthparts contaminated on one host can readily transfer organisms to the next. Bacteria causing anthrax and tuleremia as well as the protozoan *T. evansi* have been transmitted by the tabanid flies acting as mechanical vectors.

L. loa (see Chapter 9) is transmitted by African tabanids of the genus Chrysops, which include *C. silacea* and *C. dimidiata*. Microfilariae of the worm, ingested by female flies with the blood meal, develop in the flight muscles. When they reach maturity, they migrate to the mouthparts and are deposited on the skin of a new host when the fly feeds again. Infectious larvae burrow into the skin of the host after the fly has abandoned the bite wound.

Control

Tabanids are difficult to control because of their diverse breeding sites. Larvae are sensitive to DDT and other insecticides, but these compounds are seldom used. Sensitive individuals should consider using repellents to avoid bites. Mosquito repellents containing DEET are usually effective.

The House Fly and Its Relatives: Muscidae

The muscoid flies include insects important as blood-sucking pests, as vectors of diseases, and as mechanical vectors of a variety of pathogenic organisms.[28,29] Some better known members of this family are the housefly, *Musca domestica* (Fig. 38.8A–C), the stable fly, *Stomoxys*

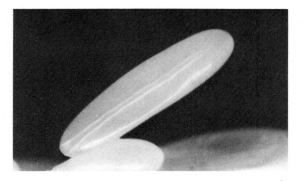

A

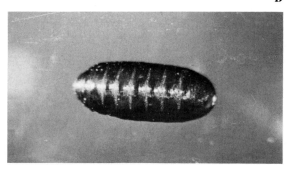

B

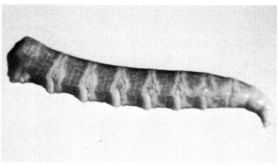

C

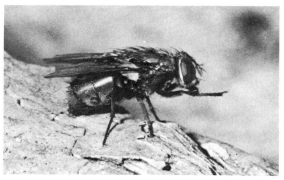

D

Figure 38.8. The egg (**A**), larva (**B**), pupa (**C**), and adult (**D**) of *Musca domestica,* the housefly. The larvae of flies are referred to as maggots. **A,** ×70; **B,** ×8; **C,** ×6; **D,** ×5.

calcitrans, and the tsetse flies of the genus Glossina.

All muscoids are fairly large, robust dipterans. They develop from eggs to maggots (larvae), nonmotile pupae, and adults by complete metamorphosis. Only the tsetse flies differ in that their larvae develop singly within the female and are deposited fully developed and ready for pupation.

Historical Information

One of the plagues of Egypt described in the Old Testament consisted of swarms of flies. It appears that man was troubled by these insects throughout his history. The role of the tsetse fly as vector of African trypanosomiasis was demonstrated by Bruce, in 1895,[30] and the importance of house flies as disseminators of various pathogens was outlined in 1898 by Veeder.[29]

Life Cycle

M. domestica lays her eggs on any matter that will serve as food for the developing maggots. Animal or human feces, garbage, decaying plant material, and sewage—all provide a suitable substrate. A single fly lays more than 1000 eggs during her life span. The development from eggs to adults requires less than 10 days at summer temperatures. As a result of this reproductive potential, given sufficient breeding sites, summer fly populations can be enormous. These flies can carry viruses, bacteria, protozoa, and eggs of parasitic worms and are thus a serious public health problem.[29] The presence of large fly populations is a clear indicator of poor sanitation.

Stable Flies

S. calcitrans is a serious biting pest usually associated with domestic animal husbandry. The fly lays her eggs in moist, decaying vegetable material (e.g., hay, alfalfa, or straw). In suburban communities, moist piles of grass clippings and weeds provide ideal sites for larval development. The egg-to-adult period in the summer lasts about 4 weeks, and a female may lay up to 400 eggs during her life span.

Although superficially similar in appearance to houseflies, stable flies possess a prominent proboscis, which both sexes use effectively for sucking blood. The bite of the stable fly is initially painful but usually causes little delayed reaction. Sensitized individuals develop allergic responses to repeated bites.

Stomoxys can serve as a mechanical vector for anthrax and some trypanosomes of animals.[29]

Tsetse Flies

Tsetse flies of the genus Glossina (Fig. 38.9) occur in sub-Saharan Africa, where they act as intermediate hosts and vectors of a number of trypanosomes infecting man and animals (see Chapter 31). Tsetse flies differ markedly from muscoid flies, and indeed from most insects, in producing only one egg at a time. This single egg is retained within the "uterus" of the female, where it hatches. The larva develops in three stages "in utero" while feeding on "milk" produced by accessory glands of the female. Eventually, a fully mature larva is deposited in a shady location; it pupates immediately. The pupal stage can last up to 30 days and the resulting adult remains inactive for 1–2 days after emerging, before seeking its first blood meal. Both male and female tsetse flies are exclusively he-

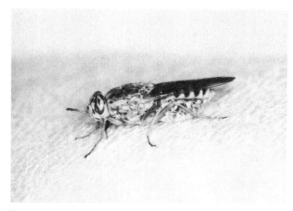

Figure 38.9. A tsetse fly of *Glossina* sp. feeding on blood. × 3. (Courtesy of Dr. J. Gingrich)

matophagous and both sexes are capable of transmitting trypanosomes.[31,32]

Female tsetse produces 10–15 larvae during her life span. Tsetse populations are relatively small and dispersed. Glossinae hunt by sight and follow animals, men, or even vehicles for long distances. They feed during the day, usually along paths or river banks. *G. palpalis* and *G. tachinoides* are the main vectors of *Trypanosoma brucei gambiense; G. morsitans, G. swynnertoni,* and *G. pallidipes* are the primary vectors of *T. b. rhodesiense.*

The Myiasis-Causing Flies: Calliphoridae, Cuterebridae, and Sarcophagidae

Not all dipterans inflict damage by the bite of adult flies seeking blood. The larvae of several families are pathogenic during their development within the tissues of the infested host. This infestation with larvae, or maggots, (Fig. 38.8B) is known as myiasis.[33] Certain species of flies are obligate parasites and require living tissue for development. Other species develop facultatively in either living or dead tissues. A third group can cause accidental myiasis when their eggs, deposited on foodstuffs, are ingested. Cheese skippers of the family Piophilidae, rat-tailed larvae of the Syrphidae, soldier fly larvae of the Stratiomyidae, and several species of the Muscidae cause gastrointestinal myiasis. Symptoms are proportional to the number of larvae developing and include nausea and vomiting. Diagnosis requires the finding of living or dead maggots in the vomitus, aspirates of gastrointestinal contents, or in stool specimens.

Species of flies that normally favor decaying flesh for larval development occasionally deposit eggs or larvae on wounds or ulcers.

The flesh flies of the family Sarcophagidae contain several members of the genera Wohlfahrtia and Sarcophaga, which cause myiasis. Female flies in this family do not lay eggs, but deposit freshly hatched first-stage larvae directly in wounds, ulcers, or even on unbroken skin. These feeding larvae may cause considerable tissue damage (Fig. 38.10).

Flies of the family Cuterebridae are obligate parasites, usually of wild and domestic animals. *Dermatobia hominis,* the human bot fly, parasitizes a number of mammals and is a serious pest of cattle in Central and South America. Flies of this species cause the infestation in a unique manner. Female Dermatobia flies capture various blood-sucking arthropods, usually mosquitoes or other flies, lay their eggs on the abdomens of

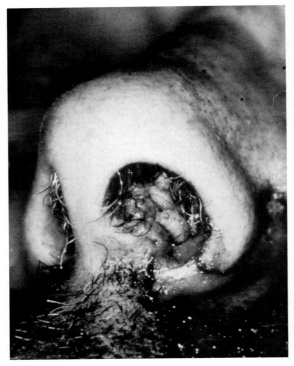

Figure 38.10. Sarcophaga larvae *in situ.* × 3

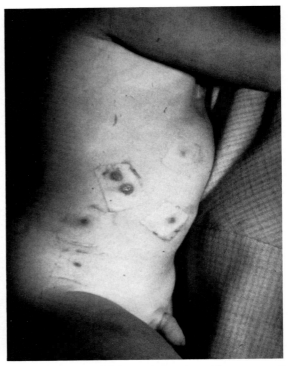

Figure 38.11. *Cordylobia anthropophaga* bites on a small child.

their prey, and release these insects. When the fly or the mosquito carrying the eggs alights on a warm-blooded host, the eggs hatch, immediately liberating larvae onto the skin of the host. These maggots penetrate the skin and develop in the subcutaneous tissue, maintaining contact with the surface through a small opening in the center of an abscess-like swelling. When the larvae complete their development after 6–12 weeks, they emerge, fall to the ground, and pupate. During the phase within the tissues the maggots can cause intermittent pain and secrete a foul-smelling material from the opening in the skin.

In human infestations, each maggot should be removed surgically. Particular care must be taken not to damage it during the procedure because the patient has usually become sensitized to the antigens of the maggot. The maggots can also be removed by coating their external spiracles with petroleum jelly, which blocks access to oxygen. They are thus forced to crawl to the surface. They may have to be removed surgically, under local anesthesia, and the wound sutured.[34]

Several species of the family Calliphoridae are obligate parasites, whereas others cause only ac-

cidental myiasis. *Cordylobia anthropophaga,* the tumbu fly, is a larval parasite of man and other animals, especially rats, in Africa. These flies lay eggs on soil contaminated with urine or feces, or on similarly soiled bedding or clothing that is set out to dry. The emerging larvae attach themselves to a host, with which they come in contact, and penetrate the skin. After penetration, larvae form individual tender abscess-like swellings from which serous fluid exudes, particularly when pressure is applied to the lesion (Fig. 38.11). Treatment consists of covering the wound with petroleum jelly to force the maggot to the surface in search of oxygen. The maggot can then be gently squeezed out. Surgical excision may be necessary in some infestations.

Another African species, the Congo floor maggot, *Auchmeromyia luteola,* is specific only for man. The fly lays eggs on the floor of the huts. The maggots come out of the soil at night to feed on blood of the inhabitants of the hut who sleep on the floor. The larvae lacerate the victim, suck blood—but do not penetrate tissues—and return into the soil.

Two species of Cochliomyia, the New World

screw worm, in North and South America occasionally cause myiasis in man, although these flies are primarily parasites of animals. Adult females lay their eggs around the edges of wounds, and the larvae invade the wounds and macerate the traumatized tissues. Large numbers of maggots can infest a single wound. Infestations of the nose can be fatal, and therefore the maggots should be removed surgically as soon as they are detected.

Flies of the genus Chrysomyia, the Old World screw worm, are important causes of human and animal myiasis throughout Asia and Africa. Larvae of these flies penetrate wounds or mucous membranes, affecting primarily areas around the eyes, ears, mouth, and nose.

The green bottle flies, *Lucilia* sp., and the blue bottle flies, *Calliphora* sp., sometimes infest wounds of man in Asia, Africa, and the Americas. The larvae of these species prefer dead tissue; in the past these maggots, reared free of pathogens, were used therapeutically for cleansing of septic wounds.

A number of flies whose larvae are primarily parasites of domestic animals occasionally infest man. Larvae of the sheep bot, *Oestrus ovis*, may invade nasal cavities of shepherds and cause severe frontal headaches. Such larvae do not complete their development, because man is an aberrant host, and usually exit spontaneously before maturation.

Cattle warbles of the genus Hypoderma occasionally infest man, causing a condition similar to creeping eruption (see Chapter 11). Larvae penetrate exposed skin and wander aimlessly, causing severe itching, pain, and sleeplessness. Surgical removal of the larvae from the ends of their burrows is recommended.

Larvae of various flies, particularly Calliphora, Phaenicia and Cochliomyia infest a cadaver in a predictable succession. The science of forensic entomology has developed using flies and to a lesser extent beetle larvae to determine manner, time and place of death, and uses entomological information to support pathology in legal proceedings.[35,36]

The Sucking Lice: Anoplura

Three species of lice infest man as obligate, blood-feeding ectoparasites. Only one of these, the body louse, is important in human medicine as the vector of the rickettsiae of epidemic typhus and trench fever, and the spirochetes of relapsing fever. Louse infestation is known as pediculosis.

The body louse, *Pediculus humanus humanus* (Fig. 38.12), and its close relative the head louse, *P. humanis capitis*, are wingless, elongate, dorsoventrally flattened insects, 2.5–4 mm long. They have three pairs of legs of about equal length. Their mouthparts are adapted for piercing flesh and sucking blood. The crab louse, *Phthirus pubis*, is shorter (0.8–1.2 mm) and, as its common name implies, resembles a crab. Crab lice have somewhat reduced front legs, with the second and third leg pairs stout and strongly clawed (Fig. 38.13). All lice undergo development characterized by incomplete metamorphosis.

Closely related species of lice now infest gorillas and monkeys. Man has certainly been aware of the discomforts of lousiness from earliest times and the condition has been recorded by poets and artists as well as by early writers on science and medicine. However, the recognition of body lice as disease vectors is more recent: transmission of typhus and relapsing fever by lice was not demonstrated until the early 1900s.

Lice have been considered variously as unwelcome pests, a sign of unclean habits (not always true), and state of saintliness. They have often been accepted as one of life's unavoidable afflictions. As vectors of diseases, body lice have on numerous occasions determined the outcome of human history. Zinsser, in 1935,[37] and Busvine, in 1976,[38] chronicled empires and even entire civilizations that were profoundly changed by epidemics of louse-borne typhus.

Historical Information

The association between man and lice is an ancient one and probably represents an evolutionary relationship begun by lice and ancestral hominids.

Life Cycle

The life cycles of the human lice are depicted in Fig. 38.14. The crab louse, *P. pubis*, sometimes referred to as *papillon d'amour*, usually inhabits

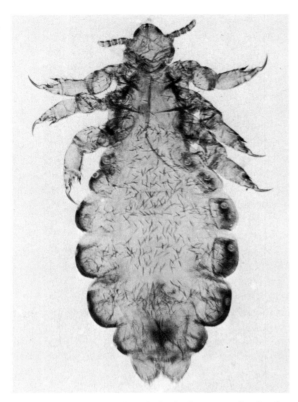

Figure 38.12. Adult female body louse, *Pediculus humanus humanus.* ×20.

the hairs of the pubic and perianal regions of the body, but can also be found on axillary hair or on moustaches, beards, eyebrows, or eyelashes. Adult crab lice are sedentary, often clutching the same hairs for days while feeding for hours at a time. Lice of all stages and both sexes feed solely on blood. They must obtain daily blood meals to survive. The female lays individual eggs or nits (approximately 0.6 mm in length) and at-

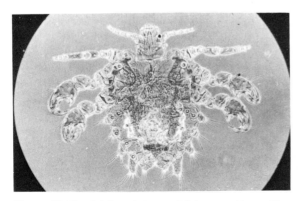

Figure 38.13. Adult crab louse, *Phthirus pubis.* ×25.

taches them to hairs of the host (Fig. 38.15). They embryonate and hatch over a 6–8 day period. The louse has three nymphal (preadult) stages lasting 15–17 days before the final molt to the adult stage. Nymphs are tiny, sexually immature versions of the adults. Adult crab lice live less than a month. The females usually lay fewer than 50 eggs during a lifetime. The entire life cycle (i.e., egg-to-egg interval) lasts 22–27 days.[39,40]

Crab lice are most frequently transmitted from one person to another by sexual contact. However, general physical contact or contact with a variety of contaminated objects such as toilet seats, clothing, or bedding can also result in infestation.

The head louse, *P. humanus capitis* (Fig. 38.16), inhabits the hairs of the head, particularly behind the ears and around the occiput. Heavy infestations may force head lice to establish themselves on other hairy parts of the body. Like the crab lice, the head lice are relatively sedentary, feeding for hours at a time while clutching firmly to hair, and, like the crab lice, they seldom leave the hairy regions voluntarily. The eggs are attached to hair shafts (Fig. 38.17) and hatch within about 7 days; the three nymphal stages are completed within less than 2 weeks. The egg-to-egg cycle lasts about 3 weeks. A head louse lays 50–150 eggs during her lifetime.

Head lice are disseminated by physical contact or by sharing of hats, scarves, combs, or brushes, or by the common storage of garments that contain nits or lice of various stages.

Although head lice have been shown capable of transmitting rickettsiae and spirochetes in the laboratory, they are usually not involved in the transmission of these organisms under natural conditions.[31]

The life cycle of the body louse, *P. humanus humanus,* differs significantly from those of the other two in that body lice spend much of their lives on the clothing of infested individuals. Body lice (commonly referred to as ''cooties'') are usually found on the clothing wherever it comes into close contact with the body. Although body lice in all stages of their development must move to the body for regular blood meals, they return to the clothing after feeding. The lice lay eggs along the seams of garments attached to cloth fibers (Fig. 38.18) and sometimes attach the eggs to some of the coarser body hairs. Eggs kept

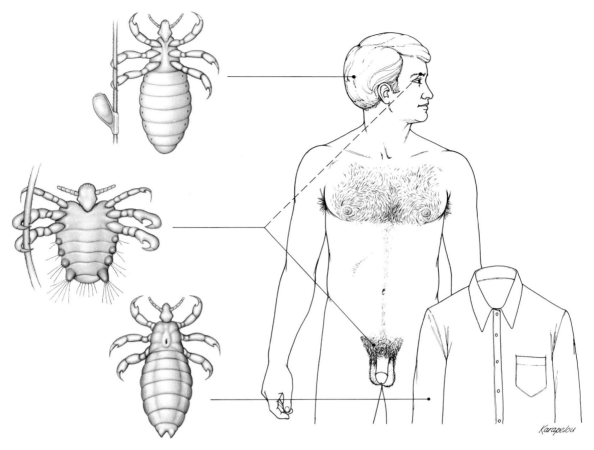

Figure 38.14. Preferred feeding and resting sites of the three species of louse affecting man. The head louse, *Pediculus humanus capitis*, resides, feeds, and reproduces on the hairs of the head. Eggs are laid individually on hair shafts. The crab louse, *Phthirus pubis*, prefers the hair of the pubic region, but may occasionally be found on the eyebrows, eyelashes, beard, or moustache. Eggs are attached to individual hairs. The body louse, *Pediculus humanus humanus*, is usually found on clothing, moving to the body of the human host only to feed. Eggs are laid in masses in the seams of the clothing of the host.

near the body hatch within 5–7 days. Nymphs require about 18 days to mature and the adult lice live for about a month. A body louse lays more than 300 eggs during her lifetime.[41]

Body lice are readily transmitted between individuals by physical contact, exchanges of clothing, or the common storage of infested garments. They are the only vectors of louse-borne relapsing fever, trench fever, and epidemic typhus.

Pathogenesis

Lice inject salivary fluids into the wound during ingestion of blood and these secretions cause varying degrees of sensitization in the human host.

Clinical Disease

Intense itching is the usual characteristic of infestation by all lice, and constant scratching can lead to secondary bacterial infection of the wound.

Crab lice produce characteristic "blue spots." These spots are often seen around the eyes of individuals with infested lashes.

The bites of head lice result in inflammatory papules and impetigenous lesions often associated with lymphadenopathy (Fig. 38.19). Heavy in-

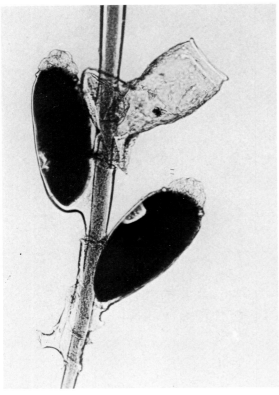

Figure 38.15. Eggs (nits) of the crab louse, *Phthirus pubis*, attached to a pubic hair. Note the two embryonating eggs and the empty shell. × 70.

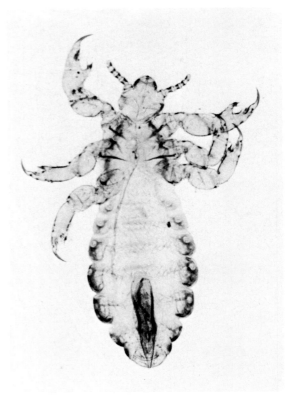

Figure 38.16. Adult male of the head louse, *Pediculus humanus capitis*. × 20.

festations with head lice can cause a condition in which hair, eggs, louse feces, and exudates of bite wounds form a cap-like mass teeming with lice. There may be secondary fungal infection within the mass.[41] Children infested with head lice are often restless.

Bites by body lice cause pinpoint macules, excoriations, and pigmentation of the skin. "Vagabond's disease" is an extreme condition caused by a combination of persistent heavy infestation and poor personal hygiene. Affected individuals show a generalized bronze pigmentation and hardening of the skin.[42]

Diagnosis

Diagnosis depends on identification of lice or eggs in the hair or in the seams of the garments; in the latter they may be difficult to find. The eggs must be identified by microscopy.

Treatment

There are several pediculocidic formulations available as dusts, shampoos, lotions, and creams; some may be obtained as over-the-counter preparations; others require a prescription. All of the effective products contain low concentrations of insecticides such as benzene hexachloride or pyrethrum.[43]

Head and crab lice can be treated similarly. Infested individuals should remove all clothing, apply the pediculocide, and put on clean clothing after treatment. The procedure should be repeated after 10 days to kill any newly hatched lice, because the treatment does not kill eggs. Clothing and bedding of infested individuals should be washed and dried by exposure to heat, or dry cleaned to prevent reinfestation. Exposure of infested clothing to temperatures of 70°C for 30 min will kill lice and eggs. Combs and brushes

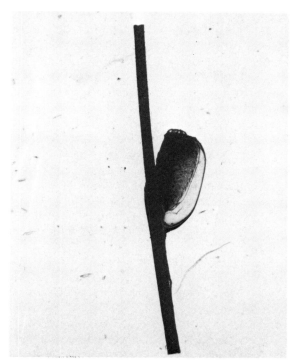

Figure 38.17. Single egg (nit) of the head louse, *Pediculus humanus capitis,* attached to the shaft of a hair. ×40.

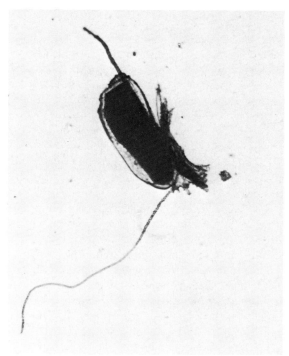

Figure 38.18. Egg (nit) of the body louse, *Pediculus humanus humanus.*

should also be treated by heat to prevent reinfestation by head lice. Simple washing of the head or affected areas with soap will not kill lice or destroy the nits.

Insecticides should not be used on crab lice infesting eyebrows or lashes. Petrolatum should be applied thickly and individual lice removed with forceps.

Because body lice inhabit and lay eggs on clothing, regular changes of underwear and garments will significantly reduce the infestation. Garments infested by lice should be treated as indicated above. Blankets, bedding, sleeping bags, and other items that might be contaminated should be similarly treated.

Various powdered formulations of pediculicides can be applied directly to clothed individuals. Several of these compounds have been used effectively in mass treatment of large groups of infested individuals in the control of epidemic typhus.

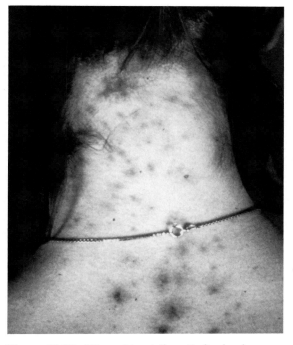

Figure 38.19. Bites of head lice, *Pediculus humanus capitis.*

Epidemiology

The three species of human lice can be considered cosmopolitan in distribution, with infestations recorded throughout tropical, temperate, and arctic regions. Absence of lice in a population is a result of social or hygienic habits rather than of geographic or climatic factors.

The rates of infestations with crab lice are usually much lower than those for head or body lice. Infestations with head lice can reach epidemic proportions, particularly among school children.[44]

Sex, age, race and socioeconomic status can affect rates of infestations with head lice. In an urban outbreak, white children were more frequently infested than black children, younger children more than older children, poorer children more than affluent ones, children from large families more than those from smaller families. Length of hair did not affect rates of infestation.[45]

Infestations with body lice are usually associated with poverty, crowded conditions, social upheavals such as wars, or natural disasters. Because body lice reside and deposit eggs on clothing, conditions that prevent the change and cleaning of garments, coupled with close contact and crowding, foster the spread of these insects.

Louse-Borne Diseases

Body lice are the only vectors involved in infecting man with *Rickettsia prowazeki*, which causes epidemic typhus; *Rochalimaea quintana*, the rickettsial agent of trench fever; and *Borrelia recurrentis*, the spirochete that causes louse-borne relapsing fever.

The rickettsiae multiply within the louse in the epithelial cells of the midgut, which ultimately rupture, releasing large numbers of these microorganisms. Human infections occur through the rubbing of infected louse feces into skin abrasions caused by the original louse bites. These abrasions are often extended by scratching. Inhalation of fomites containing rickettsiae also causes human infection. Rickettsiae survive dehydration and remain infective for more than 2 months at warm temperatures.

Man is the usual reservoir for the rickettsiae of epidemic typhus. The organism can remain latent for years, occasionally giving rise to a mild recrudescent form of typhus termed Brill-Zinsser disease. Lice feeding on people with this form of typhus can become infected with the rickettsiae and transmit them to nonimmune individuals, giving rise to the primary epidemic form of the disease.

Recent studies have demonstrated a sylvan cycle of *R. prowazeki* in flying squirrels in the United States,[46] but the importance of this rodent reservoir in the spread of typhus is yet to be determined.

Trench fever is a self-limiting disease caused by *R. quintana*. Transmission to man is similar to that of epidemic typhus. Individuals with trench fever can infect lice from the third day of illness and sometimes for months thereafter. The rickettsiae develop only within the cuticular margin of the louse (i.e., not intracellularly) and cause no disease in the insect. Infected feces and crushed lice are the usual sources of infection. Man is the only animal in which this rickettsia causes disease.

Louse-borne relapsing fever is caused by the spirochete *B. recurrentis*. The body louse is the only vector of *B. recurrentis*, although similar spirochetes cause tick-borne relapsing fevers. Lice are infected when feeding on infected individuals during febrile periods. The spirochetes invade the epithelium of the gut and ultimately the blood of the louse. Transmission can occur only when crushed lice are rubbed into a wound or are inhaled. Lice do not pass the spirochete by bite and do not excrete it in feces.[47]

The Fleas: Siphonaptera

The fleas comprise a small order of insects of generally similar appearance and habits. The adult fleas exist as ectoparasites on warm-blooded animals. The typical adult flea (Fig. 38.20) is a brown, laterally compressed, wingless insect less than 3 mm long. It has a tough skin. Its third

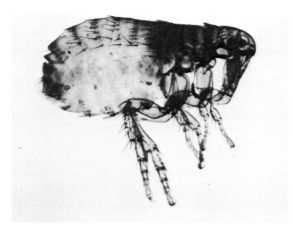

Figure 38.20. Adult female cat flea *Ctenocephalides felis.* ×20.

pair of legs is adapted for jumping and its mouthparts are designed for blood-sucking.

Fleas undergo complete metamorphosis in their development, exhibiting markedly different larval, pupal, and adult stages (Fig. 38.3). The larvae are delicate, motile, vermiform creatures; the pupae are encapsulated and quiescent.

Fleas cause diseases of man both as serious biting pests and as vectors of a number of infectious agents, most notably, *Yersinia pestis.* They usually feed quickly and to repletion at a single site.

Historical Information

Man has evolved with these "lair" parasites of domestic animals and fellow cave dwellers. Literature is replete with songs, poems, and stories extolling the virtues and vices of fleas and the miseries they cause. The importance of fleas as vectors was not recognized until the final years of the 19th century, when they were implicated in the transmission of plague. The historical impact of flea-borne bubonic plague, the Black Death, in the development of civilization has been well documented.[37]

Life Cycle

The life cycle of a typical flea is shown in Fig. 38.3. Fleas are usually parasites of animals inhabiting nests, dens, or caves. The adult flea is an obligate parasite of its warm-blooded host, feeding only on blood. The flea scatters its eggs in and around the nest of its host. Larval fleas are active, yellowish-white creatures with biting mouthparts. They feed on host feces or dried blood defecated by adult fleas.[48]

Under ideal conditions of temperature and humidity, eggs can complete embryonation and hatch within less than a week; larvae develop to adults within less than 2 weeks. After the flea has completed its development through three larval stages, it spins a cocoon and forms a quiescent pupa. The pupal period, during which the insect gradually develops its adult characteristics, may last from a week to a year depending on the species and the environmental conditions. Pupae encased in a cocoon may remain dormant for months, until they are stimulated by vibrations to emerge and give rise to a mass of hungry fleas.

Although many species of fleas bite man if the insects are sufficiently hungry, only a small number are consistent pests of man. The combless fleas, so called because they lack prominent spines or ctenidia on their heads, include four species that regularly feed on man.

The human flea, *Pulex irritans,* is an ectoparasite of man and animals, particularly swine. *P. irritans* is cosmopolitan in distribution and is the most common flea of man. A closely related species, *P. simulans,* is restricted to the New World. Both species are capable of transmitting plague, but are considered minor vectors of this disease.

The oriental rat flea *Xenopsylla cheopis* (Fig. 38.21), as the vector of *Y. pestis,* has long been considered one of the great killers of man. It is an ectoparasite of rats, feeding on man only when its customary host is unavailable. Classically, human bubonic plague is a consequence of an epizootic of plague in the rat population. As rats die in massive numbers, infected fleas leave their dead hosts and seek fresh sources of blood. Under these circumstances man is readily attacked and infected.

Xenopsylla acts as an efficient vector because of its association with reservoir rats and its readiness to feed on man. Moreover, when a flea takes a blood meal from an infected rat, the plague organism rapidly multiplies within the flea's proventriculus, an organ of the intestinal

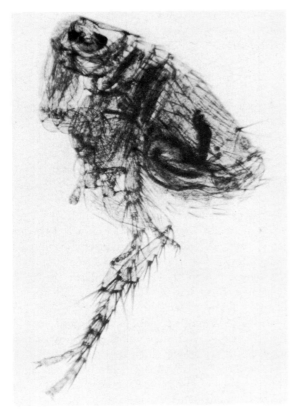

Figure 38.21. Adult of the oriental rat flea *Xenopsylla cheopis*. × 20.

tract, lined with spiny projections. Within 3 days the proventriculus becomes blocked by a gelatinous mass of partially digested blood and bacteria. When the flea feeds again, it is unable to engorge and is forced to regurgitate blood and the bacteria from the proventriculus into the host. Because the flea is unable to feed to satisfaction, it moves rapidly from host to host seeking a meal and transmitting the plague organism. The flea eventually dies of starvation, but not before its role as vector of plague has been discharged.

The combed fleas include four species that affect man. The dog and cat fleas, *Ctenocephalides canis* and *C. felis* (Fig. 38.20), are closely related, morphologically similar species with two sets of prominent combs on the head. Both species feed equally well on dogs and cats, and both bite man if given the opportunity. Their larvae and pupae are usually found in the places where the animals rest. The fleas can prove particularly annoying when the pet leaves the household and the fleas have man as the only source of blood. Raccoons can also bring cat fleas into homes.[49]

The northern rat flea, *Nosopsyllus fasciatus,* and the squirrel flea, *Diamanus montanus,* are common combed fleas of rodents in North America. They readily bite man and may be involved in transmission of plague from wild rodents to rats or to man.

The jigger flea, or chigoe, *Tunga penetrans* (Fig. 38.22), is a serious pest in the tropical and subtropical regions of the Americas, Africa, and the Indian subcontinent. This flea originated in South America and was introduced into Africa during the late 19th century. Adult chigoes are less than 1 mm long. Both sexes feed regularly on blood. After insemination, the female flea attaches itself to the skin of the toes, soles of the feet, or legs and becomes enveloped by host tissue (Fig. 38.23). Thus protected, the female swells to the size of a pea, produces 150–200 eggs, and dies still embedded in the tissue.[50,51]

The infested tissue can become ulcerated and infected by bacteria, which may include the clostridia, and cause tetanus or gas gangrene. Autoamputation of toes is not uncommon. Infection can be avoided by wearing shoes in areas where *T. penetrans* occurs. Treatment consists of removing the flea with a sterile instrument and treating the wound locally to prevent infection.

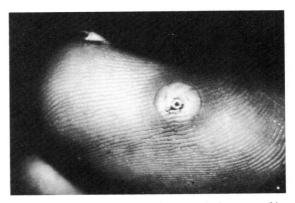

Figure 38.22. White papule with central pit on toe of individual infested with the chigoe flea, *Tunga penetrans.* The adult female flea is embedded in the tissue of the epidermis and eggs are extruded through the central pit. × 2. (Courtesy of Dr. G. Zalar)

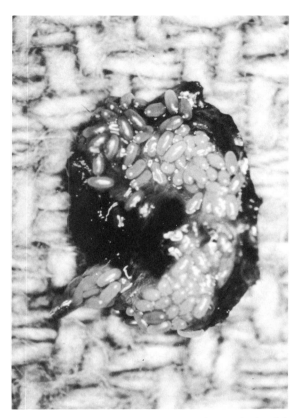

Figure 38.23. Eggs of *Tunga penetrans* from a single adult flea. × 20. (Courtesy of Dr. G. Zalar)

Pathogenesis

The response to repeated flea bites is typical of reactions to most insect bites. Initial exposure produces little or no reaction, but after an individual is sensitized to the salivary antigens of the flea, first delayed, then primary reactions develop.

Clinical Disease

Intense irritation that leads to scratching and secondary bacterial infections[52] is the main manifestation of flea bites. The major health problem caused by fleas is the transmission of infectious agents for which the fleas are vectors.

Diagnosis

The typical flea bite first appears as a single papule. However, with heavy flea infestations, pa-

pules may be grouped along the arms and legs, on the face and neck, or where clothing fits snugly.

Precise incrimination of fleas requires capture of one of the offending insects. The species of the flea can be determined with the aid of a dissecting microscope and a key to identification of fleas affecting man.

Treatment

Pruritus can be treated symptomatically; secondary bacterial infection, as appropriate.

Control

Fleas can be controlled at the source of the infestation by various commercially available insecticides. Dusts should be applied to the fur and nestings of dogs and cats. These dusts are particularly effective against the fleas that dwell in nests, whose larvae feed on particles. Space sprays can be effective against adult fleas. Flea collars on pets are also effective in preventing infestation. A number of topically applied repellents can protect individuals against flea bites for short periods.

Epidemiology of Flea-Borne Diseases

Fleas serve as primary vectors of *Y. pestis*, the agent of the plague and *Rickettsia mooseri*, which causes murine or endemic typhus. Moreover, fleas can serve as intermediate hosts of various cestodes and nematodes that infect mammals including man.

Y. pestis persists in nature in a so-called sylvan or campestral cycle in which wild rodents are constantly infected by various species of fleas. Foci of naturally infected rodents occur in central Asia, South Africa, South America, and the Russian steppe. In western North America, plague is maintained in a ground squirrel reservoir with the squirrel flea, Diamanus, the vector. A number of other rodent species and flea vectors may also be involved. The U.S. reports 5–10 autochthonous cases of bubonic plague each year, usually among campers, hunters, and farmers in the western states.

As long as plague exists as a disease of field rodents, human cases are rare. However, when the plague organism is transferred from wild rodents to peridomestic rats and becomes established in a rat-rat-flea cycle, the potential for human infection increases markedly.

The epidemiology of murine typhus has been clarified with the demonstration that *R. mooseri* can be transmitted transovarially from an infected flea to her progeny.[53]

The Bugs: Heteroptera

Heteroptera are known as true bugs. This large order contains two families of medical importance. Adults of most heteropterans are winged; the wingless bedbugs, the Cimicidae, are an exception. Bugs have mouthparts modified for piercing and sucking. Their long, slender, segmented beak is usually held along the ventral surface of the body when it is not in use. Most heteropterans are plant feeders, some are predaceous on other insects, and the ones causing human diseases, which are members of the Reduviidae and Cimicidae, are hematophagous. Heteroptera develop by incomplete metamorphosis.

The Bedbugs: Cimicidae

Three closely related species of bedbugs are blood-feeding ectoparasites of man. The common bedbug, *Cimex lectularius,* and the tropical bedbugs, *C. hemipterus* and *C. boueti,* are morphologically similar, i.e., are oval, flattened, reddish-brown insects with mouthparts well adapted for piercing flesh and sucking blood. Adult bedbugs (Fig. 38.24) have non-functional reduced wings. They are approximately 5 mm long and 3 mm wide. Their five nymphal stages are smaller, sexually immature copies of the adults.[38,54]

Bedbugs are cosmopolitan in distribution. *C. lectularius* is widespread throughout temperate and tropical regions. The Indian bedbug, *C. hemipterus,* is restricted to tropical and subtropical climates, and *C. boueti* is found in the tropical regions of Africa and South America.

Historical Information

Bedbugs evolved from ectoparasites of cave-dwelling mammals, probably bats, at the time when man was a cave dweller. They were first recorded as a problem in the Mediterranean region by early Greek and Roman writers. In

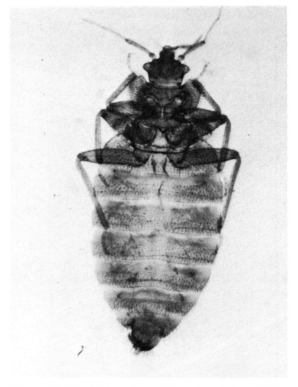

Figure 38.24. Adult bedbug, *Cimex lectularius.* ×15.

northern Europe they were identified much later, e.g., during the 11th century in Germany, 13th century in France, and 16th century in England.[38] Although bedbugs have been suspected of transmitting a number of human diseases, they have only recently been implicated in the mechanical transmission of hepatitis B virus.[55]

Life Cycle

Bedbugs are found in a variety of human habitations including homes, hotels, dormitories, prisons, barracks, and hospitals. They remain hidden in cracks and crevices in walls, floors, and furniture, usually appearing at night or in dim light to feed on a sleeping host. Man is the preferred source of blood, but bedbugs feed on a variety of animals if man is unavailable. They characteristically bite two or three times in succession over a period of a few minutes to engorge themselves.

Adult females lay 2–3 eggs per day for a total of 200–500 during a lifetime. The pearly white eggs are 1 mm long. They are laid individually in crevices, behind loose wallpaper, in cracks in woodwork or furniture, or in mattresses. Hatching is dependent on temperature but usually occurs after 9–10 days of embryonation. There are five nymphal stages, each requiring a blood meal before molting to the next. The egg-to-egg period, depending on temperature, varies from 7 to 19 weeks, which allows the development of several generations of bugs within a year. Availability of a blood source also influences generation time. Adult bugs feed weekly during the summer, less frequently in the cooler months, and starve during the winter, reappearing to feed again in the spring.

Pathogenesis

Feeding bedbugs inject salivary fluids and sensitize the host. Primary exposure produces little or no reaction. After repeated exposures a severe delayed reaction may develop; continued exposure produces an additional primary reaction. Finally, after a course of regular exposures to bites, the host can become desensitized.

Clinical Disease

Reactions to bites can be mild or severe; large hemorrhagic bullae (Fig. 38.25A) form on some sensitized individuals; others develop erythema and local edema and experience severe and prolonged pruritus. Scratching can lead to secondary bacterial infections. Heavy bedbug infestations can interfere with sleep.

Diagnosis

The bite wounds are firm, closely spaced papules, appearing as two or three lesions together (Fig. 38.25B). This grouping can be used to differentiate predation by bedbugs from the typically single bites of other insects. The final de-

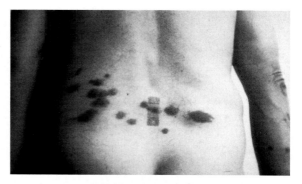

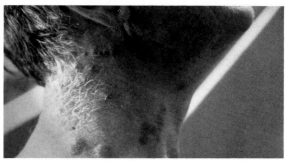

Figure 38.25A. Hemorrhagic bullae caused by the bites of *Cimex lectularius*.

Figure 38.25B. *C. lectularius* bites in groups of two or three are common for this insect.

termination that bedbugs are involved depends on finding living or dead bugs, or the circumstantial evidence of a characteristically pungent odor associated with the alarm glands of these insects, and trails of blood droplets near the hiding places of the bugs.

Treatment

The itching associated with bedbug bites responds to symptomatic therapy.

Control

Control in dwellings is best achieved with chemical insecticides. Residual compounds such as DDT and BHC are very effective and long lasting. Resistance to these compounds has been reported in a number of areas, particularly in the tropics. Diazinon has been used successfully to treat infested surfaces. Removal of old furniture, mattresses, loose wallpaper, and the patching of wall cracks can deny the bugs resting and breeding places.

The Assassin Bugs: Reduviidae

Reduviidae is a large family of predaceous insects collectively referred to as assassin bugs, most members of which are insectivorous. One subfamily, the Triatominae, is found mainly in the New World and is of particular importance because its members are hematophagous and are vectors of Chagas disease.

Bugs of the Triatominae (Fig. 38.26), the so-called kissing bugs, cone-nosed bugs, or *vinchucas,* are large insects with distinct elongate cone-shaped heads. They possess a long, three-segment proboscis well developed for piercing skin; all developmental stages are exclusively blood-feeding. Adults are winged and good fliers, whereas the nymphal stages are wingless, sexually immature miniatures of the adults, developing through the various stages by incomplete metamorphorsis.

Historical Information

The Triatominae received little attention from entomologists before 1909, when Chagas identified them as vectors of *Trypanosoma cruzi.*[56]

Life Cycle

Three species of Triatominae serve as major vectors of Chagas disease, although several species are important as vectors in restricted areas and a large number of species have been found naturally infected with the parasite. *Panstrongylus megistus, Triatoma infestans,* and *Rhodnius prolixus* are large bugs that feed on man but will also feed on wild or domestic animals whenever they are available. These insects abound in the cracks and crevices of the mud and timber houses typical of rural areas in the Latin American tropics.[57] Kissing bugs are usually found in resting places near their source of blood meals. Domestic or peridomestic species that prey on man are found in cracks and crevices of walls and floors, particularly in sleeping areas.

Adult females require a blood meal before producing a clutch of eggs. They lay eggs singly within the same cracks that harbor the nymphs and adults. The eggs hatch within 10–30 days and each of the five nymphal stages requires a full blood meal before molting to the next one. Kissing bugs are prodigious feeders. First-stage nymphs can imbibe 12 times their weight in blood; subsequent stages drink relatively less. Fifth-stage nymphs of *R. prolixus* may suck in more than 300 μl of blood and adult females more than 200 μl for each egg batch. The five nymphal stages may last several months before their final molt to the adult stage. Most species have one generation per year.[58]

Pathogenesis

Intense and persistent pain is associated with the bites of some insectivorous assassin bugs, a result of injection of various toxins. The bites of most of the blood-feeding Triatominae are notably painless, thereby enabling these insects to feed undisturbed on sleeping individuals. The habit of feeding around the mouth or eyes of a sleeper accounts for the designation ''kissing bug.'' After sensitization to the salivary fluids of feeding bugs, individuals can develop delayed reactions characterized by itching, swelling, redness, nausea, and in rare cases, anaphylaxis. Anaphylactic responses to xenodiagnosis, usually with *R. prolixus,* have been reported.[59]

Both nymphs and adult bugs act as vectors of *T. cruzi.* Although bugs may be infected by feeding on human hosts and can transmit the organism from man to man, the usual sources of bug infection are wild and peridomestic animals such as dogs, cats, mice, armadillos, and opos-

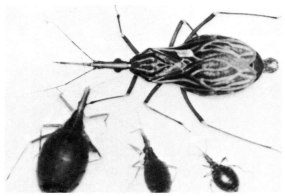

Figure 38.26. Adult (*top*) and three nymphs of the kissing bug, *Rhodnius prolixus.* Note fully formed wings on the adult. × 1.

sums. *T. cruzi* develops in the hindgut of the bug and does not invade the salivary glands. Thus the bite of the bug causes no infection. Rather, infectious parasites are passed in the feces of the bug while it feeds. The victim reacts to the irritation of the bite, then rubs infected feces into the eyes, mouth, or the wound made by the bite. Various triatomine species regularly feed on infected animals, support growth of the parasite, but do not defecate until they leave the host. These species usually are not involved in transmission to man, but may serve to maintain the parasite in an animal reservoir where infected bugs may be eaten by the animal host, which thus becomes infected. *T. cruzi* is naturally maintained in wood rats in southern California by such a cycle. Although transmission of *T. cruzi* to man is rare in the United States, infected animals are found regularly, and autochthonous cases have been reported.

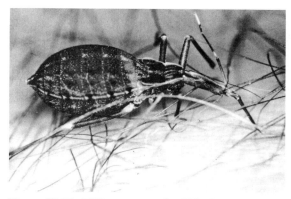

Figure 38.27. Fifth-stage nymph of *Rhodnius prolixus* in typical feeding pose. Note immature wing pads on thorax. Abdomen is distended with blood. × 5.

Clinical Disease

Except for the allergic reaction to the bite, the bite itself is innocuous. The importance of these bugs lies in their acting as vectors in Chagas disease (see Chapter 30).

Diagnosis

The night-feeding kissing bugs are insidious (Fig. 38.27), leaving little initial evidence of their blood meal. Kissing bugs normally feed from one puncture, leaving a single papule. This distinguishes the lesion from those caused by bedbugs, which also feed at night, because the latter are usually clustered in groups of two or three.

Most of the entomophagous bugs likely to bite man are large insects; the wheel bug, a common offender, with a distinctive cog-like crest on its thorax, is more than 30 mm long. Because they bite during the day, usually when handled, they can be readily identified.

Treatment

Reactions to the bites of kissing bugs require, at most, local symptomatic therapy.

Control

Insecticides have proved generally ineffective for the control of kissing bugs.

The Stinging Insects: Hymenoptera

The stinging insects, including the bees, wasps, hornets (Fig. 38.28), and ants, are members of the Hymenoptera, a large order of highly developed species. It is among the Hymenoptera that complex social systems, castes, and elaborate hive and nest structures have evolved. The only other insect group to achieve such a level of social development is the termites. In the Hymenoptera, the ovipositor, the apparatus for egg laying, has been modified to serve as a stinging organ and is used by adult females for the capture of prey for food or for defense.

The stinging apparati of honeybees, bumblebees, wasps, and hornets are generally similar in structure. They consist of paired acid glands, a single alkaline gland, a poison sac with muscular neck, and the piercing apparatus itself, which includes a stylet sheath and paired stylets.

The stylets or darts of the honeybee stinger are barbed (Fig. 38.29A) and once inserted by the

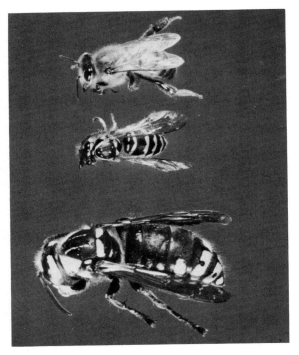

Figure 38.28. Three common species of stinging hymenoptera: honey bee (*top*), yellow jacket (*center*) and hornet (*bottom*). ×3. (Courtesy of Dr. J. Pisano)

insect cannot be withdrawn. Consequently, when a honeybee stings and attempts to fly away, it leaves behind the complete stinging apparatus, virtually disemboweling itself and suffering a mortal wound. The self-contained stinger with its attached poison sac and musculature continues to pump venom into the wound long after the bee has departed.[60] The stingers of most hymenopterans are not barbed (Fig. 38.29B) and are removed after stinging. Wasps, hornets, bumblebees, and ants are capable of multiple stings without losing the apparatus.

It is estimated that in the U.S. 50–100 people die each year from reactions to stings of the hymenopterans; there is probably substantial underreporting and some misdiagnosis. Yellow jackets and honeybees are the major causes of these reactions.

Certain behavioral characteristics of bees and yellow jackets result in increase of aggressiveness. Honeybees are generally benign, unless they are individually molested or provoked to defend their hive. Their venom contains the pheromone isopentyl acetate, which acts as an alarm signal and draws other bees to the site of the original

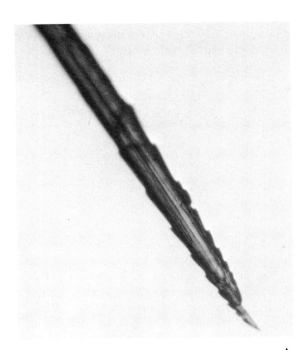

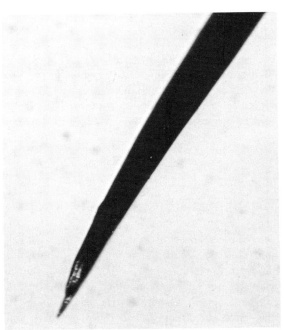

A   B

Figure 38.29. Stinging darts of honeybee (**A**) and hornet (**B**). Note the barbs on the honeybee dart. **A** and **B**, ×100. (Courtesy of Dr. J. Pisano)

sting. This leads to multiple stings.[61] Dramatic reports of the so-called African killer bees are exaggerations of reality, although these bees tend to be more aggressive and less predictable than the common bees found in most domestic hives.[62]

Yellow jackets are particularly aggressive when their nest areas are approached, and they sting without provocation or warning. Their aggressive behavior increases during the late summer and early fall. Gardeners and picnickers are particularly at risk.

Historical Information

The honeybee, *Apis mellifera,* was one of the first insects recorded by man in his writings and in his art (Fig. 38.30). Bees have long been recognized as sources of honey, and their role as plant pollinators is crucial to agriculture.

Life Cycle

Hymenopterans develop by complete metamorphosis with distinct larval, pupal, and adult stages. Larvae are vermiform and look like maggots. They are dependent on adults for food. Pupae, encased in a cocoon, represent an inactive, nonfeeding transitional phase. The adults usually have wings and are good fliers. Certain groups with highly developed social systems have evolved nonreproducing worker and soldier castes. Other groups, such as the ants, are wingless as adults except during reproductive periods.

Four families of the Hymenoptera contain

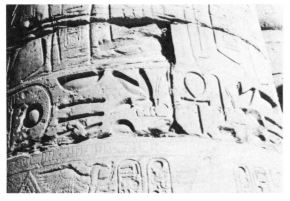

Figure 38.30. Honeybee carved over 3000 years ago on a pillar, Temple of Karnak, Egypt.

medically important species, the stings of which can cause severe reactions in man.

The bees, Apidae, include some species that live in complex social organizations such as hives, or in less structured subterranean nests, although most species in this family live as solitary insects. Only the honeybees and bumblebees among the Apidae are of concern to man because of their ability to sting.

The honeybee, *A. mellifera,* originally an Old World species is now found worldwide in domestic and wild hives. Bees of this species are raised commercially for their honey and for their role as pollinators of a wide range of plants including most fruits and legume crops. They construct elaborate hives wherein a single nonforaging queen lays eggs in wax cells. Larvae develop within these cells while being fed by nonreproductive female workers. Adult workers tend the hives and forage for nectar and pollen. The bees tend to sting when individual insects or their hive is disturbed.

Bumblebees of the genus Bombus are large, hairy, ungainly, less organized social bees, which build simple underground nests. They sting under the same circumstances as do honeybees.

The Vespidae include the wasps, hornets, and yellow jackets; all are capable of inflicting painful stings. Many species in this family build elaborate nests of masticated wood fibers or mud, whereas others construct simple nests underground. The yellow jackets are social hymenopterans with distinctive yellow and black bands on the abdomen, which are often mistaken for bees. They are aggressive insects and a major cause of stings in man.[63]

Ants belong to the family Formicidae, some members of which can cause damage by bite or by stinging. They have a variety of complex social systems, with elaborate behavior patterns, intricate nests, and castes of workers, soldiers, and reproducing insects. Two groups of ants are of concern in the United States.

The harvester ants of the genus Pogonomyrmex readily attack man and other animals and are capable of inflicting painful stings. They build underground nests, topped by mounds, in warm, dry sandy areas. When a nest is disturbed, ants come out, swarm over the invader, and sting him repeatedly and vigorously.

Fire ants (Fig. 38.31) of the genus Solenopsis

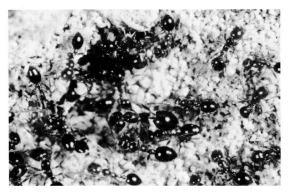

Figure 38.31. Fire ants of the genus Solenopis capable of mass attacks and inflicting repeated painful stings. ×1.5. (Courtesy of United Stages Department of Agriculture)

are so named because of their sharp fiery sting. Several native U.S. species are of medical importance, but the imported fire ant, *Solenopsis invicta* (Fig. 38.32), is a particularly dangerous species.[64] It was introduced into the United States around 1930 and since then has spread throughout the southeastern states, where it presents a serious hazard to man and livestock. They build large, hard-crusted mounds, well camouflaged, and often not seen until they are disturbed. When fire ants attack, they first bite their victim with strong mandibles and then sting repeatedly. This results in a circle of painful stings around a central bite.

Certain species of tropical ants are notorious for their ability to ravage plants and animals alike as they travel from place to place in colonies or armies numbering millions of individuals.

The so-called velvet ants are not true ants, but wingless wasps of the family Mutillidae. These large, hairy, often brightly colored insects are capable of inflicting a painful sting if they are disturbed. A large black mutillid with scarlet hairs is common in the central United States, where it can cause considerable distress by stinging barefoot bathers.

Several other groups of the Hymenoptera have the capacity for stinging and may be occasional pests.

Pathogenesis

In the act of stinging, the aroused insect first inserts the sheath to open the wound, then follows immediately with the inward thrust of the stylets and the injection of the venom. The combination of the acid and alkaline venom fluids, designed to kill insect prey, causes extreme pain and inflammation. Venom from 500 stings received within a few minutes can cause a man's death. The inhabitants of a single disturbed beehive can inflict at least that number of stings in a matter of minutes. Sensitization to the venom can result in severe allergic reactions. A number of antigenically active compounds has been identified in venom, phospholipase A being the most important. Others include hyaluronidase, melittin, and apamin.[65]

Clinical Disease

The primary manifestations of the sting are due to mechanical damage and the direct action of the venom. They include pain, edema, pruritus, and warmth at the site of the sting, but these symptoms are transitory. Severe toxic reactions can be caused by as few as 10 stings within a period of a few minutes. Muscle cramps, drowsiness, fever, and headache are characteristic.

Allergic reactions are by far the most serious consequence of the stings of hymenopterans. They may develop in previously sensitized individuals and include three patterns of symptoms. There is urticaria, associated with pruritus. The skin and mucous membranes become edematous. There may be simultaneous bronchospasm and

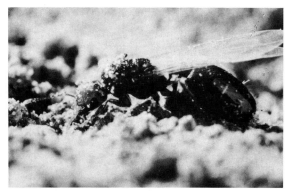

Figure 38.32. Winged reproductive stage of the fire ant, *Solenopis invicta*. ×6. (Courtesy of United States Department of Agriculture)

anaphylaxis, and death may follow. In sensitized individuals, even a single sting may bring the most severe reaction. A delayed reaction characterized by urticaria, fever, and arthralgia may occur hours or weeks after a sting.

Although the stinging hymenopterans share a number of common antigens, each possesses one or more unique ones. Sensitization to stings of one species does not always produce sensitivity to those of other species.[66-68]

Diagnosis

Individuals with suspected sting sensitivities can undergo skin testing with specific venoms to determine the level of risk.

Treatment

Initial treatment for a honeybee sting must include removal of its stinger and the attached venom sac. This can be done with a knife blade, a needle, or a fingernail. It is important not to squeeze the site, because such pressure releases more venom from the sac. A nonallergic primary reaction may be treated with ice to lessen edema and pain, and with various local antipruritics.

Individuals with known sting sensitivity must be prepared to act quickly to prevent serious reactions. On being stung, the individual should remove the stinger immediately and, if the sting is on an arm or leg, apply a tourniquet above it.

Emergency kits are available by prescription and sensitive individuals should be familiar with their use. Such kits contain epinephrine in a syringe, antihistamine tablets, and a tourniquet.

Emergency treatment consists of injections of epinephrine, half of the calculated dose intramuscularly and half intravenously, and an antihistaminic. Obviously, this presupposes planning and the sensitized person and his or her next of kin must be prepared to carry out at least the intramuscular injection of epinephrine. In addition, the potential victim must carry isoproteranol for sublingual administration and an oral, nonenteric coated antihistaminic.

Desensitization using whole body extracts of the insects has been attempted, but is ineffective. Purified venoms have been used successfully for desensitization.[69]

Control

Wasp, hornet, and ant nests can be destroyed with a number of commercially available insecticidal compounds, such as carbamates, malathion, and resmithrin. Aerial nests can be destroyed at night, when the insects are quiescent. General avoidance of areas where stinging hymenopterans occur should be a rule for sensitive individuals. There are no effective repellents against these insects.

References

1. Spielman A, Wilson ML, Levine JF, et al.: Ecology of *Ixodes damiminii* borne human babesiosis and Lyme disease. Ann Rev Entomol 30:439–460, 1985
2. Hawley WA, Reiter P, Copeland PS, et al.: *Aedes albopictus* in North America: Probable introduction in used tires from northern Asia. Science 236:1114–1116, 1987
3. Piat P, Schofield CJ: No evidence for for arthropod transmission of AIDS. Parasitol Today 2:294–295, 1986
4. Jongi BS: Centipede venoms and poisoning. In: Insect poisons, allergens, and other invertebrate venoms. Tu AT (ed): Marcel Dekker, Inc New York, 1984, pp 333–368
5. Lyell A: Delusions of parasitosis. In Orkin M, Maibach HI (eds): Cutaneous Infestations and Insect Bites, New York, Marcel Dekker; 1985, pp 131–137
6. Blanton FS, Wirth WW: The sand flies (*Culicoides*) of Florida. Arthropods Florida 10:1–204, 1979
7. Downes JA: The ecology of blood-sucking diptera: An evolutionary perspective. In Fallis AM (ed): Ecology and Physiology of Parasites. Toronto, University of Toronto Press, 1971, pp 2–258
8. Kettle, DS: The biology and bionomics of bloodsucking ceratopogonids. Annu Rev Entomol 22:33–51, 1977
9. Kettle DS: The bionomics and control of *Culicoides* and *Leptoconops*. Ann Rev Entomol 7:401–418, 1962
10. Wenyon CM: Some recent advances in. our knowledge of leishmaniasis. J Lond Sch Trop Med 1:93–98, 1912
11. Lewis DJ: The biology of Phlebotomidae in relation to leishmaniasis. Ann Rev Entomol 19:363–384, 1974
12. Sambon LW: Progress report of investigations of pellagra. J Trop Med 13:271–287, 1910
13. Blacklock DB: The development of *Onchocerca*

volvulus in *Simulium damnosum*. Ann Trop Med Parasitol 20:1–48, 1926

14. Dalmat HT: The Black Flies (Diptera, Simuliidae) of Guatemala and Their Role as Vectors of Onchocerciasis. Washington, D.C., Smithsonian Institution, 1955

15. Mattingly PF: The Science of Biology, Series 1. The Biology of Mosquito-borne Disease. London, George Allen and Unwin, 1969

16. Harrison G: Mosquitoes, Malaria and Man: A History of the Hostilities Since 1880. New York, E.P. Dutton, 1978

17. Ross R: Memoirs. London, John Murray, 1923

18. Reed W, Carroll J, Agremonte A, et al.: Etiology of yellow fever, a preliminary note. Phil Med J 6:790–796, 1900

19. Clements AN: Physiology of Mosquitoes. Oxford, Pergamon Press, 1963

20. Bates M: The Natural History of Mosquitoes. New York, Harper & Row, 1965

21. Christophers SR: *Aedes Aegypti*. the Yellow Fever Mosquito: Its Life History, Bionomics, and Structure. Cambridge, Cambridge University Press, 1960

22. Mellanby K: Man's reaction to mosquito bites. Nature 158:554, 1946

23. Beard RL: Insect toxins and venoms. Annu Rev Entomol 8:1–18, 1963

24. Wilson AB, Clements AN: The nature of the skin reaction to mosquito bites in laboratory animals. Int Arch Allergy 26:294–314, 1965

25. Feingold BF, Benjamini E, Micheali D: The allergic responses to insect bites. Ann Rev Entomol 13:137–158, 1968

26. Russell PF, West LS, Manwell RD, et al.: Practical Malariology. London, Oxford University Press, 1963

27. Leiper RT: Report of the helminthologist for the half year ending 30 April, 1913. Report Adv Commis Trop Dis Res Fund, 1913–1914

28. Linday DR, Scudder HI: Non-biting flies and disease. Annu Rev Entomol 1:323–346, 1956

29. Greenberg B: Flies and Disease, Vol. II. Princeton, Princeton University Press, 1973

30. Bruce D: Further report on sleeping sickness in Uganda. Report of the Sleeping Sickness Commission. R Soc Lond 1:1–88, 1897

31. Buxton PA: The Natural History of Tsetse Flies. London, H. K. Lewis and Co., 1955

32. Ford J: The Role of the Trypanosomiases in African Ecology. The Study of the Tse-Tse Fly Problem. Oxford, Clarendon Press, 1971

33. Zumpt F: Myiasis. London, Butterworths, 1965

34. Catts EP: Biology of New World Bot Flies: Cuterebridae. Annu Rev Entomol 27:313–338, 1982

35. Greenberg B: Forensic entomology: case studies. Bull Entomol Soc Am 31:25–28, 1985

36. Lord WD, Burger JF: Collection and preservation of forensically important entomological materials. J. Forensic Sci 28:936–944, 1983

37. Zinsser H: Rats, Lice and History. Boston, Little, Brown 1935

38. Busvine JR: Insects, Hygiene, and History. London, Athlone Press 1976

39. Buxton PA: The Louse. Baltimore, Williams & Wilkins, 1946

40. Ackerman, AB: Crabs—The resurgence of *Phthirus pubis*. N Engl J Med 278:950–951, 1968

41. Morley WM: Body infestations. Scot Med J 22:211–216, 1977

42. Epstein E Sr, Orkin M: Pediculosis: clinical aspects. In Orkin M, Maibach HI (eds): Cutaneous Infestations and Insect Bites. New York, Marcel Dekker, 1985, pp 175–186

43. Orkin M, Maibach HI: Treatment of today's pediculosis. In Orkin M, Maibach HI (eds): Cutaneous Infestations and Insect Bites. New York, Marcel Dekker, 1985, pp 213–217

44. Juranek DD: *Pediculus capitis* in school children. In Orkin M, Maibach HI (eds: Cutaneous Infestations and Insect Bites. New York, Marcel Dekker, 1985, pp 199–211

45. Slonka GF, Fleisner ML, Berlin J et al.: An epidemic of pediculosis capitis. J Parasitol 63:377–383, 1977

46. Sonenshine DE, Bozman FM, Williams MS, et al.: Epizootiology of epidemic typhus (*Rickettsia prowazekii*) in flying squirrels. Am J Trop Med Hyg 27:339–349, 1978

47. Burgdorfer W: The epidemiology of relapsing fevers. In Johnson RC (ed): The Biology of Parasitic Spirochetes. New York, Academic Press, 1976, pp 191–200

48. Jellison WL: Fleas and disease. Ann Rev Entomol 4:389–414, 1959

49. Hunter KW Jr, Campbell AR, Sayles PC: Human infestation by cat fleas. *Ctenocephalides felis* (Siphonaptera: Pulicidae) J Med Entomol 16:547, 1979

50. Goldman L: Tungiasis in travellers from tropical Africa. JAMA 236:1386, 1976

51. Zalar GL, Walther, RR: Infestation by *Tunga penetrans*. Arch Dermatol 116:80–81, 1980

52. Benjamini E, Feingold BF, Kartman L: Skin reactivity in guinea pigs sensitized to flea bites. The sequence of reactions. Proc Soc Exp Biol Med 108:700–702, 1961

53. Farhang-Azad A, Traub R, Baqar S: Transovarial transmission of murine typhus rickettsiae in *Xenopsylla* cheopis fleas. Science 227:543–545, 1985

54. Usinger RL: Monograph of Cimicidae, Vol. VII. Thomas Say Foundation, Washington, DC, Entomology Society of America, 1966

55. Jupp.
56. Chagas C: Nova trypanozomiaze humana. Estudos sobre a morfolojia e o ciclo evalutivo do *Schizotripanum cruzi*. n. genl., n. sp., ajente etiolojico de nova entidade morbida do homen. Mem Inst Oswaldo Cruz 1:159–218, 1909
57. Usinger RL: The Triatominae of North and Central America and the West Indies and their public health significance. Pub Health Bull 288:1–88, 1944
58. Buxton PA: Biology of a blood-sucking bug, *Rhodnius prolixus*. Trans Entomol Soc Lond 78:227–236, 1930
59. Costa ZHN, Costa MT, Weber JN, et al.: Skin reactions to bites as a result of xenodiagnosis. Trans R Soc Trop Med Hyg 75:405–408, 1981
60. Maschwitz UW, Kloft W: Morphology and function of the venom apparatus of insects—bees, wasps, ants, and caterpillars. In Bucherl W, Buckley EE (eds): Venomous Animals and Their Venom. Vol. III. Venomous Invertebrates. New York, Academic Press, 1971, pp 1–60
61. Koeniger N, Weiss, J, Maschwitz U: Alarm pheromones of the sting in the genus *Apis*. J Insect Physiol 25:467–476, 1979
62. Taylor OR Jr: African bees: potential impact in the United States. Bull Entomol Soc Am 31:14–24, 1985
63. Akre RP, Davis HG: Biology and pest status of venomous wasps. Ann Rev Entomol 23:215–238, 1978
64. Lofgren CS, Banks WA, Glancy BM: Biology and control of imported fire ants. Ann Rev Entomol 20:1–30, 1975
65. Hoffman DR: Insect Venom Allergy, Immunology and Immunotherapy. In: Insect Poisons, Allergens, and Other Invertebrate Venoms. Tu AT (ed), Marcel Dekker, Inc. New York, 1984, pp 187–223
66. Shulman S: Allergic responses to insects. Ann Rev Entomol 12:323–346, 1967
67. Lockey RF: Systemic reaction to stinging ants. J Allergy Clin Immunol 54:132–146, 1974
68. Rhoades RB, Schafer WL, Schmid WH, et al.: Hypersensitivity to the imported fire ant. J Allergy Clin Immunol 56:84–93, 1976
69. Hunt KJ, Valentine MD, Sobotka AK, et al.: A controlled trial of immunotherapy in insect hypersensitivity. N Eng J Med 299:157–161, 1978

39. The Arachnids

The arachnids are a class of arthropods that includes the ticks, mites, scorpions, and spiders. Its characteristics clearly differentiate it from the class Insecta. All arachnids are wingless, have four pairs of legs as adults, and usually show only two distinct body regions, a cephalothorax and an abdomen. Metamorphosis in the arachnids is of the incomplete type (Fig. 39.1). The im-

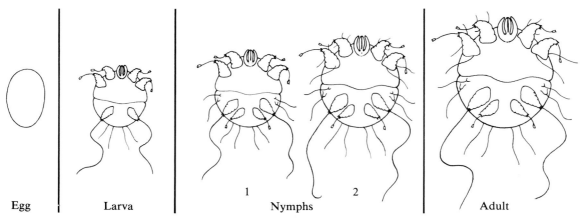

Egg | Larva | Nymphs | Adult

Figure 39.1. Incomplete metamorphosis in the arachnida. Ticks and mites undergo incomplete metamorphosis as typified by the itch mite, *Sarcoptes scabiei*. Larvae have three pairs of legs; adults and nymphal stages have four pairs of legs.

mature nonreproductive stages are smaller but morphologically similar to the adults. In many groups, arachnids in the first, or larval, stage may have only three pairs of legs.

This class comprises three orders: Acarina, Araneida, and Scorpionida. The order Acarina includes mites and ticks. Ticks are exclusively hematophagous; mites feed on a variety of substances including cells and blood. The spiders (order Araneida) are mainly insectivorous, feeding on body fluids of captured insects. Scorpions (order Scorpionida) feed on arthropods or small

a bovine protozoan parasite, *Babesia bigemina,* a serious pathogen of cattle in the western United States. They further demonstrated that the parasite was not passed from cow to cow by a single infected tick, but rather that it was transmitted from an infected cow through a female tick to the tick's offspring transovarially. This resulted in infection of larval ticks capable of transmitting the parasite at the time of the first feeding. They reported these findings in 1893, four years before Ross completed his studies on transmission of malaria by mosquitoes.

Acarina

Ticks

The ticks comprise two large families, the Ixodidae, or hard ticks, and the Argasidae, or soft ticks. They are responsible for damage to livestock, causing considerable weight loss and providing opportunities for secondary infection by bacteria or infestation by flies (Chapter 38). Many species are capable of transmitting pathogens to domestic animals and to man. The salivary secretions of some species can cause paralysis (tick paralysis) and even death in man or animals.

The consequences of infestations by ticks are enormous in terms of yearly losses in milk and beef production, which are especially serious in those areas of the world where sources of protein are already scarce.

It should be noted that man is not the natural host for any species of tick, but many species feed on human blood if given the opportunity and thus become vectors of human infections.

Historical Information

The feeding of ticks on man was recorded by Homer in the 9th century B.C. and later by Aristotle in the 4th century B.C. One of the earliest references to ticks as a possible cause of disease was the suggestion by a 12th-century Persian physician that a fever (probably Crimean-Congo hemorrhagic fever) was transmitted by ticks.[1]

Smith and co-workers were the first to demonstrate that ticks could transmit disease.[2] They showed that the tick *Boophilus annulatus* carried a bovine protozoan parasite, *Babesia bigemina,* a

serious pathogen of cattle in the western United States. They further demonstrated that the parasite was not passed from cow to cow by a single infected tick, but rather that it was transmitted from an infected cow through a female tick to the tick's offspring transovarially. This resulted in infection of larval ticks capable of transmitting the parasite at the time of the first feeding. They reported these findings in 1893, four years before Ross completed his studies on transmission of malaria by mosquitoes.

The role of ticks as vectors of spirochetes was shown first with an avian parasite by Marchoux and Salimbeni, in 1903,[3] and a year later with the spirochete causing human relapsing fever by Ross and Milne.[4]

Hard Ticks: The Ixodidae

Hard ticks (Fig. 39.2A and B) (family Ixodidae) are found throughout the world as ectoparasites of a variety of animals. Their name derives from the characteristic tough, leather-like integument covering most of the body. Their mouthparts are included in a capitulum (Fig. 39.3), but there is no defined head. Members of both sexes feed exclusively on blood.

Life Cycle

The typical hard tick develops by gradual metamorphosis from the egg through the larva and nymph to the adult (Fig. 39.1). Larvae have three pairs of legs; the nymphs and adults have four pairs. Each stage takes a single blood meal. The larvae and nymphs feed prior to molting, the

Table 39.1. Arthropods of Medical Importance and the Pathology They Cause

Order and Representative Species	Common Name	Geographical Distribution	Effects on Man
ARACHNIDA Scorpionida (scorpions)			
Various genera and species	Scorpion	Tropics and subtropics	Initially painful sting often followed by systemic reactions
Araneidae (spiders)			
Latrodectus mactans	Black widow spider	Americas	Bite usually painless delayed systemic reaction
Latrodectus spp.	Widow spider	Worldwide	
Loxoceles reclusa	Brown recluse spider	North America	Initial blister at wound site followed by sometimes exten-
Loxoceles laeta	South American brown spider	South America	sive necrosis and slow healing
Acarina (ticks and mites)			
Argasidae Various genera and species	Soft ticks	Worldwide	Skin reactions to bite, tick paralysis, vec- tors of relapsing fever
Ixodidae Various genera and species	Hard ticks	Worldwide	Skin reactions to bite, tick paralysis, vec- tors of rickettsia viruses, bacteria and protozoa
Dermanyssidae *Allodermanyssus sanguineus*	House mouse mite	Worldwide	Vector of *Rickettsia akari*, the cause of rickettsial pox
Various genera and species	Mites	Worldwide	Occasional dermatitis from bites
Demodicidae *Demodex folliculorum*	Follicle mite	Worldwide	Found in sebaceous glands and hair fol- licles, occasional skin reactions
Trombiculidae *Trombicula* spp.	Chigger, red bug	Worldwide	Intense itching at site of attachment
Trombicula akamushi		Southeast Asia, India, Pacific Islands	Vector of *Rickettsia tsutsugamushi*, the cause of scrub typhus
Sarcoptiae *Sarcoptes scabiei*	Human itch mite	Worldwide	Burrows in skin causing severe itching

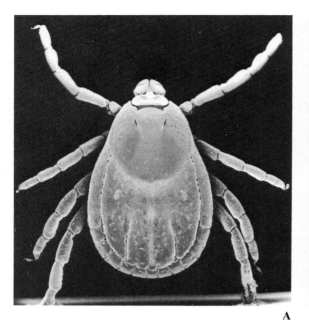
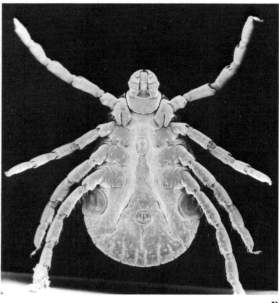

A   B

Figure 39.2. Scanning electron micrographs of female American dog tick, *Dermacentor variabilis*. **A.** Dorsal view; **B.** ventral view. ×7. (Courtesy of Dr. C. Clifford)

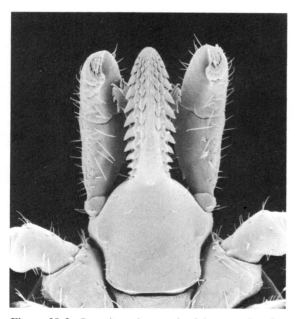

Figure 39.3. Scanning micrograph of the ventral surface of the mouthparts of *Ixodes scapularis*. Note the strongly barbed central hypostome and the lateral palps. The hypostome anchors the tick during feeding. ×80. (Courtesy of Dr. C. Clifford)

adult females prior to producing a single batch of eggs. Death occurs after oviposition.[5]

Hard ticks exhibit one of three life cycles and may be classified as one-, two-, or three-host ticks. A one-host tick spends its life on a single animal, where it attaches to the skin as a larva, feeds and molts to the nymphal stage, feeds again, molts to the adult, and mates, after which the female engorges with blood, falls to the ground, and lays eggs. Larvae begin to hatch within 30 days and await a new host to begin the cycle anew.

Two-host ticks usually spend their larval and nymphal stages on one host, drop to the ground, molt, and await the second host of another species for the completion of the adult phase of the cycle. Each of the three stages of a three-host tick develops on a separate host. The immature stages are usually found on small rodents. The adults feed and mate on larger mammals.

Hard ticks display remarkable longevity, adults of many species surviving up to 2 years without a blood meal. One-host ticks have the shortest egg-to-egg life cycles, sometimes lasting less than a year. Three-host ticks require 2 or even 3 years to complete their life cycles.

Hard ticks feed slowly, taking 7–9 days to become completely engorged. After attaching to a suitable host, the tick searches for a feeding site often well concealed by hair. Once in place, it inserts its mouthparts, armed with recurved teeth, secretes a cement, and begins to feed. After engorging, it easily detaches and moves away. In general, the act of feeding is painless to the host, who is often unaware of the tick.[5,6]

Hard Ticks of Medical Importance

There are at least 11 genera within the Ixodidae, which include species of ticks that feed on man.

Ambylomma americanum and *A. cajennense* prey on a variety of animals, feed avidly on man, and are serious pests in the southern and southwestern states of the United States and in Mexico. They are capable of transmitting rickettsiae of Rocky Mountain spotted fever.

Dermacentor variabilis (Fig. 39.4), the American dog tick, is the major vector of Rocky Mountain spotted fever in the eastern and central United States, is involved in the transmission of tularemia, and can cause tick paralysis in man and dogs. *D. variabilis* is a three-host tick. The larval and nymphal stages feed on small rodents; the adults feed and mate on larger mammals. The dog is the most common host for adults of this species, but man is readily attacked.

D. andersoni (Fig. 39.5), the Rocky Mountain wood tick, is a common species in western and

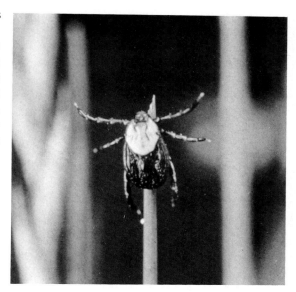

Figure 39.5. Adult female *Dermacentor andersoni* on vegetation, awaiting host. ×3. (Courtesy of Dr. W. Burgdorfer)

northern United States. It transmits Rocky Mountain spotted fever and Colorado tick fever, and causes tick paralysis in man. This three-host tick feeds on a variety of small mammals as a larva or nymph. As an adult, it feeds on large wild or domestic animals and man. Both nymphs and adults are capable of overwintering, and therefore the life cycle of this species usually extends over 2 years.

D. albipictus and *D. occidentalis* are two species found in the Western United States that are capable of transmitting Rocky Mountain spotted fever and Colorado tick fever, but attack man only infrequently.

Ixodes scapularis and *Ixodes dammini* (Fig. 39.6) are three host ticks common on the east coast of the United States. Both species readily attack man and can inflict painful bites. *I. dammini* has been incriminated as the vector of *Babesia microti* and Lyme disease. *I. dammini* has extended its range throughout the northeastern U.S., and elsewhere. It is now being found in Wisconsin, Virginia, and eastern Canada. The rapid spread has been probably facilitated by migratory birds.[7] *I. pacificus* is a common pest of deer and cattle in California. It frequently bites man and is a vector of Lyme disease,[8] in addi-

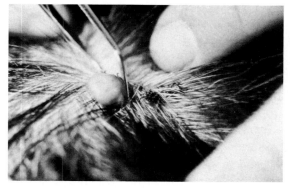

Figure 39.4. Blood-engorged adult female American dog tick, *Dermacentor variabilis.* ×1. (Courtesy of Dr. W. Burgdorfer)

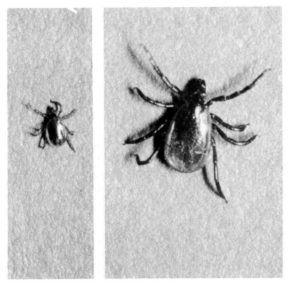

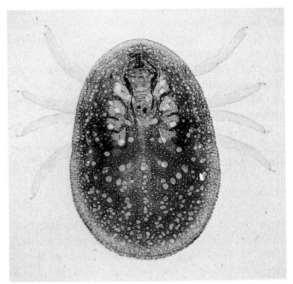

Figure 39.6. Adult female and nymph of *Ixodes dammini*. × 5. (Courtesy of Drs. A. Spielman and P. Rossignol)

Figure 39.7. Adult fowl tick, *Argas persicus*. The mouthparts are not visible from above in soft ticks. × 15. (Courtesy Armed Forces Institute of Pathology, Neg. no. 33311–7)

tion to being a serious pest. *I. holocyclus* is an important cause of tick paralysis in Australia.

Rhipicephalus sanguineus, the brown dog tick, is a cosmopolitan ectoparasite of dogs. Although this species does not readily bite man, it can be a serious nuisance around homes. Female ticks recently engorged on pet dogs drop off and deposit eggs in houses or kennels. The newly hatched larvae tend to crawl up vertical surfaces, literally covering walls or furniture. *R. sanguineus* is considered the major vector of the rickettsia that causes boutonneuse fever.

Hyalomma and Boophilus are genera of ticks whose members are ectoparasites of animals and play important roles in transmitting pathogens in animal populations. Occasionally, these ticks act as vectors of human diseases.

Soft Ticks: The Argasidae

Ticks of the family Argasidae are soft-bodied arthropods covered by a wrinkled, often granulated tegument (Fig. 39.7). They do not have a distinct head region and their mouthparts are located on the ventral surface, not visible from above. Soft ticks are found throughout the world, usually as ectoparasites of birds, although some species normally feed on bats and other small mammals. Several species attack man if given the opportunity.

Argasidae differ from the ixodid hard ticks in their feeding behavior, habitat, and life cycles. Soft ticks normally inhabit the nesting site of their hosts, moving on to the host to feed and returning to the nest when satisfied. They complete engorgement in a matter of minutes or, at most, a few hours, feeding usually at night while the host is asleep.

The typical life cycle of a soft tick consists of a single six-legged larval stage, two or more eight-legged nymphal stages, and the eight-legged adult stage. Some species require several blood meals before each molt and adult females feed repeatedly, producing a small batch of eggs after each meal.

Soft Ticks of Medical Importance

Three genera of the Argasidae affect man as pests or as vectors of pathogens. The fowl tick, *Argas persicus* (Fig. 39.7), is an important cosmopolitan ectoparasite preying on poultry. It does bite man, particularly if the normal fowl hosts are no longer available. Ticks of the genus Otobius may occasionally infest human ears.

Ticks of the genus Ornithodorus are important pests and vectors of the spirochetes causing tick-borne relapsing fevers. *O. moubata* attacks a number of wild and domestic animals, but man is its major host. This tick inhabits huts, feeding at night on the sleeping inhabitants. It is found throughout southern and central Africa reaching as far north as Ethiopia and is the major vector of African relapsing fever. *O. moubata,* the tampon tick, has been implicated in the mechanical spread of Hepatitis B virus in Africa.[9]

Several species of ornithodorus are vectors of relapsing fevers in both the New and Old World; however, most of these are ectoparasites of rodents and other mammals, feeding on man only occasionally.

Pathogenesis and Treatment of Tick Bites

Most ticks firmly attach themselves to the skin of the host before beginning the blood meal. The mouthparts and injected salivary secretions provoke inflammation of the surrounding tissue characterized by local hyperemia, edema, hemorrhage, and thickening of the stratum corneum.[10] Although the initial bite and insertion of the mouthparts may be painless, irritation often develops later and is followed by necrosis and secondary infection at the wound site.

It is important to remove ticks from the skin of the host as soon as they are detected. Early removal will often prevent firm attachment and make transmission of the pathogens less likely. It will also limit the infusion of toxins that cause tick paralysis, because they are released slowly.

Numerous methods have been suggested for the removal of firmly attached ticks. Traditionally, ticks have been treated with chloroform, ether, benzene, turpentine, or petrolatum, which irritate it so that it withdraws. However, the U.S. Public Health Service recommends mechanical removal without any chemical aids. Many genera of ticks, especially Dermacentor, may be removed by gentle but firm pulling of the tick. Ixodes and Amblyomma, which have longer mouthparts that do not detach easily, may require the use of instruments for removal. These ticks should be pulled gently away from the host so that the skin surrounding the mouthparts forms a tent. A sterile needle or scalpel can then be inserted under the mouthparts and used to tease them away from the tissue. In all cases care should be taken to avoid leaving any tissue of the tick, because it will induce an intense inflammation. The tick should not be crushed or damaged, to prevent the release of pathogenic organisms onto the wound site. Subsequent thorough cleansing of the wound is recommended.

Tick Paralysis

More than 40 species in 10 genera of both hard and soft ticks secrete salivary toxins that cause paralysis in man and in a number of other animals. However, this is not a universal property of any one species, suggesting that salivary secretions are characteristic of individual ticks.[11]

The affected patient becomes irritable, is restless, and experiences numbness and tingling in the extremities, face, lips, and throat. Soon the patient develops symmetrical, flaccid paralysis, which is ascending in nature and can lead to bulbar palsy. Sensory loss is rare. There is no fever. Death results from respiratory paralysis. The laboratory findings, i.e., CBC, urinalysis, and cerebrospinal fluid examination, are normal. Differential diagnosis includes poliomyelitis, Guillain-Barré syndrome, transverse myelitis, and spinal cord tumors. Diagnosis depends on clinical history and finding of the tick. Treatment consists of removal of the feeding tick. Rapid recovery follows.

In the United States, *D. andersoni* and *D. variabilis* and, in Australia, *I. holocyclus* are the usual causes of human tick paralysis. A number of species of Dermacentor, Ixodes, Amblyomma, Rhipicephalus, Argas, and Ornithodorus often cause paralysis in animals, but may occasionally affect man.

Tick-Borne Diseases of Man

Ticks transmit a broad array of viruses, rickettsiae, protozoa, and spirochetes.

Viral Diseases

In the United States, Colorado tick fever is the only tick-borne viral disease of man. It is a benign disease transmitted by the bite of *D. andersoni* and maintained in nature as an enzootic infection of rodents spread by the same vector. Transovarial transmission of the virus has not been demonstrated. Colorado tick fever is characterized by sudden onset of chills, headache, severe myalgia, and fever.[12] In the Old World, hard ticks are vectors of a number of viral diseases grouped as hemorrhagic fevers or tick-borne encephalitides. Among these are Russian spring-summer encephalitis, Kyasanur Forest disease, Crimean-Congo hemorrhagic fever, and Omsk hemorrhagic fever.[12,13]

Bacterial Diseases

Tularemia is a bacterial disease caused by *Franciscella tularensis* and characterized by a focal ulcer at the site of entry of the organism, enlargement of regional lymph nodes, fever, prostration, myalgia, and headache. *D. andersoni* and *D. variabilis* are the ticks most frequently involved in the transmission of this infection from small mammals, particularly rabbits, to man; a number of tick species maintain the infection in the reservoir population.

Spirochetal Diseases

The relapsing fevers are a group of diseases with a similar clinical pattern, caused by spirochetes of the genus Borelia, all of which are transmitted by arthropod vectors. Lice transmit epidemic louse-borne relapsing fever; and soft ticks, endemic tick-borne relapsing fever.

The human relapsing fevers are described as acute infections with toxemia and febrile periods that subside and recur over a period of weeks. Tick-borne relapsing fevers occur throughout the Old and New Worlds and are transmitted by ticks of the genus Ornithodoros. In the Western Hemisphere, *O. hermsi*, *O. turicata*, and *O. rudis* are the most important vectors. A close association, usually in a rural setting, between man, vector ticks, and rodents infected with spirochetes is the typical condition necessary for human infections. In Africa, *O. moubata*, which feeds primarily on man and lives within human dwellings, maintains transmission of relapsing fever from man to man.[14]

Protozoal Diseases

Babesiosis is a disease of a variety of animals and rarely of man. (For details see Chapter 36.)

Rickettsial Diseases

Rocky Mountain spotted fever is an acute, sometimes fatal, febrile, exanthematous disease caused by *Rickettsia rickettsii*. It most frequently affects children and is characterized by fever, headache, musculoskeletal pains, and a generalized rash that appears first on the wrists and ankles and often becomes hemorrhagic.

Although initially described from the Rocky Mountain region of the United States and distributed throughout much of North and South America, the infection is of particular importance in the "tick belt" states of Maryland, Virginia, North Carolina, South Carolina, and Georgia. In these states the incidence of the disease has been steadily rising. The main vector in the eastern states is *D. variabilis*, the American dog tick, and in the western states *D. andersoni*. Other tick species considered minor vectors have the capacity to transmit the organism to man, but may be primarily important as vectors that infect reservoir hosts.

In areas where Rocky Mountain spotted fever is prevalent, regular inspection for ticks should be undertaken. Children especially should be examined twice daily. The tick must be attached to the host for several hours before transmission of the pathogen takes place. Therefore, expeditious removal of it can prevent infection. No vaccine against Rocky Mountain spotted fever is currently available.[15]

Old World tick-borne typhus has different regional names: boutonneuse fever, Kenya typhus, and South African tick bite fever. It is a relatively mild disease, presenting with chills, fever, and generalized body rash. *Rhipicephalus sanguineus*, the brown dog tick, is the main vector of boutonneuse fever in the Mediterranean region; other hard ticks are involved elsewhere.

Q fever is a self-limited infection. The disease consists of fever, headache, constitutional symptoms, often with pneumonitis, caused by the rickettsia, *Coxiella burnetti*. It is usually contracted through inhalation. Ticks are involved in maintaining the infection in the animal reservoir host and can transmit the organism to man.

Lyme Disease

Lyme arthritis, erythema chronicum migrans, or—as these conditions are known collectively—Lyme disease is caused by the spirochete *Borrelia burgdorferi*,[16] transmitted by a number of Ixodid ticks. *I. dammini*[17] is the primary vector in the eastern U.S.; *I. pacificus*, on the West Coast; and *I. ricinus*, in Europe.[18]

The spirochete is commonly found in rodents,

especially white-footed deer mice. The tick vector, *I. dammini* in its immature stages feeds on this rodent reservoir host and in its adult state, on deer. The range of the tick is limited by the range of the deer populations.

Human infection with this spirochete usually results from a bite of the nymphal tick, although adult ticks are also capable of transmitting it. Before the tick has fed, the spirochete is found in its gut. After the tick has attached to a host and has begun feeding, the spirochetes disseminate throughout the haemocoel, invade the salivary glands and infect the host. This process takes a day or so and therefore prompt removal of the tick reduces the chance of infection.[19]

Mites

Within the Acarina, the term mite is applied to members of several large families of minute arthropods, most free-living but many existing as ecto- or endoparasites of vertebrates and invertebrates alike. Mites affect man by causing dermatitis, serving as vectors of a number of diseases, and as a source of allergens that can lead to serious hypersensitivity reactions.

Historical Information

Mites, described by Aristotle, were well known to ancient man. Their function as ectoparasites was not recognized until about the year 1000 A.D., when scabies was first recorded. Although scabies continued to be described in the early medical literature and the association of a mite with this skin condition was repeatedly noted by physicians and naturalists, the causal relationship was largely ignored by the medical profession. The unequivocal demonstration that a mite was indeed the cause of scabies took place in 1834 when a Corsican medical student recovered mites from affected individuals.[20]

The Human Itch Mite: *Sarcoptes scabiei*
Scabies is a human skin disease caused by the mite *Sarcoptes scabiei* (Fig. 39.8). It is usually associated with crowded living conditions, and its outbreaks often accompany wars, famine, and human migrations. Currently, scabies has reached pandemic proportions.[21]

Prevention and Control

The best measure of tick control for individuals is avoidance of areas where ticks are known to occur. Wide-scale chemical control of tick populations is impractical although various compounds have been used.

Tick control on dogs can be achieved with commercially available tick collars; dusts have proved useful in preventing introduction of brown or American dog ticks into homes.

Diethyltoluamide (DEET) applied to clothing is an effective tick repellent. However, careful examination for ticks is still necessary after traveling through infested areas.

The condition first presents as nocturnal itching, usually on the webbing and sides of the fingers, later spreading to the wrists, elbows, and the rest of the body. The buttocks, women's breasts, and external genitalia of men are also occasionally affected. Lesions appear as short, sinuous, slightly raised, cutaneous burrows.

Infections begin when fertile female mites are transferred from infected individuals by direct contact. The female mite (Fig. 39.9) finds a suitable site, burrows into the skin, and tunnels through the upper layers of the epidermis, depositing fertile eggs. Six-legged larvae hatch from these eggs, leave the tunnel, and wander about the skin before reinvading it and starting new burrows. Once in place the larvae eat, molt, and transform into eight-legged nymphs. Larvae destined to become females molt again to a second nymphal stage; those destined to become males molt directly to the adult form. After fertilization, young adult females begin construction of a new tunnel. The egg-to-egg life cycle may be as short as 2 weeks. A typical infection usually involves only 10–15 adult female mites.[22]

In primary infections, itching and skin eruption are usually delayed for several weeks. As sensitization develops, the typical scabies rash appears on various parts of the body that do not necessarily correspond to the location of active adult female mites, but represent a generalized response to the allergens.

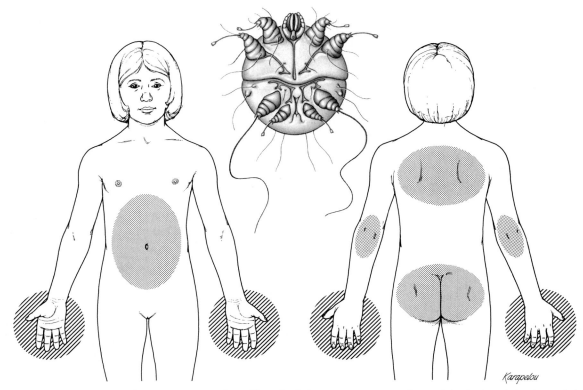

Figure 39.8. The itch mite, *Sarcoptes scabiei*. The stippled areas represent regions of the body where the rash is found. The mites themselves are found predominantly between the fingers and on the wrists (*hatched areas*).

In infants and children the face and scalp may be affected, whereas adults seldom show lesions in these areas. A rare condition, known as Norwegian or crusted scabies, may result from hyperinfection with thousands to millions of mites. The consequence is a crusted dermatosis of the

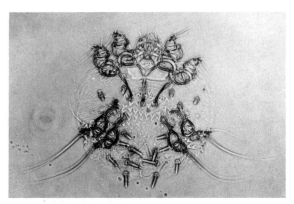

Figure 39.9. Adult female itch mite, *Sarcoptes scabiei*. × 100.

hands and feet and often much of the body. (Fig. 39.10). This condition is characteristic of infected individuals who cannot take care of themselves and is often reported in custodial institutions, such as mental hospitals.[23] It is highly contagious because of the large numbers of loosely attached, easily transferred mites present in the exfoliating skin. Crusted scabies has also been reported in individuals treated with immunosuppressive drugs (Fig. 39.11).

Secondary infections of lesions, particularly as a result of scratching, are common and poststreptococcal glomerulonephritis has been reported.[24]

Diagnosis

A diagnosis of scabies can be confirmed by picking up adult female mites at the ends of their burrows or by scraping the affected skin lightly covered with mineral oil. The scrapings are then examined under a microscope in search for im-

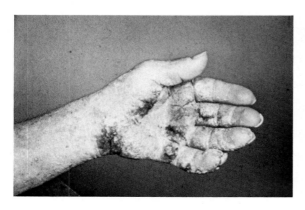

Figure 39.10. Norwegian scabies showing numerous lesions. Many mites are present in this patient.

mature or adult mites, or for eggs. Skin biopsy reveals mites in tissue sections. Presence of infection in several members of a family is reasonable circumstantial evidence for a diagnosis of scabies in those not yet examined.

Treatment

Lindane, the gamma isomer of benzene hexachloride, is the most effective compound available for treatment of scabies. It is available in the form of a lotion or cream, which is applied once to the affected areas. Benzyl benzoate in a 25% emulsion is an alternative drug, but must be applied to the whole body. Treatment of all members of a family group may be necessary to prevent reinfection.[25]

Animal Scabies

The itch and mange mites of various domestic animals, such as horses, pigs, dogs, cats, and camels, can infest man. These mites are often morphologically indistinguishable from the human parasites and are fully capable of penetrating human skin. However, the infection is usually self-limited, because the mites do not form tunnels and cannot complete their life cycles. Nevertheless, man may react with severe papular urticaria to these transitory infestations.

Chigger Mites

The chiggers, or redbugs (Fig. 39.12), of the family Trombiculidae are an important group of annoying human ectoparasites, which in some areas act as vectors of the rickettsiae causing scrub typhus.

In the United States, they include three species of trombicula. Among the chiggers, only the six-legged larvae feed on man and other mammals, whereas the nymphs and adults usually feed on arthropods or arthropod eggs. Chigger larvae are usually picked up in brush frequented by rodents

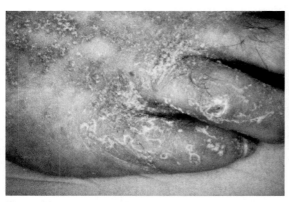

Figure 39.11. Large numbers of scabies mites and lesions in an immunosuppressed patient.

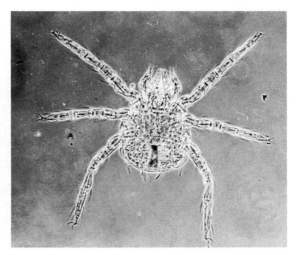

Figure 39.12. Larval stage of the common chigger, *Trombicula alfreddugesi.* It is the larva, with three pairs of legs, that feeds on vertebrates. × 50.

or other small mammals, which serve as normal hosts of larvae. These mites tend to attach to the skin where clothing is tight or restricted. The ankles, waistline, armpits, and perineal skin are common areas of infestation. Chiggers insert their capitula, but do not burrow into the skin. The host reacts to the mouthparts and the injected saliva by forming a tube-like ''stylosome'' partially engulfing the feeding mites. The chigger does not feed on blood, but ingests a mixture of partially digested cells and fluids formed within the stylosome. After feeding for several days, the engorged chigger withdraws and drops to the ground.[26]

The intense itching and discomfort associated with chigger ''bites'' often begins after the chiggers have withdrawn and departed. Irritation may be so severe as to cause fever and loss of sleep. Local anesthetics may be useful in relieving itching, and antibiotics may be needed to treat secondary bacterial skin infections.

In areas where chiggers are common, repellents containing DEET applied to skin and clothing can be very effective. Scrubbing exposed or infected areas of the body with soap and water removes even well-attached chiggers.

Scrub typhus (tsutsugamushi fever) is a chigger-borne rickettsial disease found in southeast Asia, certain islands in the Indian and Pacific Oceans, and in Australia. The causative agent is *Rickettsia tsutsugamushi* and the usual vectors are larvae of the chigger *Trombicula akamushi* and *T. deliensis*. Rodents are the normal reservoir hosts for this pathogen.[27]

Follicle Mites
The follicle mites, *Demodex folliculorum,* inhabit sebaceous glands and hair follicles of infected people, particularly around the nose and eyelids. Follicle mites are minute (less than 0.4 mm long), atypically vermiform arthropods that cause little or no discomfort. In rare cases the skin of the scalp may become heavily infected. Treatment consists of single application of gamma benzene hexachloride.

Closely related species of Demodex, which cause mange in dogs and other mammals, may cause a transitory burning reaction in people handling heavily infected animals.

Mites and Dermatitis
A number of species of mites either parasitic for animals or free living, occasionally infest man and cause dermatitis. Mites associated with straw, flour, grain, dried fruits, vanilla, copra, and cheese can produce serious but transitory skin irritation in persons contracting large numbers of these acarines. Bird and rodent mites may also cause serious annoyance when they occasionally attempt to feed on man. Bird mites may be particularly bothersome if their normal avian hosts depart and the insects are forced to forage for food.

The tropical rat mite, *Ornithonyssus bacoti* is a parasite of rodents, which can attack man and cause dermatitis.[28] The house mite, *Allodermanyssus sanguineus,* is a common ectoparasite of the mice, but readily feeds on man. These mites have been shown to transmit rickettsial pox, a mild exanthematous disease related to Rocky Mountain spotted fever found in the eastern United States and the Soviet Union. The pathogen involved in this infection is *Rickettsia akari.*[29]

Allergies Caused by Mites
Certain mites of the genus Dermatophagoides have been incriminated as sources of antigens associated with allergies to house dust.[30] These house dust mite allergens commonly precipitate asthma in sensitized individuals, particularly children. Desensitization has been successful.[31]

Scorpionida

The scorpions belong to an order of the Arachnida, with all members generally similar in appearance (Fig. 39.13). The typical scorpion is an elongate arthropod with stout crab-like claws (pedipalps), four pairs of walking legs, and a distinctly segmented abdomen ending in a hooked stinger.

Scorpions are shy, nocturnal animals that feed primarily on other arthropods and sometimes on small rodents. In feeding the scorpion holds its

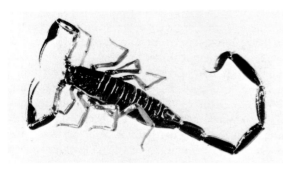

Figure 39.13. Scorpion. ×0.5.

second produces intense pain at the site of the sting and causes chills, cold perspiration, thirst, excessive salivation, and vomiting. Other systemic symptoms may include generalized numbness, difficulties in speech and swallowing, paralysis, convulsions, tachycardia, and myocarditis. Death may result from respiratory paralysis, often within 2 h of the sting.[34]

Children under 5 years of age are particularly sensitive to scorpion stings, and case fatality rates of 5% in Mexico, 25% in Trinidad, and 60% in the Sudan have been reported. Multiple stings, stings around the head, and stings of debilitated individuals are also particularly serious.

prey with its pedipalps and repeatedly stings its victim with over-the-back thrusts of its stinger. When the scorpion is disturbed, it will use the stinger for defense. This is the manner in which man is affected.[32] However, most species of scorpions are unable either to penetrate human skin or inject sufficient toxin to cause damage. The few species that do sting man are capable of inflicting a painful wound, precipitating a severe reaction and sometimes causing death. These species present a significant hazard to public health in many tropical and subtropical regions.[33]

Scorpions produce two types of venoms, hemolytic and neurotoxic. The first induces local reactions characterized by a burning sensation, swelling, and necrosis at the wound site. The

Treatment

Initial treatment of scorpion stings should be designed to delay absorption of the toxin. A tourniquet should be applied above the wound with care taken to release pressure every 20–30 min. Ice should be applied to the wound site and the patient kept quiet.

Specific scorpion antisera are available in areas where stings are common.

Programs to reduce scorpion populations with wide-scale or focal application of persistent chemical pesticides have met with limited success. Elimination of rubbish piles around dwellings can reduce favored hiding and breeding places of scorpions.

Araneida (Spiders)

The spiders constitute a large, distinctive order of arachnids whose bodies are divided into two regions, cephalothorax and abdomen. Four pairs of walking legs, pedipalps, and chelicerae with poison fangs all arise from the celphalothorax.

All spiders produce a venom in anterior venom glands which is capable of immobilizing prey. However, most species are unable to pierce human skin. Several groups of spiders do occasionally bite man. The consequences of these bites may include transitory pain, necrotic lesions, systemic reactions, or even death.

Tarantulas

The name tarantula is loosely applied to a number of large, hairy spiders, some of which belong to the family Theraphosidae. These spiders are common in tropical and subtropical regions. Although they are much feared, few tarantulas bite man. Those that do may inflict a painful wound, but the symptoms are short lasting and no fatalities have been reported.[35]

Black Widow Spiders

Spiders of the genus Latrodectus are found throughout the world, primarily in warmer climates. At least six species that bite man have been reported. They inflict painful and sometimes fatal wounds.

Latrodectus mactans, the black widow, hourglass, or shoe-button spider, is widespread through the United States and southern Canada. Related species are found throughout the temperate and tropical regions of all continents. The adult female black widow spider is usually black in color with a characteristic crimson hourglass marking on the underside of its globose abdomen. Both the coloration (variation shades of black, gray, or brown) and shape of the hourglass may vary. The typical mature female is about 40 mm long with its legs extended.[36]

Black widow spiders are normally shy, but females bite if disturbed and are particularly aggressive when they are gravid, or when they defend their egg cases. These spiders frequent wood and brush piles, old wooden buildings, cellars, hollow logs, and vacant rodent burrows. Privies have long been a preferred site for webs, and a significant number of human spider bites have taken place in these locations.

Bites of the black widow spider may be initially painless, sometimes appearing only as two small red puncture marks at the site. Thereafter, pain at the site increases and spreads, reaching a maximum within 1–3 h and later subsiding. Within an hour of the bite, general muscle pain, rigid abdomen, tightness in the chest, difficulty in breathing and speech, nausea, and sweating may occur. Most symptoms pass without treatment after 2–3 days. However, in severe cases, paralysis and coma may precede cardiac or respiratory failure.

The toxin has been identified as a low molecular weight protein[37,38] that prevents the depolarization of synapses by interfering with the fusion of neurotransmitter vesicles with the membranes.

Treatment usually consists of measures designed to relieve pain and reduce muscle spasms. An antivenom is available in areas where bites are common.

Control of black widow spiders with the use of insecticides, such as malathion, particularly in privies, is effective.

Necrotic Arachnidism

Four species of the genus Loxoceles in the New World attack when they are disturbed. Their bites may produce severe tissue reaction. *Loxoceles reclusa* (Fig. 39.14) is found in the south and central United States, *L. unicolor* and *L. arizonica* are found in the western states, and *L. laeta* in South America. These are medium-size spiders, yellow to brown in color, with body length of 10–15 mm.

L. reclusa, the brown recluse spider of the United States, is a timid, passive creature found outdoors in wood piles and debris in warmer climates and in basements or storage areas in cooler regions. Man is bitten only by the disturbed spiders, often in sleeping bags, shoes, or clothing that harbor these spiders.[39]

The South American brown spider, *L. laeta,* is a common domestic species found in closets, corners of rooms, or behind pictures. Man is

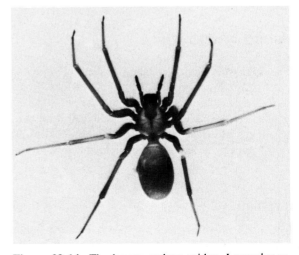

Figure 39.14. The brown recluse spider, *Loxoceles reclusa.* ×2.5.

bitten often while sleeping or dressing, but only when the spider is threatened or disturbed. This species has been introduced into the United States on at least one occasion.[40]

The bite of Loxoceles tends to be initially painless. Several hours later, itching, swelling, and tenderness may develop in the area of the bite. The wound site may turn violaceous and then black and dry. In other cases, a blister may form over the bite. Necrosis may begin within 3–4 days and tissue destruction may be extensive. Healing may take 8 weeks or longer. Some of the more serious lesions may require surgery and skin grafts.[41] The venom of Loxoceles appears to work by inactivating hemolytic components of complement.[42]

Loxoceles spiders may be controlled in dwellings with insecticide compounds containing gamma benzene hexachloride or malathion.

Chiracanthium mildei (Fig. 39.15) is the most common spider found in houses in the eastern United States, usually in bathrooms, kitchens, and bedrooms. It attacks when disturbed and its bite can cause a mild necrotizing skin lesion.[43]

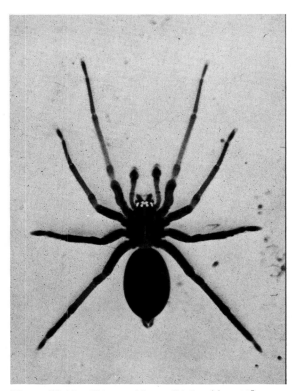

Figure 39.15. *Chiracanthium mildei*, spider. × 8.

Spiders of the genera Phoneutria in Brazil and Chile and Atrax in Australia are capable of inflicting severe bites, sometimes with fatal results. Only the male Atrax spider is capable of inflicting a lethal bite in man. The venom is neurotoxic and causes nausea, vomiting, abdominal pain, diarrhea, profuse sweating, salivation, and lacrimation. There can be severe hypertension and cardiac arrest.[44]

References

1. Hoogstraal H: The epidemiology of tick-borne Crimean-Congo hemorrhagic fever in Asia, Europe, and Africa. J Med Entomol 15:307–417, 1979
2. Smith T, Kilbourne FL: Investigations into the nature, causation, and prevention of Texas, or southern cattle fever. USDA Bureau Anim Ind Bull 1:1–301, 1893
3. Marchoux E, Salimbeni A: La spirillose des poules. Ann Inst Pasteur, Paris 17:569–580, 1903
4. Ross PH, Milne AO: Tick fever. Br Med J 2:1453–1454, 1904
5. Arthur DR: Ticks and Disease. Evanston, Illinois, Row, Peterson, 1961
6. Sen SK: The mechanism of feeding in ticks. Parasitol 27:355–368, 1935
7. Spielman A, Wilson ML, Levitne JF, et al.: Ecology of *Ixodes dammini*-borne human babesiosis and Lyme disease. Ann Rev Entomol 30:439–460, 1985
8. Burgdorfer W, Lane RS, Barbour AG, et al.: The western black-legged tick, *Ixodes pacificus:* a vector of *Borrelia burgdorferi.* Amer Jour Trop Med Hyg 34:925–930, 1985
9. Jupp PG, Joubert JJ, Cornell ??, et al.: An experimental assesment of the tampon tick, *Ornithodorus moubata* Murray, a vector of Hepatitis B virus. Med Vet Entomol 1:----, 1987
10. Nelson WA, Bell, JF, Clifford CM, et al.: Interaction of ectoparasites and their hosts. J Med Entomol 13:389–428, 1977
11. Gothe R, Kunze K, Hoogstraal H: The mechanisms of pathogenicity in the tick paralyses. J Med Entomol 16:357–369, 1979
12. Burgdorfer W: Tick-borne diseases in the United States: Rocky Mountain spotted fever and Colorado tick fever. Acta Trop 34:103–126, 1977
13. Hoogstrall H: Ticks in relation to human diseases caused by viruses. Ann Rev Entomol 11:261–308, 1966
14. Burgdorfer W: The epidemiology of the relapsing fevers. In Russell C, Johnson C (eds): The Biology of Parasitic Spirochetes. New York, Academic Press, 1976, pp 191–200

15. Burgdorfer W: A review of Rocky Mountain spotted fever (tick-borne typhus), its agent, and its tick vectors in the United States. J Med Entomol 12:269–278, 1975

16. Burgdorfer W, Barbour AG, Hayes SF, et al: Lyme disease—a tick borne spirochetosis? Science 216:1317–1319, 1982

17. Basler EM, Coleman JL, Benach Jl, et al: Natural distribution of *Ixodes dammini* spirochete. Science 220:321–322, 1983

18. Burgdorfer W, Barbour AG, Hayes SF, et al: Erythema chronicum, migrans—a tick borne spirochetosis. Acta Trop 40:79–83, 1983

19. Steere AC, Grodzicki RL, Kornblatt AN, et al: The spirochetal etiology of Lyme disease. N Eng J Med 308:733–740, 1983

20. Busvine JR: Insects, Hygiene, and History. London, Athlone Press, 1976

21. Orkin M, Maibach HI: This scabies pandemic. N Eng J Med 298:496–498, 1978

22. Mellanby K: Biology of the parasite. In Orkin M, Maibach HI, Parish LC, et al. (eds): Scabies and Pediculosis. Philadelphia, J.B. Lippincott, 1977, pp 8–16

23. Epstein E, Sr, Orkin M: Scabies: Clinical aspects. In Orkin M, Maibach HI, Parish LC et al. (eds): Scabies and Pediculosis. Philadelphia, J.B. Lippincott, 1977, pp 17–22

24. Potter EV, Earle OP, Mayon-White R, et al.: Acute Glomerulonephritis as a Complication of Scabies. In: Cutaneous Infestations and Insect Bites, Orkin M, Maibach HI (eds), Marcell Dekker, Inc, New York, 1985, pp 49–61

25. Orkin M, and Maibach HI: Treatment of Today's Scabies. In: Cutaneous Infestations and Insect Bites, Orkin M, Maibach HI (eds), Marcel Dekker, Inc, New York, 1985, pp 103–108

26. Sasa M: Biology of chiggers. Annu Rev Entomol 6:221–244, 1961.

27. Audy JR: Red Mites and Typhus. London, Athlone Press, 1968

28. Busvine JR: Dermatoses due to arthropods other than the scabies mite. In Orkin M, Maibach, HI, Parish LC et al. (eds): Scabies and Pediculosis. Philadelphia, J.B. Lippincott, 1977, pp 132–138

29. Fuller HS: Studies of rickettsial pox III. Life cycle of the mite vector, *Allodermanyssus sanguineus*. Am J Hyg 59:236–239, 1954

30. Wharton GW: House dust mites. J Med Entomol 12:577–621, 1976

31. Warner JO, Price JF, Soothill JF, et al.: Controlled trial of hyposensitisation to *Dermatophagoides pteronyssinus* in children with asthma. Lancet 2:912–915, 1978

32. Bucherl W: Classification, biology, and venom extraction of scorpions. In Bucherl W, Buckley EE (eds): Venomous Animals and Their Venoms. Vol. III, Venomous Invertebrates. New York, Academic Press, 1971, pp 317–347

33. Balozet L: Scorpionism in the old world. In Bucherl W, Buckley EE (eds): Venomous Animals and Their Venoms. Vol. III, Venomous Invertebrates. New York, Academic Press, 1971, pp 317–347

34. Possani LD, Fletcher PL, Jr, Alagon ABC, et al.: Purification and characterization of a mammalian toxin from venom of the Mexican scorpion *Centruroides limpidus tecomanus* Hoffman. Toxicon 18:175–183, 1980

35. Bucherl W: Spiders. In Bucherl W, Buckley EE (eds): Venomous Animals and Their Venoms. Vol. III, Venomous Invertebrates. New York, Academic Press, 1971, pp 197–277

36. Maretic Z: Latrodectism in Mediterranean countries, including south Russia, Israel, and north Africa. In Bucherl W, Buckley EE (eds): Venomous Animals and Their Venoms. Vol III, Venomous Invertebrates. New York, Academic Press, 1971, pp 299–309

37. McCrone JD, Hatala RJ: Isolation and characterization of a lethal component from the venom of *Latrodectus mactans mactans*. In Russell FE, Saunders PR (eds): Animal Toxins. New York, Pergamon Press, 1967, pp 29–34

38. Russell FE: Venom poisoning. Ration Drug Ther 5:1–7, 1971

39. Foil LD, Norment BR: Envenomation by *Loxosceles reclusa*. J Med Entomol 16: 18–25, 1979

40. Levi HW, Spielman A: The biology and control of the South American brown spider *Loxosceles laeta* (Nicolet), in a North American focus. Am J Trop Med Hyg 13:132–136, 1964

41. Hufford DC: The brown recluse spider and necrotic arachnidism: A current review. J Arkans Med Soc 74:126–129, 1977

42. Gebel HM, Fink JH, Elgert KD, et al.: Inactivation of complement by *Loxosceles reclusa* spider venom. Am J Trop Med Hyg 28:756–762, 1979

43. Spielman A, Levy HW: Probable envenomation by *Chiracanthium mildei*; a spider found in houses. Am J Trop Med Hyg 19:729–732, 1970

44. Ori M: Biology and Poisonings by Spiders. In: Insect Poisons, Allergens, and Other Invertebrate Venoms. Tu AT (ed), Marcel Dekker, Inc, New York, 1984, pp 397–440

40. Arthropods of Minor Medical Importance

Butterflies and Moths: Lepidoptera

Larvae or caterpillars of several species of Lepidoptera are covered with hollow, sharp-pointed hairs containing a toxin that may cause a severe dermatitis. Contact occurs when man handles the caterpillars or inhales the "hairs" that are blown about after the larva molts (Table 40.1). In the Northeastern US, the gypsy moth, *Hymantria dispar,* has been responsible for defoliation of enormous areas forests. The "population explosion" of the caterpillars of this species has led to

Table 40.1. Arthropods of Minor Medical Importance and the Pathology They Cause

Order and Representative Species	Common Name	Geographical Distribution	Effects on Man
INSECTA Orthoptera (cockroaches, grasshoppers and their relatives)			
Blatella germanica	German cockroach	Worldwide	Mechanical disseminator
Periplaneta americana	American cockroach	Worldwide	of pathogens,
Various genera	Cockroach	Some worldwide, some local	intermediate host of certain helminths
Coleoptera (beetles)			
Various genera and species	Beetles	Worldwide	Mechanical disseminators of pathogens
Various species of the family Meloidae	Blister beetles	Worldwide	Blistering of skin after contact with adult beetles
Tenebrio spp.	Grain beetles	Worldwide	Intermediate hosts of tapeworms
Lepidoptera (moths and butterflies)			
Various genera and species	Caterpillar	Worldwide	Urticating spines and hairs may cause reaction when handled or inhaled
CRUSTACEA *Cyclops* spp. *Diaptomus* spp.	Copepod	Worldwide	Intermediate hosts of guinea worm and broad fish tapeworm
CHILOPODA *Scolopendra* spp.	Centipede	Tropics and subtropics	Painful bite
PENTASTOMIDA *Linguatula serrata*	Tongue worm	Tropics	Endoparasitic in internal organs

periodic outbreaks to pruritic dermatitis, primarily among school children. Similar outbreaks of dermatitis have been reported from the Southeastern and South-central states, attributed to the caterpillars of the puss moth, *Megalopyge operculis*.[1,2]

Individuals working with lepidopterans may become sensitized to the scales of adult moths or butterflies. Repeated exposure may produce severe bronchospasm and even asthma.[3]

Beetles: Coleoptera

Within the Coleoptera, a large order of insects, only a few families contain members of medical importance.

Certain scavenger beetles of the family Dermestidae, Silphidae, and Staphylinidae feed on feces and carrion and mechanically transmit pathogenic organisms. Adult beetles of the Meloidae, the blister beetles, produce a vesicating substance (cantharidin) that may cause blistering or a severe burning sensation on contact with the skin or mucous membranes.

Inadvertent ingestion of beetle larvae, a condi-

tion termed canthariasis, may produce transient gastrointestinal discomfort.

Many beetles, particularly those that feed on feces, act as intermediate hosts for helminth parasites of man and other animals. Members of the family Scarabaeidae are intermediate hosts of the spiny-headed worm *Macracanthorhynchus hirudinaceus,* a parasite of pigs, which very rarely infects man. *Hymenolepis nana* and *H. diminuta* (Chapter 17) develop in grain beetles of the Tenebrionidae.

Cockroaches: Orthoptera

Orthoptera is a large, diverse order of primitive, very successful insects including the grasshoppers and crickets. The cockroaches are included in a single family, the Blattidae, with several members closely associated with human habitations.

The female cockroach encloses her eggs in a bean-shaped case called on ootheca. Some species retain the ootheca internally until the eggs hatch; some carry it externally for several weeks, and some drop the ootheca soon after it is formed. After hatching, the young wingless feeding nymphs begin to undergo staged development. Some species progress through as many as 13 nymphal stages, each being wingless and somewhat larger than its predecessor, until the final molt produces the winged adult. With its series of wingless nymphal stages, the cockroach is a classic example of an insect developing by incomplete metamorphosis (Fig. 38.1).

Most cockroach species do not invade homes, confining themselves to outdoor habitats. In the United States, five species of cockroaches do invade houses. The most common is the German cockroach or croton bug, *Blatella germanica,* a small (less than 16 mm), light brown species. The American cockroach or palmetto bug, *Periplaneta americana,* is, in fact, an African species

now found worldwide. It is a large (30–40 mm) reddish-brown insect with long wings. It is found in and around homes, farms, restaurants, stores, and warehouses. Other species that may infest homes are the Oriental cockroach, *Blatta orientalis;* the Australian cockroach, *P. australasiae;* and the brown-banded cockroach, *Supella supellectilium.*

Most of these species are cosmopolitan, having been distributed by ship traffic starting with the earliest voyages. In general, domestic species are omnivorous. They feed on a wide variety of nutrients, paper, and bookbindings, and on human and animal feces. They serve as mechanical vectors of pathogens, carrying infectious agents from feces to food.[4,5]

The presence of cockroaches is usually associated with a breakdown of general sanitation. Exposed foods, or poor packaging and storage, open garbage, darkness, and moisture are all conducive to development of large cockroach populations. Initial infestations may be introduced with foodstuffs or from adjoining dwellings. In apartment buildings, the insecticide treatment of one apartment may cause the migration of cockroaches to adjoining, untreated apartments.

Although cockroaches can be resistant to a

number of insecticides in some areas, compounds are commercially available for control. Coupled with improved housekeeping, these can be sufficient. However, heavy infestations require repeated treatments by professional exterminators.

Chilopoda

The centipedes are worm-like, segmented creatures with a distinct head and paired appendages on each of 15–100 or more segments. They have a pair of poisonous claws, the maxillipeds, on the first segment after the head, which are used for capturing prey. Most centipedes are predaceous insectivores, but man is sometimes bitten accidentally. Centipede bites may be locally painful, causing transient swelling at the site of the bite. No complications are associated with these bites.[4]

Crustacea

The Crustacea include many species serving as intermediate hosts of parasites of man and animals. These organisms are discussed in the other, relevant chapters.

Pentastomida

The Pentastomids, or tongue worms, are a small group of parasites of uncertain origin and affinity. Because their larvae superficially resemble the larvae of mites, they have been included among the Arthropoda, but they probably evolved early from annelid or arthropod ancestral stocks. They were first noted in the nasal cavities of dogs and horses in the 18th century and later described in human autopsy material as insect larvae.

Life Cycle

The adult tongue worms are blood-sucking, endoparasitic, legless vermiform inhabitants of the respiratory system of reptiles, birds, and mammals. Eggs fertilized within the host emerge through the respiratory tract. After being eaten by an intermediate host, they hatch in the gut, yielding a migratory larva, which pierces the stomach wall and encysts in host tissue. When the intermediate host is eaten by the definitive host, the larvae mature.

In man, encysted larvae have been found at autopsy in lung, liver, intestine, spleen, and other internal organs.

Pathogenesis

There is no evidence that any human disease results from infection with tongue worms.[5] They are usually identified at autopsy.

References

1. Kawamoto F, and Kumada N: Biology of and Venoms of Lepidoptera. In: Insect Pioisons, Allergens and Other Invertebrate Venoms, Tu AT (Ed), Marcel dekker, Inc, New York, 1984, pp 291–330.
2. Wirtz RA: Allergic and toxic reactions to non-stinging arthropods. Ann Rev Entomol 29:47–69, 1984
3. Pesce H, Delgado A: Poisoning from adult moths and caterpillars. In Bucherl W, Buckley EE (eds): Venomous Animals and Their Venoms. Vol. III, Venomous Invertebrates. New York, Academic Press, 1971, pp 119–156
4. Cornwell PB: The Cockroach. London, Hutchinson, 1968
4. Jongi BS: Centipede Venoms and Poisoning. In: Insect Poisons, Allergens, and Other Invertebrate Venoms, Tu AT (ed), Marcel Dekker, Inc. New York, 1984, pp 333–368
5. Guthrie DM, Tindall AR: The Biology of the Cockroach. New York, St. Martin's Press, 1968
5. Cannon DA: Linguatulid infestation of man. Ann Trop Med Parasitol 36:160–166, 1942

Appendix I

Procedures Suggested for Use in Examination of Clinical Specimens for Parasitic Infection*

There is no general agreement about diagnostic laboratory procedures in clinical parasitology. Certain minimum standards have been established. They utilize techniques that can be employed even in smaller clinical laboratories. However, technicians who are not experienced in diagnostic parasitology and who do not have frequent exposure to these techniques will not be able to carry out these tests reliably. It is far better under such circumstances to utilize the resources of regional reference laboratories. Nevertheless, the small laboratories can be helpful in situations when speed is of the essence, as, for example, in making the diagnosis of malaria. A permanent collection of identified stained fecal and blood smears, as well as formalinized specimens of adult worms, eggs, larvae, and cysts may be purchased initially and added to over the years, to be used as reference material.

Collection of Stool Specimens

Collection of satisfactory specimens is essential for reliability, whether the tests are done locally or elsewhere. The following procedures are suggested for proper collection of stool specimens:

1. Fresh, unpreserved feces should be obtained and transported to the laboratory immediately. Fresh specimens are preferred for examinations for trophozoites, and are necessary when con-

centrations for strongyloides larvae are to be performed.
2. Unpreserved feces should be examined within 1 h after passage, especially if the stool is loose or watery and might contain protozoan trophozoites. Examination of formed feces may be delayed for a short time, but must be completed on the day on which the specimen is received in the laboratory. If prompt examination or proper fixation cannot be carried out, formed specimens may be refrigerated for 1 or 2 days.
3. If specimens are delayed in reaching the laboratory or if they cannot be examined promptly (such as those received at night, on weekends, or when no parasitologist is available), portions should be preserved in fixatives such as 8% aqueous formalin or formol-saline, and polyvinyl alcohol (PVA)-fixative. Formalin preserves cysts, eggs, and larvae for subsequent wet-mount examination or for concentration; PVA-fixative preserves trophozoites, cysts, and eggs for subsequent permanent staining. A ratio of one part of feces to three parts of fixative is recommended. The specimen may be placed in fixatives in the laboratory, or the patient may be provided with fixatives and instructions for collection and preservation of his own specimens.

Methods of Stool Examination and Related Procedures

Stool specimens may be examined by the three complementary methods listed below. The advantages and limitations of each technique must be recognized.

1. Saline mounts are of value primarily for demonstration of the characteristic motility of certain amebae and flagellates. These may be

---

*Modified from a statement by the Council of the American Society of Parasitologists, the American Society for Medical Technologists, the Board of Scientific Advisors of the American Association of Bioanalysis, and the Board of Directors of the International Society for Clinical Laboratory Technology.

found in fresh unformed stools, or at times in bloody mucus adhering to the surface of formed stools. Material should be obtained from several different parts of the specimen. An iodine stain (a drop of 1% iodine in 2% potassium iodide) mixed with a stool suspension in saline solution will facilitate identification of protozoan cysts, but will kill and distort trophozoites.

2. Concentration techniques, useful in detecting small numbers of cysts and helminth eggs, may be used on unpreserved stool specimens, those preserved in aqueous formalin or formol-saline, or on PVA-fixed material.

3. Stained fecal films should be made if possible on all specimens obtained fresh or fixed in PVA. If properly prepared they are the single most productive means of stool examination for protozoa. Films may be stained with trichrome solution or with iron-hematoxylin. Stained slides of positive specimens should be placed in a permanent file, analogous to those used for surgical and cytologic specimens.

Number of Specimens To Be Examined and Appropriate Intervals

1. For the detection of amebae, a minimum of 3 specimens should be examined; if these (obtained preferably at intervals of 2 to 3 days) are negative and amebic infection remains a diagnostic consideration, additional specimens should be examined.

2. In suspected giardiasis, initially 3 specimens should be examined. If they are negative, additional specimens should be obtained at weekly intervals for three weeks. Duodenal aspiration or the enteric string test may also be of value in occult infections.

3. A single concentrate from one stool specimen is frequently sufficient to detect intestinal helminthic infections of clinical importance. In very light *Schistosoma* spp. infections, few or no eggs may be found in the feces or urine. Strongyloides may also require concentration of the specimen for diagnosis, but this is not always reliable; various fecal culture methods or the enteric string test may also be used.

4. Examination after treatment should under most circumstances be delayed until 1 month after completion of therapy; 3 months after treatment for schistosomiasis; and 3 months after treatment for tapeworms.

Examination of Blood

1. Smears for malaria should consist of both thick and thin films. It is important that all involved laboratory personnel be aware of the technique for making thick films; if improperly made, they are useless. Smears should be stained with Giemsa solution, and a minimum of 100 microscopic fields examined before a specimen is reported as negative. If the first specimen is negative, additional thick and thin films should be taken every 6 h for 24 h.

2. In examination for filarial infection one must consider the possibility of diurnal or nocturnal periodicity of microfilariae in the peripheral blood, and obtain specimens accordingly. Thick smears or blood concentration methods are most likely to demonstrate infection.

Serologic Methods

A large variety of immunodiagnostic methods may serve as useful adjuncts to the clinical diagnosis of parasitic infections. In some cases, serologic methods may be the only laboratory recourse in making a diagnosis. Certain serologic tests provide a high degree of diagnostic accuracy; however, mixed infections, antigen-sharing by related and unrelated parasites, and other diseases or physiologic conditions in man may interfere with this diagnostic accuracy.

Most serum specimens may be shipped frozen, or preserved with thimerosal to a final concentration of 1:10,000, to a state public health laboratory for forwarding to the Centers for Disease Control in Atlanta, Georgia. The vial, containing at least 2 ml of serum, should indicate preservative used.

Appendix II

Table of Drugs for Parasitic Infections

Comment

Indications for therapy are given in the text. In this table drugs are listed in alphabetical order; route of administration is expressed as PO (oral), IM (intramuscular), IV (intravenous), T (topical); doses are expressed in units per 24 h or per kg of body weight per 24 h and followed by fraction of the total dose, frequency of administration of the fraction, and number of days of treatment. Maximum 24-h dose is indicated in the last column.

Before prescribing any drug, it is important to check the latest information about it, because textbooks cannot be brought up to date as frequently as new information about drugs becomes available. It is especially important to familiarize oneself with undesirable side effects of the drugs and with their potential synergistic toxicity or interference with one another.

Drug	Route	Adult Dose	Pediatric Dose	Maximum/24 h
Amphotericin B (primary amebic meningo-encephalitis)	IV	1 mg/kg 1/1 × qd (duration unknown)	Same	
Bithionol	PO	40 mg/kg 1/1 once alternate days × 15 doses	Ditto	
Chloroquine phosphate (malaria therapy)	PO	600 mg base 1/1 stat and 300 mg base 6 h later and qd × 2	10 mg base/kg 1/1 stat and 5 mg base/kg 6 h later and qd × 2	600 mg 300 mg
(malaria prophylaxis)	PO	300 mg base 1/1 q 1 week; start 2 weeks before arrival, continue until 6 weeks after departure	5 mg base/kg 1/1 q 1 week; start 2 weeks before arrival, continue until 6 weeks after departure	300 mg
Chloroquine HCl	IM	800 mg base 1/4 q6h	Not appropriate for children	
Crotamiton	T	10% cream	Ditto	
Dehydroemetine	IM	1.5 mg/kg 1/1 × 5	1.5 mg/kg 1/2 bid × 5	60 mg

Drug	Route	Adult Dose	Pediatric Dose	Maximum/24 h
Diethylcarbamazine citrate (all filariae except Onchocerca)	PO	50 mg 1/1 × 1 150 mg 1/3 tid × 1 300 mg 1/3 tid × 1 6 mg/kg 1/3 tid × 18	35 mg 1/1 × 1 105 mg 1/3 tid × 1 225 mg 1/3 tid × 1 6 mg/kg 1/3 tid × 18	
(Onchocerca)	PO	25 mg 1/1 × 3 50 mg 1/1 × 5 150 mg 1/1 × 12	1.5 mg/kg 1/3 tid × 3 3 mg/kg 1/3 tid × 4 4.5 mg/kg 1/3 tid × 4 6 mg/kg 1/3 tid × 21	25 mg 50 mg 100 mg 150 mg
Diloxanide furoate	PO	1500 mg 1/3 tid × 10	20 mg/kg 1/3 tid × 20	1500 mg
Emetine	IM	1 mg/kg 1/1 qd × 5	1 mg/kg 1/1 qd × 5	60 mg
Furazolidone	PO	400 mg 1/4 qid × 7	5 mg/kg 1/4 qid × 7	400 mg
Iodoquinol (Diiodohydroxyquin)	PO	1950 mg 1/3 tid × 20	40 mg/kg 1/3 tid × 20	1950 mg
Ivermectin	PO	150 μg/kg 1/1 once; repeat q 6–12 months	150 μg/kg 1/1 once	
Lindane	T	Apply once, repeat in 7 d	Apply once, repeat in 7 d	
Mebendazole (all indications except Enterobius)	PO	200 mg 1/2 bid × 3	200 mg 1/2 bid × 3	
(Enterobius)	PO	100 mg 1/1 once	100 mg 1/1 once	
Melarsoprol	IV	3 mg/kg 1/1 qd × 3 no drug × 7 3.6 mg/kg 1/1 qd × 3 no drug × 15 3.6 mg/kg 1/1 qd × 3	See note 1	
Metronidazole (Entamoeba)	PO	2250 mg 1/3 tid × 5	40 mg/kg 1/3 tid × 5	2250 mg

Drug	Route	Adult Dose	Pediatric Dose	Maximum/24 h
(Giardia and Trichomonas)	PO	750 mg 1/3 tid × 5	15 mg/kg 1/3 tid × 5	750 mg
Niclosamide	PO	2 gm 1/1 qd × 5	1 gm 34 kg and under 1.5 gm 35 kg and over 1/1 qd × 5	
Nifurtimox	PO	See note 2	Not established	
Oxamniquine	PO	15 mg/kg 1/1 once	Ditto	
(in East Africa)	PO	30 mg/kg 1/1 once	Ditto	
(in Egypt and South Africa)	PO	30 mg/kg 1/1 qd × 2	Ditto	
Pentamidine isethionate	IM	4 mg/kg 1/1 qd × 14	Ditto	
Piperazine citrate	PO	75 mg/kg 1/1 qd × 2	Ditto	3500 mg
Praziquantel (*Schistosoma mansoni* and *S. haematobium*)	PO	40 mg/kg 1/1 once	Ditto	
(*S. japonicum*)	PO	60 mg/kg 1/2 bid × 1	Ditto	
(other flukes except Fasciola)	PO	75 mg/kg 1/3 tid × 1	Ditto	
Primaquine phosphate	PO	15 mg base 1/1 qd × 14	0.3 mg base/kg 1/1 qd × 14	
Pyrantel pamoate	PO	11 mg/kg 1/1 once	Ditto	1000 mg
Pyrimethamine	PO	25 mg 1/1 qd × 28	2 mg/kg 1/1 qd × 3 1 mg/kg 1/1 qd × 28	
Pyrimethamine with sulfadoxide (R)				
Fansidar (each tablet contains 25 mg pyrimethamine and 500 mg sulfadioxine)	PO	Single dose of 3 tablets for selfadministration in case of fever and before medical help becomes available	(ditto, as follows) < yr: 1/4 tab. 1–3 yrs: 1/2 tab. 4–8 yrs: 1 tab. 9–14 yrs: 2 tab. >14 yrs: 3 tab.	

Drug	Route	Adult Dose	Pediatric Dose	Maximum/24 h
Quinacrine HCl	PO	300 mg 1/3 tid × 5	6 mg/kg 1/3 tid × 5	300 mg
Quinine sulfate	PO	1950 mg 1/3 tid × 3	25 mg/kg 1/3 tid × 3	1950 mg
Quinine dihydrochloride	IV	See note 3	See note 3	1800 mg
Spiramycin	PO	3 gm 1/3 tid. × 14 days	not known	
Sulfadiazine	PO	2000 mg 1/4 qid × 4 wks	120 mg/kg 1/4 qid × 4 wks	4000 mg
Sulfadoxine	PO	500 mg 1/1 q 1 week	Not established	
Suramin	IV	100 mg test dose, then 1000 mg on days 1,3,7 14,21	2 mg/kg test dose, then 20 mg/kg on days 1,3,7 14,21	
Stibogluconate	IM or IV	600 mg 1/1 qd × 7	10 mg/kg 1/1 qd × 7	600 mg
Tetracycline (Balantidium)	PO	2000 mg 1/4 qid × 10	10 mg/kg 1/4 qid × 10	2000 mg
(*P. falciparum*)	PO	1000 mg 1/4 qid × 7	5 mg/kg 1/4 qid × 7	1000 mg
Thiabendazole	PO	50 mg 1/2 bid × 3	Ditto	
Trimethoprim sulfamethoxazole	PO or IV	20 mg/kg (tr.) 100 mg/kg (s.) 1/4 qid × 14	Ditto	

[1]Melarsoprol pediatric dose: Calculate total dose as 20 mg/kg to be delivered over 1 month; begin with 0.36 mg/kg increasing gradually to 3.6 mg/kg at intervals of 1 to 5 days, depending on the reaction, until the total dose has been administered.

[2]Nifurtimox must be prescribed in gradually increasing doses, beginning with the dose of 5 mg/kg, 1/4 qid × 14, and increasing it by 2 mg/kg q 14 days, until the dose of 15 mg/kg is reached and completed in 14 days.

[3]For adults 600 mg in 300 cc saline solution is infused over 1 h; it is repeated in 6 h, if PO therapy cannot be initiated. Pediatric dose is 12.5 mg/kg dissolved in saline solution in the same proportion as the adult dose; it is infused over 1 h and repeated in 6 h, if PO therapy cannot be initiated.

Appendix III

Laboratory Diagnostic Methods*

This section presents the most effective tests for the identification of protozoan and helminthic parasites. The first part deals with unpreserved and the second with preserved specimens. There is no single method for diagnosing all stages of all parasites. Therefore, often several different tests must be performed to obtain optimal results.

Unpreserved Specimens

For best results the specimens should be less than 1 hour old when first examined, but this may not always be possible. Specimens that are up to 24 hours old may still be useful for recovering protozoan cysts and helminthic larvae and eggs, but trophozoites rarely survive that long. A confounding factor in examining specimens left at room temperature for more than 24 hours is that the living organisms can grow and develop. Refrigeration will help to prevent this problem. The specimen should not be frozen, because this will alter morphology of the objects examined.

Stool

Because of the daily variability in the quantity of various stages of parasites shed by the infected individual, they may be missed in a single casual specimen, particularly when the infection is light. Multiple samples—generally considered a total of 3 specimens collected on consecutive days—may be needed to detect most infections. Some parasites, for example, the schistosomes and giardia, tend to require more specimens for detection.

Barium or mineral oil interferes with the identification of parasites. Therefore patients should not be subjected to radiographic studies involving barium or given laxatives containing mineral oil until the stool specimens have been obtained.

Direct Examination

- *Gross examination:*
- Observe and record the appearance of the entire specimen, noting color, consistency, and odor.

- Examine for the presence of living parasites.
- *Microscopic examination*
- *Direct smear*

This test is most effective for the diagnosis of living parasites (e.g., *Entamoeba histolytica*, *Giardia lamblia*, and *Strongyloides stercoralis*, and should be used on loose, diarrheic, or purged stool. When motile amebae are found on a direct smear a stained preparation should also be examined for the definitive diagnosis. (If the ameba contains erythrocytes within the cytoplasm it is *E. histolytica;* a stained specimen is not necessary for further identification.)

If the specimen appears negative, as may happen in light infections, it is necessary to concentrate the sample.

1. Dip a wooden applicator stick into the specimen to coat the tip of it with stool.
2. Smear the stool onto a clear glass microscope slide on which a drop of normal saline solution has been placed and overlay with a coverslip. (Smears must be thin enough to facilitate microscopic observation.)

*Text: Judith Despommier.
  Photographs: Dickson D. Despommier.

Staining the Direct Smear

In the Wheatly–Gomori Trichrome stain the protozoan nuclei stain red to dark blue, the cytoplasm stains a lighter blue, and the background material stains green. Furthermore, trophozoites and cysts tend to shrink away from the background material and are therefore relatively easy to locate.

This stain is applied to a thin smear of stool on a coverslip and the coverslip is immersed sequentially in the solutions enumerated below for the prescribed lengths of time.

	Solution	*Time*
1.	Schaudinn's fixative	5 min at 50 + °C or 1 h at room temperature
2.	70% Ethanol–iodine	1 min
3.	70% Ethanol	1 min
4.	70% Ethanol	1 min
5.	Trichrome stain	2–8 min
6.	90% Ethanol (acidified)	10–20 sec

Destaining Solution

Dip the coverslip in the destaining solution once or twice. Rinse in 90% ethanol to stop the destaining process. Thin smears will destain quickly; thicker ones may require 3 or 4 dips to obtain optimal differentiation.

7.	95% or 100% Ethanol	Two rinses
8.	100% Ethanol	1 min
9.	Xylol	1 min
10.	Mount the stained coverslip.	
11.	Examine under a microscope.	

Concentration Methods

Sedimentation by Centrifugation
The Formaldehyde Ether Method

This test concentrates cysts and eggs of parasites by centrifugation, but debris and ether-soluble materials localize in the formaldehyde–ether interface or the ether layer in the top of the tube. (This process destroys trophozoites, because they disintegrate in ether.)

1. Mix stool 1:10 with water.
2. Strain through a single layer of gauze into a 15-ml centrifuge tube.
3. Centifuge the stained stool (1 min at 2,000 rpm) and discard the supernatant.
4. Wash the sediment once with water.
5. Repeat steps 3 and 4.
6. Discard the supernatant and save the sediment.
7. Add 10 ml of 7.5% formaldehyde to the sediment.
8. Let stand 10 to 30 min.
9. Add approximately 3 ml of ether, plug the tubes with stoppers, and agitate the mixture vigorously.
10. Remove the stoppers and centrifuge the tubes at 1,500 rpm for 1 min.
11. Gently loosen the debris from the tube wall with an applicator stick, being careful not to disturb the pellet.
12. Discard the supernatant.
13. Examine the sediment under a microscope.
14. Add a drop of 70% ethanol–iodine solution (Lugol's solution) and examine again if internal structures of cysts are not recognized on first examination.

Many facilities have difficulty meeting the safety requirements for the use of ether. As an alternative ethyl acetate can be used as a substitute for ether.

Sedimentation by Gravity
Water Sedimentation

This test is used primarily for the concentration and recovery of *Schistosoma mansoni* and *Schistosoma japonicum* eggs, and is also effective for determining their viability. An entire day's worth of stool should be examined in a single test, because schistosome eggs are shed sporadically.

1. Emulsify the entire stool sample in water.
2. Strain the specimen through a single layer of gauze into conical sedimentation flasks.
3. Allow the sediment to settle (approximately 20 min) and discard the supernatant.
4. Resuspend the sediment in water.
5. Repeat steps 3 and 4 until the supernatant is clear.
6. Discard the final supernatant and save the sediment.
7. Examine under a microscope *the entire* sediment.
8. If schistosome eggs are present, determine their viability by examination under oil immersion or high magnification (40×) to determine the activity of flame cells.

The entire water sedimentation procedure should be done within 2 hours of starting the procedure, because prolonged exposure of the eggs to water will stimulate them to hatch. If hatching occurs, the empty shells remain in the sediment and the ciliated miracidia are be seen moving about rapidly.

Baerman Sedimentation Method

This method is specific for concentrating and recovering the larvae of *Strongyloides stercoralis*. The test requires a funnel with a piece of rubber tubing attached to it. An adjustable clamp is applied across the tubing and the entire apparatus is suspended from a ring stand in a 37°C incubator. Because strongyloides larvae cannot swim against gravity, they concentrate in the sediment that accumulates in the base of the rubber tube connected to the funnel, and can then be expressed into a test tube for microscopic identification.

1. Break apart 5–15 g of a stool sample.
2. Place the sample in gauze and rest it in a funnel filled with water at 37°C so that most of the sample is submerged.
3. Let it sit 1 hour, then drain 4 ml of the sediment into a 15-ml tube.
4. Centrifuge the sediment at 1,000 rpm for 5 min.
5. Decant the supernatant.
6. Examine the pellet under a microscope.

Flotation by Centrifugation

These methods concentrate the parasites by taking advantage of their specific gravity. The unwanted debris sediments to the bottom of the tube during centrifugation, but the diagnostic forms float to the surface. Cysts and most eggs can be recovered in large quantities by this method, but trophozoites, operculated eggs, and schistosome eggs are either destroyed or sediment to the bottom of the tube.

Zinc Sulfate Flotation

1. Mix 1 part stool in 15 ml of water in a 15-ml centrifuge tube.
2. Centrifuge for 1 min at 2,500 rpm, then decant the supernatant.
3. Add zinc sulfate solution (specific gravity = 1.18) until the tube is half full and resuspend the sediment with a wooden applicator stick.
4. Fill the tube to the top with more zinc sulfate solution.
5. Centrifuge the suspension for 1 min at 2,500 rpm. Do not apply the brake to the centrifuge or jar the tube, because either will cause any eggs or cysts accumulated at the liquid–surface interface to sink.
6. Using a bacteriological loop, remove two loopfuls of material from the surface and place them on a clean glass slide.
7. Examine under a microscope. (A small drop of Lugol's iodine may be added to provide more contrast.)

Sugar (Sheather's Method) Flotation

This method is designed specifically for the recovery of *Cryptosporidium spp.* oocysts.

1. Filter stool through three pieces of cheesecloth.
2. Place 2 ml of stool filtrate in a conical tube.
3. Fill tube to the top with sucrose solution.
4. Place coverslip on top of tube.
5. Centrifuge at 1,000 rpm for 5 min. (If the stool sample is watery, no centrifugation is necessary.) Let the coverslip rest on the top of sucrose solution for 20 min.
6. Examine the coverslip under a microscope under magnification of $400\times$. The focal plane is important, because the oocysts are located on the inner surface of the coverslip, rather than on the slide itself.

The oocysts appear slightly pink in color without the addition of any stain. They are ovoid to spherical in shape, range in size from 5–6 μm in diameter and are usually not sporulated.

There are no useful staining techniques.

Blood

Fresh, heparinized or citrated blood samples are best for these examinations.

Delays will reduce the chances of finding the parasites.

Place a drop of blood on a slide, overlay with a coverslip, and examine under a microscope for living microfilariae or trypanosomes. Both groups of parasites are motile and can be seen swimming among the formed blood elements. Motility will be significantly decreased if the blood sample is refrigerated. If an organism is seen, the specimen should be stained, preferably with Giemsa solution. (see Section).

Urine

Gross Examination

Observe and record the degree of turbidity and color of the specimen.

Microscopic Examination

1. Take a drop of urine with a Pasteur pipette, preferably from the bottom of the container, and transfer it to a glass slide.
2. Examine under a microscope.

If one is searching for *Trichomonas vaginalis,* the specimen must be fresh (less than 1 hour old), because the trophozoites quickly lose their characteristic morphology and motility.

Sedimentation by Centrifugation

1. Divide the entire urine specimen into 15-ml conical glass centrifuge tubes.
2. Sediment at 1,000 rpm for 5 min.
3. Discard the supernatant.
4. Resuspend the pellets with a Pasteur pipette and examine them under a microscope.

Sputum

Gross Examination

Observe and record the appearance of the specimen.

Microscopic Examination

1. Transfer a small amount of sputum with a wooden applicator stick to a clean glass slide.
2. Add a drop of normal saline solution.
3. Examine under a microscope.

Sedimentation by Centrifugation

1. Mix sputum with equal parts of 3% NaOH.
2. Let stand 5 min.
3. Sediment at 1,000 rpm for 5 min and examine under a microscope.

Tissues

Tissues

Place a small piece (1–3 mm^3) of tissue between two clean glass slides using forceps, press to flatten, then examine under a microspce.

Skin Scrapings

1. Place the scrapings on a clean glass slide.
2. Add a drop of normal saline solution and overlay with a coverslip.
3. Let stand 30 min.
4. Press the coverslip gently to break up the skin pieces, then examine under a microscope.

Tapeworm proglottids must be carefully examined for the identification of a scolex. It is located at the narrowest end of the strobila. The scolex can adhere to toilet paper and must be sought there. The uterus in the proglottids is injected with India ink using a 25-gauge needle. A proglottid is then placed between two glass slides, compressed, and examined under the microscope to count the lateral branches on one side of the main uterine stem.

Arthropods are best identified preserved. The specimen should be placed in 70% ethanol and when it is no longer motile transferred to a Petri dish for examination.

Aspirated Fluids

Sedimentation by Centrifugation

1. Centrifuge clear fluid aspirates at 1,000 rpm for 5 min in a conical centrifuge tube.

2. Decant supernatant.
3. Examine the pellet under a microscope.
4. Stain by the Wheatly–Gomori Trichrome procedure.

Miscellaneous

Examination for Pinworms

Clear tape preparations of various types, available commercially, are routinely used for this purpose. The tape is placed with the sticky side down on the perineum and eggs or adult worms are thus picked up. The tape is then examined under a low power lens of a microscope.

Adult pinworms are also occasionally found on the surface of formed stool samples.

Preserved Specimens

Whenever a delay of 24 hours or longer is anticipated, it is advisable to preserve the specimen. The kind of preservative to be employed depends on the type of test selected.

Stool

Direct Smear

Merthiolate–iodine–formaldehyde (MIF) Method
A solution of merthiolate, iodine, and formaldehyde (MIF) preserves and stains trophozoites and cysts. The organisms develop an orange color. A permanent stain should also be done on the same stool sample. At present, there is no permanent staining procedure that can be carried out on an MIF-treated specimen. For example, if the Wheatly–Gomori Trichrome stain is run on such a sample, the material peels off the coverslip.

1. Emulsify 1 g of stool sample in 10 ml of MIF solution.
2. Place a drop of stool–MIF emulsion on a clean glass slide and examine under a microscope.

Stools preserved in MIF can be concentrated by sedimentation using the formaldehyde ether method (_____ pp.).

Stool specimens preserved in polyvinyl alcohol (PVA) can be stained by the Wheatly–Gomori Trichrome solution in the same manner as described previously for unpreserved stool. The technique is the same as the one used on unpreserved stools except that Schaudinn's Fixative is not necessary and the staining time differs.

Wheatly–Gomori Trichrome Stain for Polyvinyl Alcohol-Preserved Stool

Procedure

Solution	Time
1. 70% Ethanol-iodine	10–20 min
2. 70% Ethanol	3–5 min
3. 70% Ethanol	3–5 min
4. Trichrome stain	8–10 min
5. 90% Ethanol (acidified)	1–10 sec

Dip the coverslip in the destaining solution once or twice. Rinse in the 95% alcohol to stop the destaining process. Thin smears will destain quickly; thicker smears require 3 to 5 dips.

6. 95% Ethanol	Rinse
7. 95% Ethanol	5 min
8. Xylol	10 min
9. Mount the stained coverslip.	
10. Examine under a microscope.	

Blood

Microscopic Examination

A thick smear consists of several drops of blood on a slide, dried in air, and hemolyzed by immersion in a hypotonic solution. This concentrates the parasites. A thin smear is prepared by making a film of blood analogous to that used for a differential count of the white cells. Both must be stained.

Giemsa Stain Method
1. Immerse the slide in 100% ethanol or methanol for 2–3 min.
2. Make a solution consisting of 1 drop of concentrated Giemsa stain per 1 ml of distilled water (pH 7.4) and fill a Copeland jar with 50 ml of the mixture.
3. Stain for 10–30 min.
4. Wash in distilled water.
5. Air dry the slide.
6. Examine under an oil immersion lens of a microscope. View 100 fields of a thin smear.

Concentration by Sedimentation.

The Knott technique concentrates and preserves microfilariae, which can be stained by the Giemsa solution and identified morphologically.

The Knott Technique
1. Mix 1 ml of heparinized blood with 9 ml of 2% formaldehyde.
2. Centrifuge at 2,000 rpm for 10 minutes.
3. Decant the supernatant.
4. Examine the sediment under a microscope.

If microfilariae are present, the material can then be stained as follows:

1. Spread the sediment on clean glass slide.
2. Dry overnight.
3. Stain with Giemsa solution (1 ml of concentrated Giemsa stain in 50 ml of distilled water at pH 7.4).
4. Destain 10–15 min. in water.
5. Air dry.
6. Examine under a microscope.

Solutions

Schaudinn's Fixative

Saturated aqueous solution of $HgCl_2$	666 ml
95% Ethyl alcohol	333 ml

Saturated Solution $HgCl_2$

Add 80 g $HgCl_2$ to 1 liter deionized water; stir 3–4 h, then filter.

70% Ethanol–Iodine Solution

Add enough crystalline iodine to 70% ethanol to turn the solution deep amber-brown color. Filter before using.

Wheatly–Gomori Trichrome Stain

Chromotrope 2R	0.6 g
Light green SF	0.3 g
Phosphotungstic acid	0.7 g

Mix with 1 ml of glacial acetic acid and stir gently for 20 min. Add 100 ml of distilled water, then store in dark brown bottle.

Buffered Formaldehyde

37%–40% Formaldehyde solution	100 ml
Solium phosphate (monobasic, anhydrous)	4.0 g
Sodium phosphate (dibasic, anhydrous)	6.5 g
H_2O	900 ml

Adjust the pH of the solution to 7.0.

Zinc Sulfate

Zinc sulfate	333 g
Water (50–55 + °C)	1,000 ml

Adjust the specific gravity to 1.18 by adding either more water or zinc sulfate crystals.

Sugar Solution (Sheather's Method)

Sucrose	500 g
Water	320 ml
Phenol	6.5 g

Merthiolate–Iodine–Formaldehyde (MIF) Solution

Stock solution	2.35 ml
Lugol's iodine	0.15 ml

Stock Solution

Tincture Merthiolate No. 99 (Lilly) 1:1000	100 ml
37–40% Formaldehyde solution	25 ml
Glycerol	5 ml

Water	250 ml

Store solution in dark bottle.

Lugol's iodine

Iodine	5 g
Potassium iodide	10 g
Water	100 ml

Polyvinyl Alcohol

Schaudinn's fixative	935 ml
Glycerol	15 ml
Glacial acetic acid	50 ml
Polyvinyl alcohol (powder)	50 g
Water	1,000 ml

I
The Nematodes

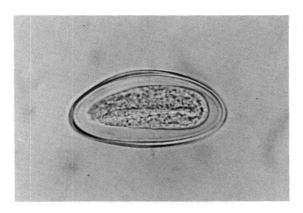

Figure A.1. *Enterobius vermicularis.* × 760

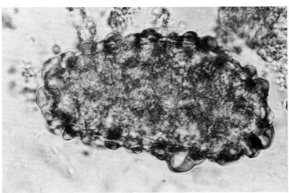

Figure A.3. *Ascaris lumbricoides* (unfertilized). × 760

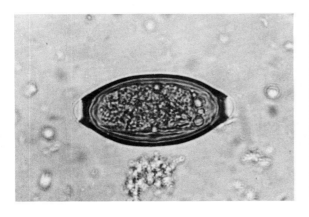

Figure A.2. *Trichuris trichiura.* × 760

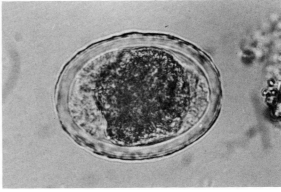

Figure A.4. *Ascaris lumbricoides* (decorticated). × 760

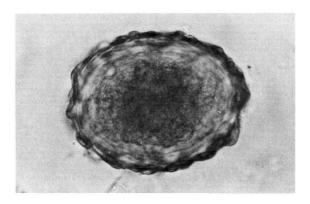

Figure A.5.   *Ascaris lumbricoides* (fertilized). ×760

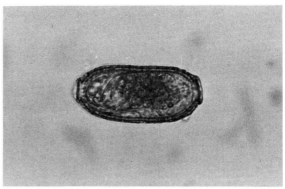

Figure A.8.   *Capillaria philippinensis.* ×760

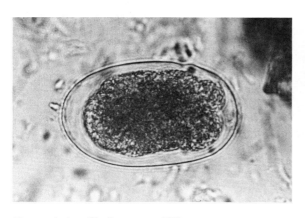

Figure A.6.   Hookworm. ×760

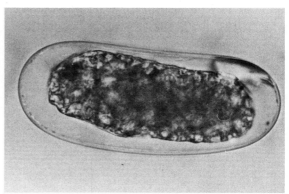

Figure A.9.   *Herterodera* (Plant nematode). ×480

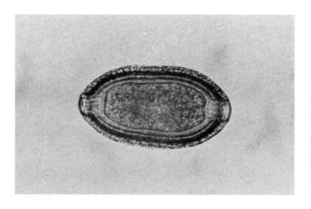

Figure A.7.   *Capillaria hepatica.* ×760

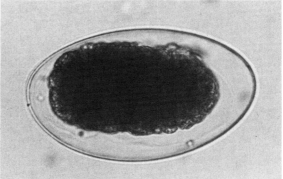

Figure A.10. *Trichonstrongylus sp.* × 480

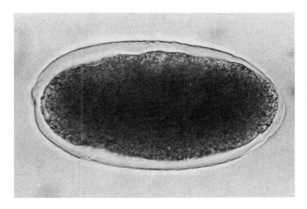

Figure A.11. *Oesophagostomum sp.* ×480

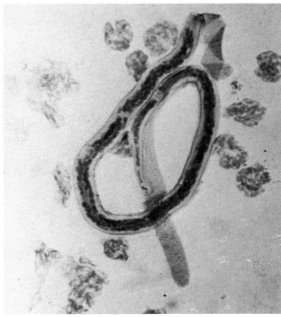

Figure A.14. *Brugia malayi.* ×600

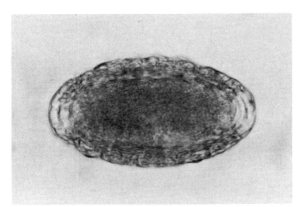

Figure A.12. *Dioctophyma renale.* ×760

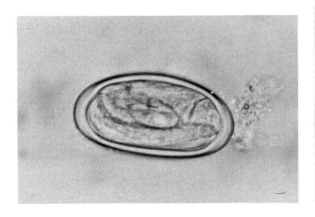

Figure A.13. *Gongylonema pulchrum.* ×760

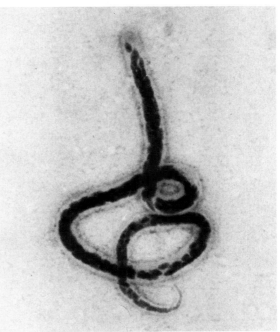

Figure A.15. *Mansonella ozzardi.* ×600

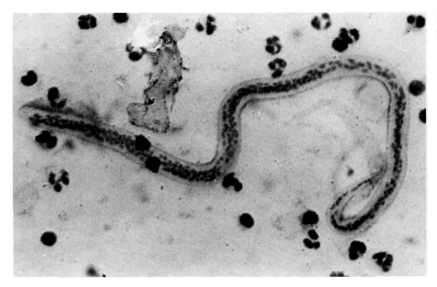

Figure A.16.
Wuchereria bancrofti.   ×600

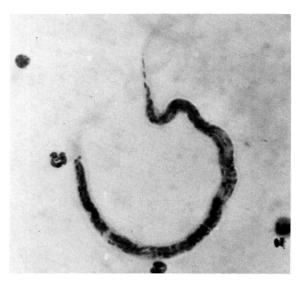

Figure A.17. *Loa loa.* ×600

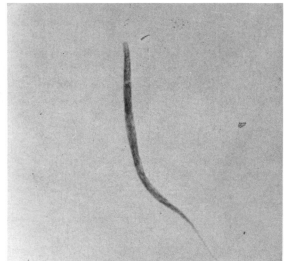

Figure A.19. *Dracunculus medinensis.* ×600

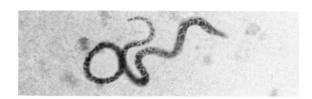

Figure A.18. *Dipetalonema perstans.* ×600

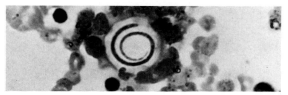

Figure A.20. *Helicosporum* (plant artifact). ×600

II
The Cestodes

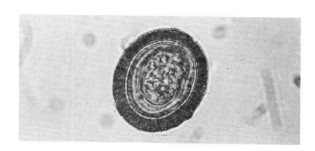

Figure A.21. *Taenia sp.* ×760

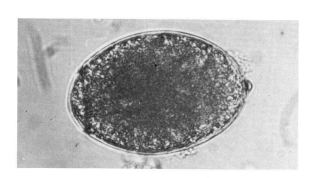

Figure A.22. *Diphyllobothrium latum.* ×475

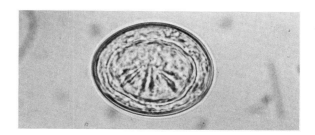

Figure A.23. *Hymenolepis nana.* ×760

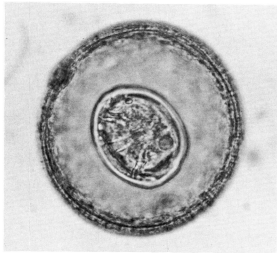

Figure A.24. *Hymenolepis diminuta.* ×760

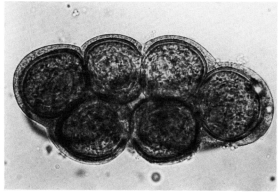

Figure A.25. *Dipylidium caninum.* ×360

III
The Trematodes

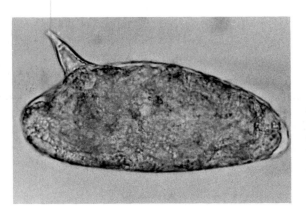

Figure A.26. *Schistosoma mansoni.* × 340

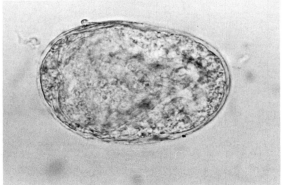

Figure A.28. *Schistosoma japonicum* (Japan). × 340

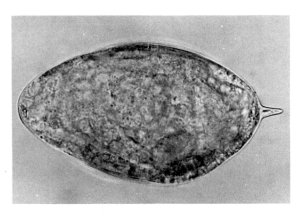

Figure A.27. *Schistosoma haematobium.* × 340

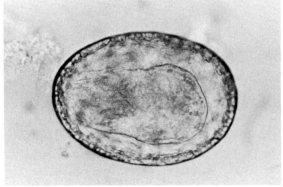

Figure A.29. *Schistosoma japonicum.* × 340

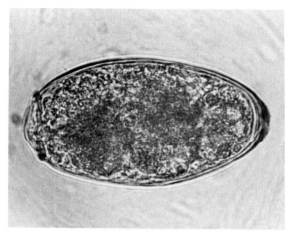

Figure A.30. *Paragonimus westermani.* ×440

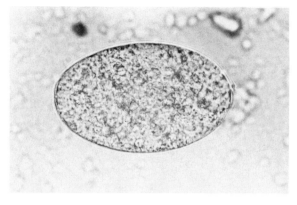

Figure A.33. *Echinostoma ilocanum.* ×450

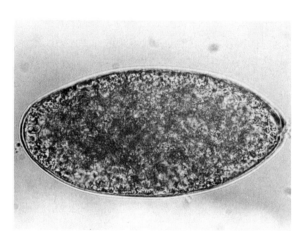

Figure A.31. *Fasciola hepatica.* ×450

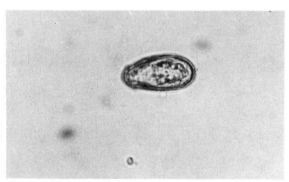

Figure A.34. *Clonorchis sinensis.* ×760

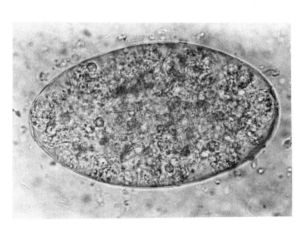

Figure A.32. *Fasciolopsis buski.* ×450

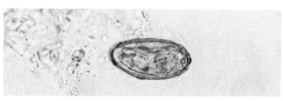

Figure A.35. *Metagonimus yokogawai.* ×760

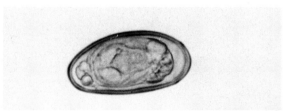

Figure A.36. *Dicrocoelium dendriticum.* ×760

IV
The Protozoa

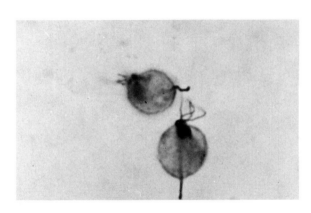

Figure A.37. *Trichomonas tenax* (Two Trophozoites). × 1,600

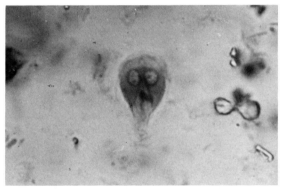

Figure A.39. *Giardia lamblia* (Binucleate trophozoite). × 1,000

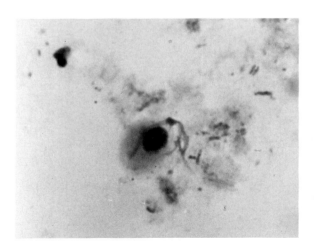

Figure A.38. *Trichomonas vaginalis* (Trophozoite). × 1,200

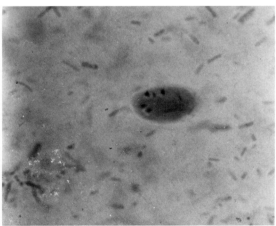

Figure A.40. *Giardia lamblia* (Quadrinucleate cyst).

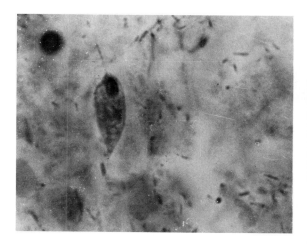

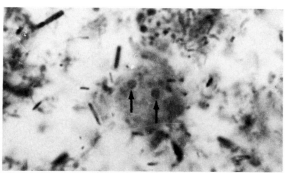

Figure A.44. *Dientamoeba fragilis* (Binucleate tropho-zoite. arrows = nuclei). ×2,200

Figure A.41. *Chilomastix mesnili* (Trophozoite). ×1,770

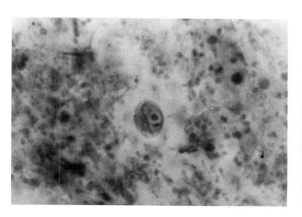

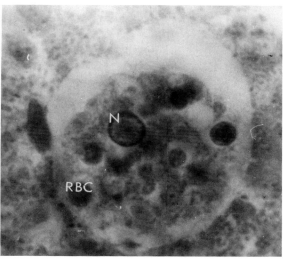

Figure A.42. *Chilomastix mesnili* (Cyst). ×1,500

Figure A.45. *Entamoeba histolytica*. (Trophozoite. N = nucleus, RBC = red blood cells). ×2,800

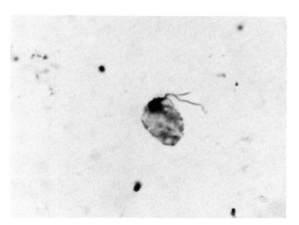

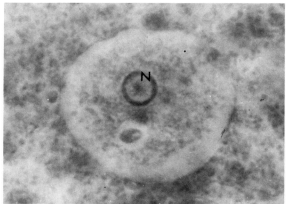

Figure A.43 *Retortamonas sp.* (Trophozoite). ×1,000

Figure A.46. *Entamoeba histolytica*. (Trophozoite. N = nucleus). ×2,800

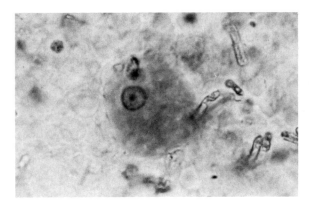

Figure A.47 *Entamoeba histolytica* (trophozoite). × 2,800

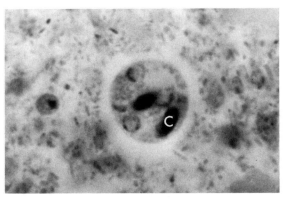

Figure A.50 *Entamoeba histolytica* (Quadrinucleate cyst. C = Chromatoidal bar). × 600

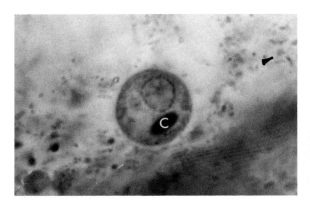

Figure A.48. *Entamoeba histolytica* (Uninucleate cyst. C = chromatoidal bar). × 600

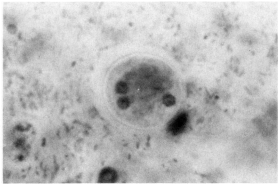

Figure A.51. *Entamoeba histolytica* (Quadrinucleate cyst). Only three nuclei are visible in this view. × 600.

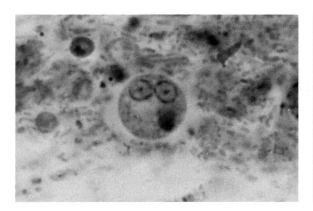

Figure A.49. *Entamoeba histolytica* (Binucleate cyst). × 600

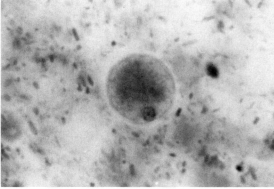

Figure A.52. *Entamoeba histolytica* (Quadrinucleate cyst). Same as above, different focal plane. One nucleus is visible in this view. × 600.

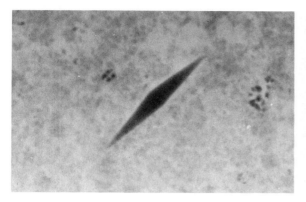

Figure A.53. Charcot–Leyden crystal. ×1,400

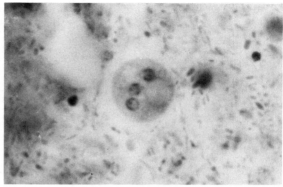

Figure A.56. *Entamoeba coli* (Quadrinucleate cyst). Same figure as A.55, different focal plane. Three nuclei are visible.

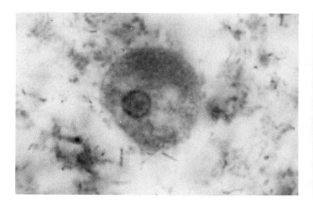

Figure A.54. *Entamoeba coli* (Trophozoite). ×600

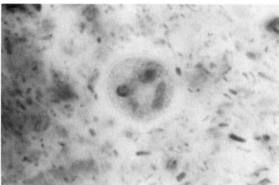

Figure A.57. *Entamoeba coli* (Octanucleate cyst). Same figure as A.55, different focal plane. Two nuclei are visible in this view. ×500.

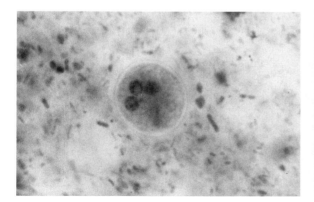

Figure A.55. *Entamoeba coli* (Octanucleate cyst). Three nuclei are visible in this view. ×500.

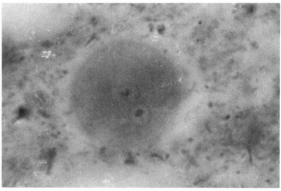

Figure A.58. *Entamoeba coli* (Octanucleate cyst). Same figure as A.55, different focal plane. Two nuclei are visible in this view. ×500.

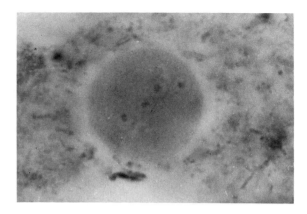

Figure A.59. *Entamoeba coli* (Octanucleate cyst). Same figure as A.55, different focal plane. Two nuclei are visible in this view. ×500.

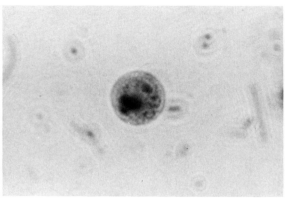

Figure A.62. *Entamoeba hartmanni* (Quadrinucleate cyst). ×1,500

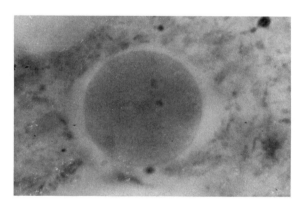

Figure A.60. *Entamoeba coli* (Octanucleate cyst). Same figure as A.55, different focal plane. Two nuclei are visible in this view.

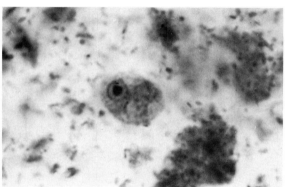

Figure A.63. *Iodamoeba butschlii* (Trophozoite). ×1,800

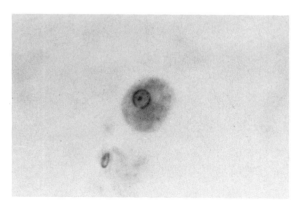

Figure A.61. *Entamoeba hartmanni* (Trophozoite). ×1,500

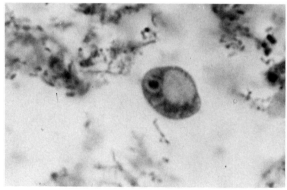

Figure A.64. *Iodamoeba butschlii* (Cyst). ×1,800

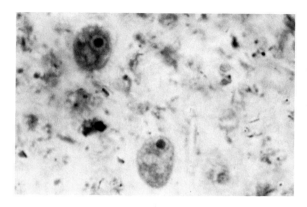

Figure A.65. *Endolimax nana* (Two trophozoites). ×1,300

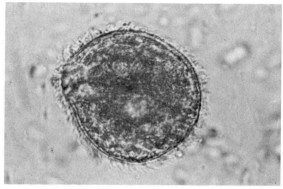

Figure A.68. *Balantidium coli* (Trophozoite). ×600

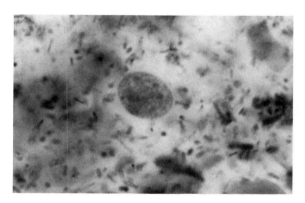

Figure A.66. *Endolimax nana* (Quadrinucleate cyst). ×1,300

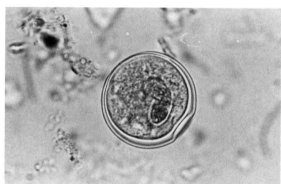

Figure A.69. *Balantidium coli* (Cyst). ×430

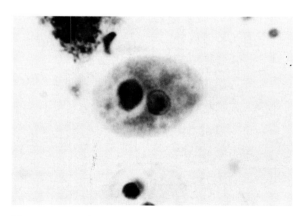

Figure A.67. *Entamoeba gingivalis* (Trophozoite). ×750

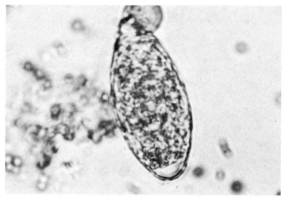

Figure A.70. *Isospora sp.* (Unsporulated oocyst). ×900

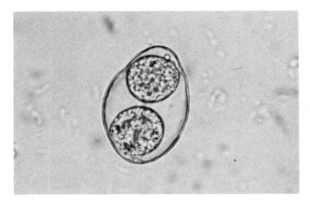

Figure A.71. *Isospora sp.* (Sporulated oocyst). × 1,000

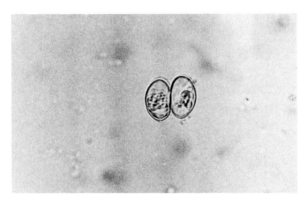

Figure A.72. *Sarcocystis bovicanus* (Sporulated oocyst). × 800

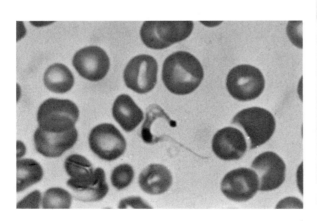

Figure A.73. *Trypanosoma cruzi* (Trypomastigote). × 1,500

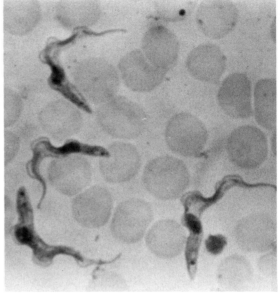

Figure A.74. *Trypanosoma brucei rhodesiense* (Trypomastigote). × 1,500

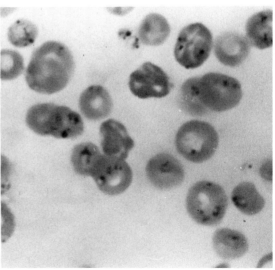

Figure A.75. *Babesia sp.* × 1,750

Index

Page numbers in *italics* refer to illustrations; page numbers followed by t refer to tables.